Stem Cell and Regenerative Medicine

By

Editor: Herman S. Cheung

Bentham Science Publishers	**Bentham Science Publishers**	**Bentham Science Publishers**
Executive Suite Y - 2	P.O. Box 446	P.O. Box 294
PO Box 7917, Saif Zone	Oak Park, IL 60301-0446	1400 AG Bussum
Sharjah, U.A.E.	USA	THE NETHERLANDS
subscriptions@benthamscience.org	subscriptions@benthamscience.org	subscriptions@benthamscience.org

CONTENTS

FOREWORD

The last decade has witnessed an explosion of new knowledge regarding cellular homeostasis throughout life. This new information essentially requires a revision of fundamental paradigms regarding the life cycle of the higher organism. Importantly these new insights have therapeutic implications.

The traditional paradigm has held that most (but importantly not all) of our crucial organ systems are terminally differentiated – in essence the cells that throughout life comprise the heart, central nervous system, islets of Langerhans, kidney are the ones that we are born with. The inevitable loss of these cells throughout life leads to permanent diminution in the function of the organ. Moreover, with widespread destruction of tissue such as due to myocardial infarction, stroke, or type I diabetes, tissue recovery does not occur.

We now know that all of our organs have greater plasticity than the initial paradigm held. The central discovery is that of adult stem cells – reservoirs of stem and precursor cells that underlie a cellular homeostatic process. In the heart estimates range that throughout adult life there is a turnover rate that ranges between 1 and 7 percent per year. Importantly this rate declines with age. Thus, endogenous repair pathways are operative and disease processes must now be viewed within the context of a homeostatic balance between cell loss and replacement.

Not only do these cells exist, but they can be accessed and amplified ex vivo, offering a major new therapeutic avenue. The book edited by Professor Herman Cheung offers a state of the art examination of this exciting new area of biology and therapeutics. The contributions cover important areas ranging from the ethics and considerations of justice in stem cell therapeutics to evaluations of crucial areas of the biology of endogenous tissue homeostasis.

The field of adult stem cells builds upon the discovery of pluripotent stem cells – embryonic and inducible. The discovery of these cells has initiated a field based upon the idea that tissue and cell loss can be replaced by exogenous cells. Work in the area of pluripotency has lead to the exciting insight that the adult mammal possesses a greater degree of plasticity than previously appreciated. The book Stem Cell and Regenerative Medicine offers a comprehensive and state of the art review of this exciting new area of biology and medicine.

Joshua M. Hare, *MD*
University of Miami
USA

PREFACE

Cellular-based therapies for regenerative medicine have evolved quite significantly in the past decades. The realization that such an endeavor requires the acquisition of an adequate stem or progenitor cell population, techniques to effectively maintain or induce the desired phenotype and efficient culturing and implantation conditions have led researchers to develop a wide variety of protocols to approach the issue. The goal of this E-Book is to review the recent advances and applications of stem cells in regenerative medicine. The book content can be generally divided into 3 sections: Ethics, Basic Biology and Clinical Applications.

ETHICS:

The ability of pluripotent stem cells to generate various replacement cells and tissues presents the potential of their application in cell-based regenerative therapies. Although human embryonic stem cells are, in principle, the most versatile source of pluripotent stem cells, ethical controversies, immunogenic rejection and spontaneous tumor formation remain major concerns for their use in transplantation.

Ritter *et al* focused largely on issues relating to the moral status of the embryo and suggest an ethically-optimized framework be established to help guide research in particular, the issues of social justice and the importance of both protecting vulnerable populations from bearing too great a burden for research while receiving too little of its benefits.

BASIC STEM CELL BIOLOGY

In contrast to ES cells, adult stem cells transplanted in pre-clinical animal models have shown no evidence of tumor formation and can be obtained mostly at all developmental stages and from numerous anatomical sites. Due to their broader clinical use, extensive research, and a more comprehensive understanding of their physiology, bone marrow-derived cells appear as the first choice for applications in regenerative medicine. Numerous environmental and trophic factors have been identified to play central roles in regulating the self-renewal, proliferation, migration, differentiation, senescence, and death of stem cells, their derived progeny, and the final differentiated cells that perform all tissue and organ functions. Besides direct differentiation of the stem cells to the desired mature cell type, other indirect mechanisms have been identified to play important roles in the overall repair of the injured tissue. These include production of paracrine factors, modulation of the host inflammatory response, host cell survival, and recruitment and activation of host tissue stem cells (Rios et al).

To deliver cellular products capable of replacing damaged tissue and/or cells, one must understand that the need for the balance between cellular proliferation and differentiation is a carefully controlled process involving a range of growth factors and cytokines produced in large part by tissue stromal cells. These stromal cells make up the tissue microenvironment and appear to be essential for normal homeostasis. McNiece and Hare hypothesize that tissue damage involves damage to the microenvironment resulting in a lack of signals through growth factor networks necessary to maintain survival and proliferation of tissue specific stem cells and progenitor cells. Therefore, optimal repair of disease tissue must account for the damage to the stromal environment. Optimal cellular therapies for regenerative medicine will require combination cellular products consisting of a stromal cell population to reconstitute the microenvironment and to support the survival, proliferation and differentiation of the tissue specific stem cells or progenitor cells.

Huang *et al* try to define the functional metrics required for engineering articular cartilage, and to situate the current state of MSC-based constructs within this framework. They examine the components and function of the native tissue, and review the progress made to date using differentiated cartilage cells (chondrocytes) for cartilage tissue engineering. This discussion includes methods of formation, biochemical formulations for enhancing *in vitro* development, as well as progress made towards using mechanical forces to further direct maturation. They then review the origins and applications of adult multi-potential stem cells, and discuss how routes towards cartilage tissue engineering with stem cells match (or fail to match) those approaches that were successful using differentiated cells. In particular, they describe new requirements to be understood for cartilage formation with MSCs, and outline several research areas that may inform this new direction in cartilage tissue engineering.

The application of biomimetic mechanical forces for stem cell differentiation is a technique that has been on the rise in recent years. The effects of these forces on stem cells are the most commonly explored combinations in functional tissue engineering. Paleaz et al summarized the current findings in functional tissue engineering, explain the importance of engineering in medical research, and describe the ways tissue engineers are attempting to understand what biochemical changes are occurring in the stem cells during the application of mechanical stress.

CLINICAL APPLICATIONS

The goal of angiogenic therapy is to activate endogenous angiogenic and arteriogenic pathways and stimulate revascularization of ischemic myocardial tissue. The feasibility of such a strategy has now been established through the results of studies over the past two decades, and clinical trials involving more than 1000 patients have been implemented. Critical evaluations reveal that neither proteins nor genes delivered by transient expression vectors provide an optimal therapy. Similarly, stem cell therapy is not achieving the level of improvement that was expected or predicted from preclinical results. The future of therapeutic angiogenesis lies in the use of permanent gene delivery vehicles expressing regulated genes and/or stem cells appropriately engineered with regulated genes (Keith A. Webster).

The use of progenitor/stem cells to modulate the sensory systems in chronic pain is a new field in translational research. Stem cells or progenitor approaches have been tested in cardiac myopathies, liver dysfunction, stroke, and genetic abnormalities, but almost none have applied progenitor cells to the relief of neuropathic, pain. Perhaps the best studied neural progenitor cell line NT2, has recently resulted in two NT2-derived cell lines: hNT2.17, secreting the inhibitory neurotransmitters GABA and glycine; and hNT2.19, secreting the neurotransmitter serotonin. Each of these NT2-lines has demonstrated antinociceptive potential in models of SCI-related neuropathic pain, in peripheral neuropathy, and diabetic neuropathic pain. These human progenitors may prove to be useful in the relief of chronic pain and open the way to other regenerative approaches to pain management (Eaton et al).

Early results of therapy with neural stem cells have been attributed to factors released by infused cells and investigator bias. The stem cell progeny identified as neurons by antigen expression and by morphology has been questioned, leading to the re-interpretation of these results by investigators who first reported them. Despite the diminished expectations, regenerative cells, or structures that mimic the function regenerative cells possess, are present in germinal areas of the adult human brain, albeit in limited numbers. Evidence does suggest that damaged brain tissue does, in some patients, regenerate with recovery of lost function. These cellular entities have not been widely studied, characterized but they may be similar to structures generated in neural tissue of primitive vertebrates which have a remarkable capability to regenerate intact, functional brain. These structures can potentially be expanded using methods that differ vastly from stem cell culture methods employed to date. Successfully expanded and stored, these structures may provide an effective means to regenerate brain tissue after stroke and traumatic brain injury in humans (English et al).

The existence of clinically successful islet transplantation for type I diabetes has stoked a keen interest in developing alternative, inexhaustible sources of insulin-producing cells. Domínguez-Bendala and Ricordi cover the state of the art in regenerative therapies for the endocrine component of the pancreas, from stem cells to transdifferentiation. They review the basics of pancreatic development, whose recapitulation remains the subject of a plethora of *in vitro* differentiation strategies using both embryonic and adult stem cells. They also examine the leading theories about the cellular and molecular mechanisms behind the *in vivo* regeneration of the organ that is observed under specific circumstances, as well as the purported ability of some tissues to turn into pancreatic endocrine cells when subjected to specific interventions (transdifferentiation). They conclude with a general overview of the remaining challenges and clinical perspectives of all the above strategies, with a special emphasis on the immunological hurdles to be overcome for these approaches to find their way to standard clinical practice.

To date, several sources of dental stem cells have been isolated and being characterized as dental epithelial stem cells, dental pulp stem cells, dental follicle precursor cells, stem cells from human exfoliated deciduous teeth, stem cells from apical papilla, and periodontal ligament stem cells. Dental stem cells have been shown to have multi-potential by their ability to differentiate into neuronal, adipogenic, myogenic, chondrogenic, osteogenic and dentinogenic cells when cultured under specific conditions. These facilitated studies to address an important property of stem cells, that is, the capacity of a given stem cell population to regenerate an organized, functional tissue following transplantation *in vivo*. Furthermore, the ready availability of tooth tissues from redundant teeth such as third molars can provide a good supply of dental stem cells that may be utilized for regenerating other body parts or organs (Zheng and Cheung).

Yam et al address the important questions regarding functions of cornea epithelial progenitor cells (CEPCs) and therapeutic strategies in health and diseases. The human cornea is a site of tissue-specific adult progenitor cells, residing between cornea and conjunctiva in the Palisade of Vogt of the limbus region. While specific molecular markers of CEPCs are still unknown, recent research provide new information to apply them for cell replacement in damaged tissues. Cultured CEPCs have been used for *ex vivo* cornea therapy with satisfactory clinical outcome. While the niche environment, i.e., the extracellular matrix, growth factors and cytokines, provide regulatory measures in the proliferation of CEPCs, the recent discovery of CEPC specific microRNAs opens a new direction of research on the biological properties of CEPC and stem cells of other resources.

Last but not the least, I like to thank Ms. Lauren L. Vernon, who spent countless hours in working with all the authors.

Herman S. Cheung, *PhD*
James L. Knight Professor of Biomedical Engineering
Senior Veteran Affairs Research Career Scientist
Professor of Medicine & Orthopedic Surgery
University of Miami
USA

CONTRIBUTORS

Akshay Anand	Dept. of Neurology, Post Graduate Institute of Medical Education and Research, Chandigarh, India
Herman S. Cheung	Dept. of Biomedical Engineering, College of Engineering, University of Miami, 1251 Memorial Drive, Coral Gables, FL & Geriatrics Research, Education and Clinical Center and Research Service, Miami VA Healthcare System, 1201 NW 16 Street, Miami, FL USA
Kevin Curtis	Departments of Medicine and Biochemistry & Molecular Biology, University of Miami Leonard M. Miller School of Medicine and Geriatric Research, Education, and Clinical Center and Research Service, Veterans Affairs Medical Center, Miami, FL. USA
Gianluca D'Ippolito	Geriatric Research, Education, and Clinical Center and Research Service, Veterans Affairs Medical Center, Miami, FL. USA
Juan Domínguez-Bendala	Diabetes Research Institute, University of Miami, Leonard M. Miller School of Medicine, 1450 NW 10th Avenue, Miami, FL. USA
M.J. Eaton	Dept. of Veterans Affairs Medical Center, Miami, FL, USA
Denis English	Dept. of Neurosurgery, Foundation for Developmental Research, University of S. Florida College of Medicine, Tampa, FL, USA
Robin N. Fiore	University of Miami Bioethics Program, University of Miami, FL USA
Elisa Garbayo	Departments of Medicine and Biochemistry & Molecular Biology, University of Miami Leonard M. Miller School of Medicine, Geriatric Research, Education, and Clinical Center and Research Service, VA Medical Center, Miami, FL, USA
Stephan Gluck	Sylvester Comprehensive Cancer Center, Division of Hematology/Oncology, Dept. of Medicine, Leonard M. Miller School of Medicine, University of Miami, Miami, FL, USA
Lourdes A. Gomez	Departments of Medicine and Biochemistry & Molecular Biology, University of Miami Leonard M. Miller School of Medicine, Geriatric Research, Education, and Clinical Center and Research Service, Veterans Affairs Medical Center, Miami, FL, USA
Kenneth W. Goodman	University of Miami Bioethics Program, University of Miami, FL, USA,
Joshua Hare	Interdisciplinary Stem Cell Institute, University of Miami, 1120 NW 14th St, Miami, FL, USA
Josh M. Hare	Interdisciplinary Stem Cell Institute, University of Miami Leonard M. Miller School of Medicine, Miami, FL 33101, USA
Alice H. Huang	McKay Orthopaedic Research Laboratory, Dept of Orthopaedic Surgery and Dept. of Bioengineering, University of Pennsylvania, Philadelphia, PA, USA
Clark T. Hung	Cellular Engineering Laboratory, Dept. of Biomedical Engineering, Columbia University, New York, NY, USA
Lim Kwong Cheung	Oral & Maxillofacial Surgery, The Prince Philip Dental Hospital, 34 Hospital Road, Hong Kong SAR, China
Robert L. Mauck	McKay Orthopaedic Research Laboratory, Dept of Orthopaedic Surgery and Dept. of Bioengineering, University of Pennsylvania, Philadelphia, PA, USA

Ian McNiece University of Miami Leonard M. Miler School of Medicine, 1120 NW 14th St, Miami, FL, USA

Daniel Pelaez Dept. of Biomedical Engineering, College of Engineering, University of Miami, 1251 Memorial Drive, Coral Gables, FL, USA

Carmen Rios Geriatric Research, Education, and Clinical Center and Research Service, Veterans Affairs Medical Center, Miami, FL, USA

Camillo Ricordi Diabetes Research Institute, University of Miami Leonard M. Miller School of Medicine, 1450 NW 10th Avenue, Miami, FL, USA

Isaac H. Ritter University of Miami Bioethics Program, University of Miami, FL, USA

Paul C. Schiller Departments of Medicine and Biochemistry & Molecular Biology, University of Miami Miller School of Medicine and Geriatric Research, Education, and Clinical Center and Research Service, VA Medical Center, Miami, FL, USA

Rama S. Verma Stem Cell and Molecular Biology Laboratory, Deptartment of Biotechnology, Institute of Technology-Madras, Chennai, India

Keith A. Webster Dept of Molecular and Cellular Pharmacology, The Vascular Biology Institute, University of Miami, Leonard M. Miller School of Medicine, Miami. FL, USA

Eva Widerström-Noga The Miami Project to Cure Paralysis, University of Miami Leonard M. Miller School of Medicine, Miami, FL, USA

Stacey Quintero Wolfe Dept. of Neurological Surgery, University of Miami Leonard M. Miller School of Medicine, Miami, FL, USA

Li Wu Zheng Oral & Maxillofacial Surgery, The Prince Philip Dental Hospital, 34 Hospital Road, Hong Kong SAR, China

Gary Hin-Fai Yam Department of Ophthalmology & Visual Sciences, The Chinese University of Hong Kong, Hong Kong

Chi Pui Pang Department of Ophthalmology & Visual Sciences, The Chinese University of Hong Kong, Hong Kong

CHAPTER 1

Justice and Vulnerability in Human Embryonic Stem Cell Research

Isaac H. Ritter*, Robin N. Fiore and Kenneth W. Goodman

University of Miami Bioethics Program, University of Miami, Florida, USA

Abstract: Human embryonic stem cell (hESC) research has been a topic of much debate within the ethics community, centering largely on issues relating to the moral status of the embryo. While this discussion has been ongoing, hESC research has progressed at an ever-quickening pace. As this research continues forward, it is imperative that an ethically-optimized framework be established to help guide research. In particular, inadequate attention has been given to issues of social justice and the importance of both protecting vulnerable populations from bearing too great a burden for research while receiving too little of its benefits.

INTRODUCTION

Human embryonic stem cell (hESC) research has been a source of intense controversy for ethicists, politicians, scientists, and religious leaders, prompting widespread and global debate. Advocates herald stem cells as a gateway to knowledge that will catapult science forward and alleviate the burden of disease for those suffering from some of nature's most debilitating conditions. Opponents argue that the potential benefits of stem cell research are over-hyped, and that the destruction of embryos necessary to create stem cell lines, the substrate for hESC research, is tantamount to murder. Despite continued debate and opposition in many places throughout the world, hESC research has blossomed into a vibrant field of research.

In the United States, the ethics debate has focused largely on the moral status of the embryo. Because the blastocyst is generally (though not necessarily) destroyed during the extraction of cells required to create a stem cell line, the question of its moral status has proven an obstacle to hESC research. Bioethicists and the public are often divided on as to whether be it morally permissible to use embryos to acquire totipotent stem cells. Arguments based on religious traditions with respect to "ensoulment" – or the point at which fertilized or re-nucleated ova acquire immortal souls – take the view that the blastocyst is a potential human life and contend that because of its trajectory it is wrong to destroy it. That is, zygotes and blastocysts ought to be afforded the same treatment and protection as persons [1,2]. The contrasting view holds that the embryo has no inherent moral status and may generally be treated like other biological material made available for research [3]. A moderate and philosophically well-founded position acknowledges the potential of an embryo but rejects the notion that it should thus be afforded the same moral consideration owed to a person. In other words, there is a moral difference between a person and a human embryo because the properties that are morally relevant – sentience and consciousness – are not available in the case of early embryos [4,5]. On this view, embryos can be used in research under certain conditions; for example, creating embryos solely for research purposes might not be permissible, but using leftover embryos that would otherwise be discarded or frozen is an acceptable source for hESC lines.

A "Post-Moral Status of the Embryo" Discussion

The moral status of the embryo has commanded most of the attention in the stem cell ethics debate, often to the detriment of many other important ethical concerns. In particular, inadequate attention has been paid to issues of social justice and appropriate protections for vulnerable populations.

One important reason to begin thinking beyond the "moral status" question is suggested by a growing body of research that has demonstrated methods for extracting stem cell lines while leaving the blastocyst unharmed. The availability of technology allowing for the derivation of hESC lines without the destruction of the blastocyst would seemingly resolve the political impasse that has hindered hESC research since its inception. A number of

---

*Address Correspondence to this Author Isaac H. Ritter:** UM Ethics Programs, P.O. Box 016960 (M-825), Miami FL 33101, USA; E-mail: ihritter@med.miami.edu

different strategies are emerging including the dedifferentiation of somatic cells into cells resembling hESCs, extraction of cells from the blastocyst without destruction of the embryo, and parthenogenesis, which sidesteps the creation, and ultimate destruction, of a viable embryo [6, 7]. The efficiency and utility of cells created by these modalities is hardly proven, but, increasingly, studies have demonstrated more efficient methods for creating hESC lines that sidestep the need to destroy the embryo.

Will these emerging technologies set the hESC debate to rest? Some argue that if these technologies prove adequate, and blastocysts are not destroyed for research, the hESC debate will ultimately fade. Without embryo destruction, they argue, there is nothing objectionable to hESC research. These solutions suggest one reason for moving beyond the "status" issue, namely, that it may not be an issue in the future.

Furthermore, despite ongoing debate, the national and global political climate has tended towards a more permissive stance for hESC research, requiring those who wish to see research performed ethically to create an ethically optimized framework in which hESC research can occur. National polling data suggest that the United States wants hESC research to move forward: a Pew Research Center poll indicates that 54% of the U.S. public supports hESC research, while only 32% oppose it [8]. The attitudes at the top of the political system are also changing. The most significant impediment to hESC research in the past decade has been the moratorium imposed by former President George Bush in 2001; this measure prohibited use of federal funds for any research to create new stem cell lines;[9] President Barack Obama has voiced support for hESC research throughout his campaign and is expected to reverse Bush's moratorium [10]. Furthermore, despite the federal government's moratorium, individual states have increasingly taken it upon themselves not only to permit hESC research, but also to provide significant state funding. California is among the best examples, having passed Proposition 71 in November 2004 establishing the California Institute for Regenerative Medicine and mandating nearly $300 million in state funds for hESC research each year over a 10-year period. California is not alone; Connecticut, Illinois, Iowa, Maryland, Massachusetts, New Jersey and New York expressly encourage stem cell research, with many allocating significant state funds for research purposes [11, 12].

The need for thoughtful and ethically motivated policies is amplified by global trends in hESC research. Despite institutional and financial advantages in the United States, significant research volume has shifted overseas, where more receptive governments hope to benefit from the influx of talent and innovation. Centers have emerged throughout the world, where more permissive policies have helped spur research and attract talent and funding [13]. The net effect of this efflux on ethical practices has proven detrimental. Among many examples, a group of leading Russian scientists petitioned the Russian Ministry of Health over concerns about stem-cell treatments that used stem cells derived from aborted fetuses, which were being administered at "beauty salons" at exorbitant rates [14]. Similarly, poor oversight has had a negative effect on public trust, damaging the credibility of good research. The South Korean debacle surrounding Dr. Hwang Woo Suk, who fabricated evidence and relied on unethical practices to acquire oocytes for experimentation, demonstrates this well [15]. The scandal significantly damaged the research community in South Korea and left the global public more suspicious of well-intentioned hESC research.

The power of United States to regulate research practices diminishes as more research moves abroad. Furthermore, by not outlining a robust and ethically-informed comprehensive hESC policy, the U.S. fails to suggest a gold standard for the international community. A growing number of ethicists, international societies, and government commissions have taken up the mantle, offering guidelines and recommendations for hESC research [16-17]. This body of work has helped inform research ethics committees and other entities invested with the responsibility of ensuring that research is conducted ethically. However, despite the Herculean effort to keep up with hESC research, ethical guidelines have at times been outstripped by the continuous flow of new research. Crucially important issues receiving inadequate attention concern protection for vulnerable populations and social justice. Generally, what must be done to protect vulnerable populations, and how ought we to ensure that the benefits of research are distributed fairly to ensure that those who have borne burdens for hESC research receive benefits in proportion to their contribution?

This chapter addresses two major categories of issues. First, what special considerations affect vulnerable populations' participation in hESC research? Second, how can an ethically-optimized system foster a just distribution of benefits derived from this research?

Vulnerability

Vulnerable populations in biomedical and behavioral research are regarded as requiring special protections; however, defining "vulnerable population" has proven a greater challenge than might be expected. To understand the concept of vulnerability, it will perhaps be instructive to discuss the history of human subjects research in general and vulnerability in particular.

The general principle that human subjects require formal protections was articulated in the Nuremberg Code, established at the end of World War II. The Nuremberg Code outlined many of the fundamental principles that form the foundation of ethical research today, including informed consent, careful experimental design, and protections for the safety and health of research subjects [18]. While the Nuremberg Code broadly discussed the importance of subjects' protection, vulnerable populations as such became a more central focus only after the war with reports of human research subject abuse. The most famous of these was the "U.S. Public Health Service Syphilis Study at Tuskegee," in which African-Americans with syphilis were studied to investigate the natural course of the disease. Research participants were not informed of their diagnosis, did not give informed consent, and later were denied access to antibiotic therapy during the course of the study when treatment with antibiotics had become the gold standard for treatment of the disease [19]. The abuses at Tuskegee were a watershed, leading to the creation of The National Commission for the Protection of Human Subjects of Biomedical and Behavioral Research and its publication of the Belmont Report, which proposed ethical principles to govern research with human subjects [20]. The Belmont Report also identified a special need to protect vulnerable populations:

> "One special instance of injustice results from the involvement of vulnerable subjects. Certain groups, such as racial minorities, the economically disadvantaged, the very sick, and the institutionalized may continually be sought as research subjects, owing to their ready availability in settings where research is conducted. Given their dependent status and their frequently compromised capacity for free consent, they should be protected against the danger of being involved in research solely for administrative convenience, or because they are easy to manipulate as a result of their illness or socioeconomic condition"[20].

This account of vulnerability focused on two major areas: the inability to give adequate informed consent and undue inducement or coercion to participate in research. In the years following the Belmont Report, vulnerability was expanded, and subsequent U.S. law included groups of people such as pregnant women, prisoners, children and others [21].

Some scholars have taken issue with the notion that vulnerability can be defined as a simple compilation of disparate subpopulations seen as needing additional protections, and have attempted to establish more useful definitions for vulnerability [22]. Some have even suggested that vulnerability, being so difficult to define precisely, is not a particularly useful idea at all, and ought to be eliminated from the research evaluation process [23]. Despite these views, vulnerability is a well-established principle in modern research ethics and in current regulatory guidelines. Moreover, the obligation to protect all human subjects requires special attention to those whose material situation or cognitive capability puts them at greater risk.

In what follows, we discuss specific issues of vulnerability and justice in stem cell research.

ACQUISITION OF MATERIALS FOR HESC RESEARCH

Informed or valid consent is widely considered among the most important, if not the most important, safeguard for protecting research participants. It is a critical piece of the Nuremberg Code, the Belmont Report and various international regulations governing human subjects research [24, 25]. Briefly, for consent to be considered valid it must fulfill three broad requirements: i) Research participants must be given an adequate full account of the research and its risks, potential benefits and alternatives, ii) they must have capacity to understand and appreciate this information and to decide whether to participate, and iii) they must not be subject to coercion or undue influence [26].

Flawed consent has already had practical repercussions for hESC research. In one analysis, none of the informed consent forms used to attain the stem cell lines that are currently funded by the US federal government fulfills the standards for informed consent set forth by the National Academy of Science [27]. This analysis demonstrated that the majority of the consent forms fail to give an adequate account of risks and potential benefits or the nature of the research. While the U.S. National Institute of Health has not planned any changes to its policies because of the report, the analysis demonstrates the challenges to proper informed consent for hESC research.

Acquiring adequate consent from vulnerable populations poses significant challenges to researchers. Studies have demonstrated that research participants with lower levels of education and poor health literacy are less likely to comprehend the risks, potential benefits and purposes of research [28]. Additionally, studies have shown that some patients who may be receiving medical treatment or regular office visits as part of a study may be unduly induced to participate [29].

The difficulty with vulnerable populations begins with adequately explaining the nature and purpose of research. Adequate consent does not require that patients understand the scientific rationale for an experiment; however, the consent process is expected to provide all relevant information that a reasonable person might find useful in deciding to participate [26]. This is particularly challenging in hESC research for two principle reasons. First, because hESC lines are by definition immortal, they can potentially be used in an indefinite number of future experiments. This means that researchers might want to obtain consent from patients for experiments not yet designed. The challenge is large: How can a prospective subject agree to research that cannot be fully described?

This is not a new issue unique to hESC research; a similar concern arises for much genetic research where information or samples attained at the beginning of an experiment may be wanted later on down the road for different purposes. Some scholars have suggested that prospective subjects could be asked to consent to broad categories of future research to be conducted on stem cell lines [30]. Whether categorical consent adequately fulfills the requirement that participants be given the opportunity to withhold participation from experiments they find objectionable seems hardly assured. There is a real concern that categories will either be too broad to adequately inform participants of how their tissues may be used, or they may be too narrow, forcing investigators to abandon their work or continue with inadequate consent.

The prospect of consenting a patient for future, unknown experiments using hESCs is all the more daunting given that many who support hESC research in general may object to certain types of experimentation; for example, many who support hESC research object to the mixing of human and non-human cells and somatic cell nuclear transfer. While in some instances researchers can bypass the need to explain the science behind experiments (generally, adequate consent requires only that prospective subjects be given access to the kind of information reasonable people would want in deciding whether to participate), hESC research involves more nuanced ethical challenges and it may prove necessary to explain these experiments in some detail.

Valid consent could also be jeopardized by expectations that participation in research may be linked to access to care, which is especially concerning where prospective subjects are recruited from cohorts of infertility patients. This was identified as a problem in five of the six stem cell lines eligible for federal funding, where consent documents did not adequately explain to patients that they had various options available to them for the disposition of leftover fertilized ova [27]. Many argue that blastocysts used in hESC research should be taken from leftover embryos unused after in vitro fertilization therapy for infertile couples. A serious complication arises if participation in research is perceived as a prerequisite for in vitro fertilization treatment. This problem is compounded in certain ethnic groups that may particularly cherish reproductive capacity and who are at the same time the most vulnerable to misunderstanding the consent process by virtue of their socioeconomic status, education level, or language.

All populations may be regarded as vulnerable to the extent both that risk is probabilistic and that some risks are unknown and hence cannot be disclosed. This is particularly relevant regarding the long term risks to future fertility associated with ovarian hyper-stimulation and ova extraction required for somatic cell nuclear transfer (SCNT). While most current research uses existing stem cell lines, SCNT requires the harvesting of eggs from fertile women. Although egg harvesting is widespread in assisted reproduction, fertility clinics typically operate as private commercial ventures, and so the procedure's risks to women have not been well studied. Also, in some research protocols, subjects are not reimbursed for medical treatment required after adverse events, and women, especially young women, are more likely than other groups to be uninsured or underinsured.

Women's health advocates have raised concerns about the potential for exploitation of young or low-income women offered high payments for eggs used in assisted reproduction. Commercial payments for eggs from young women can range from a few thousand dollars to $30,000 or more for "especially desirable" egg-donors (young, Caucasian, high IQ, talented, proven egg donor). The National Academies of Sciences has recommended that payments to oocyte donors be limited to reimbursement for direct expenses like transportation and childcare [31]. In 2006, California approved a measure defining women who provide eggs for research as "research subjects" thus triggering federal and state regulatory protections. The California approach also addresses conflicts of interest between researchers and medical personnel who conduct the egg retrieval procedures; and requires payment for treatment for study-related injuries. Like California, Massachusetts and New York (among other states) have ambitious private funding initiatives for stem cell research and have addressed the special vulnerability of egg donors.

The ethical challenge at the core of ova harvesting is based on the third requirement listed earlier for valid consent, namely that subjects not be coerced or unduly influenced. If a human subject would not – except for compensation – run a large or unknown risk, the concern is that it is the compensation and no other reason that motivates the choice. Because those other reasons might include altruism, the desire to advance biomedical science or the possibility of personal medical benefit, the supremacy of financial considerations is regarded as problematic.

These challenges can be addressed in a number of ways. One is to limit financial compensation in the hope there will be enough oocyte donors motivated by altruism and other social considerations; it is hypothesized that the likelihood of that working is greater for publicly funded studies than for profit-driven research. Another way is to require as an inclusion criterion that women who become oocyte sources have already completed their families, thus mitigating the risks to future fertility.

ETHNICALLY SKEWED ACCESS TO THERAPEUTIC BENEFITS

The requirements for special protection for vulnerable populations serve two purposes. The first is obviously protective. The less obvious aspect is that the identification and protections make it possible for vulnerable populations to be included in ethically designed research, and thus ensure that the products of research are therapeutically relevant to them as well. It is then that the question of justice arises: Will they be able to access the benefits of the research, either in proportion to their having undergone the burdens of contributing to the research or on par with others? When thinking about the potential for a just distribution of the burdens and benefits of research, it is tempting to focus on the latter, the proportional benefit. However, with respect to hESC research, a different picture emerges in which vulnerable populations are disproportionately *excluded* from research and therefore do not have the potential to receive benefits.

Among countries and international bodies supporting hESC initiatives, research is generally restricted to embryos that are left over from in vitro fertilization (IVF) [11]. Proponents argue that IVF is an effective and socially acceptable treatment modality for patients suffering from infertility. During treatment, excess embryos are fertilized to allow clinicians to evaluate the most viable ones for implantation and to retain additional embryos for future pregnancy attempts, should they be necessary or desired. Many of these excess embryos are then either discarded or stored indefinitely. These embryos provide an obvious and morally (if not scientifically) acceptable source for hESC studies [32]. Estimates regarding the number of embryos potentially available for research vary; as of 2003, there were perhaps 400,000 embryos suitable for research in the United States. Among these, 2.8% or 11,000 had been designated as available for research, which investigators believe could produce approximately 275 new stem cell lines [33].

While these leftover embryos are a seemingly viable and ethically acceptable source for hESCs, the demographic distribution of these embryos raises serious ethical questions regarding the ethnic groups that would most directly benefit from research. Data from the 2002 National Survey of Family Growth conducted by the U.S. Department of Health and Human Resources shows that nearly 90% of patients using IVF were non-Hispanic white, while

Blacks and Hispanics each comprise only 5% of IVF patients [34]. If leftover egg donations were the sole source of hESCs, Hispanics or Blacks, who make up approximately 25% of the American population, would be poorly represented by the genetic makeup of hESC cell lines [35].

Interestingly, the International Society for Stem Cell Research discussed this very issue in recent guidelines for the clinical translation of stem cell research:

> "The ISSCR seeks to maximize social good, which leads to the following considerations: (a) Stem cell collection with genetically diverse sources of cell lines should be established" [17].

If leftover blastocysts from IVF are to be the primary source of stem cell lines, and given that non-Hispanic whites disproportionately make up those who utilize IVF, it might be impossible to comply with this recommendation.

The importance of this genetic skewing could influence the diseases researchers are most likely to study using hESCs. Physicians have long known that many diseases evince significant ethnic variability; sickle cell disease is most commonly associated with African-Americans, Tay-Sachs with Aschenazi Jews, and Cystic fibrosis with those of European descent. Increasingly scientists are delineating genetic causes that account for the increased prevalence of certain diseases among certain ethnic groups.   As stem cells are increasingly used to study the progression of disease and its underlying genetic etiologies, a paucity of stem cell lines from certain ethnic groups could impede progress in the study of diseases most commonly seen in those groups.

An ethnically homogenous, and by extension genetically homogenous, supply of stem cell lines may affect the efficacy of research in many more ways. For example, among the proposed uses of stem cells is the ability to test the safety and efficacy of new drugs [36]. Some argue that hESCs provide an excellent means of evaluating how tissues will respond to certain pharmacologic interventions. At the same time, recent research has shown that some variability in the efficacy of certain drugs can depend on ethnicity; for example, studies have demonstrated a statistically significant difference in efficacy of different antihypertensive agents depending on race [37]. Other studies have shown similar relationships between ethnicity and drug efficacy, including two experiments that demonstrated differences in response to bronchodilators between Mexicans and Puerto Ricans [38, 39]. If future experiments examining drug efficacy and safety are conducted on hESC lines that are ethnically homogenous, the ability for researchers to generalize results may be limited.

JUSTICE AND THE FAILURE TO SHARE THE FRUITS OF BIOMEDICAL RESEARCH

The U.S. and international bioethics communities have generally supported the scientific community in pressing for greater freedom of and financial support for embryonic stem cell research. The strongest argument is, in brief, that even if hECSs have moral status, that status is vastly exceeded by the moral status of human beings with diabetes, Parkinson's disease, Alzheimer's disease and so on. If suffering humans can benefit from embryonic stem cell research, it is a peculiar kind of standing on ethical ceremony to suggest that blastocysts should enjoy the same status as people. Indeed, given its promise, one could argue that not only is this research morally permissible – it is morally obligatory.

But the promise of the research, the growth of regenerative medicine, the opportunity to ease the burden of terrible maladies – all of these are mitigated by a dismal track record in making the results of biomedical research available to all people. Put differently: It will be a shame, or worse, if stem cell research realizes its potential and these benefits are not fairly distributed but, rather, serve to widen health disparities. Some three decades after the Belmont Report's insistence that if a population is a source of human subjects then that population should share the benefits of discovery, we have yet to arrive at a fair system of medical resource allocation. The tension should be seen as especially acute for traditional biomedical research undertaken at academic medical centers in urban centers, especially in the United States. There, many human subjects will lack fair access to the treatments they helped develop.

This is Unacceptable

Moreover, it will be at least as unacceptable if we repeat or perpetuate this disparity with the fruits of stem cell research. If governments have resources to foster and build the new sciences of stem cell inquiry, then on pain of hypocrisy will they fail to address health care inequity and foster and build equitable health care systems.

Ultimately, distribution of the therapeutic advances and other benefits of research depend on the existing health care infrastructure. To the extent that health care is distributed on the basis of ability to pay (including payments from health insurance) the economically disadvantaged will not receive the benefits of stem cell or any other research on par with others. Given the potential of stem cell research and its translation in terms of regenerative medicine, a failure to address the distributional inequities in our current health care delivery systems will have devastating effects on the least well off, on our democratic ideals and on our most humane aspirations.

REFERENCES

[1]   Doerflinger R. Destructive stem-cell research on human embryos. Origins. 1999; (28):769-773.
[2]   George RP, Gomez-Lobo A. The moral status of the human embryo. Perspect Biol Med 2005; 48(2):201-210.
[3]   McCullough L, Chervenak F. Ethics in Obstetrics and Gynecology. New York: Oxford University Press; 1994: 103.
[4]   Kamm FM. Ethical Issues in Using and Not Using Embryonic Stem Cells. Stem Cell Reviews 2006; 1(4): 325-330.
[5]   Sandel MJ. Embryo ethics--the moral logic of stem-cell research. N Engl J Med 2004 Jul 15;351(3):207-209.
[6]   Cowan CA, Atienza J, Melton DA, *et al*. Nuclear reprogramming of somatic cells after fusion with human embryonic stem cells. Science. 2005 Aug 26; 309(5739):1369-1373.
[7]   Klimanskaya I, Chung Y, Becker S, *et al*. Human embryonic stem cell lines derived from single blastomeres. Nature. 2006 Nov 23; 444(7118):481-485.
[8]   Kohut A, Doherty C. Stable Views of Stem Cell Research. 2009. Pew Research Center :2. Available at http://people-press.org/reports/pdf/500.pdf , 4/15/2010.
[9]   Wertz DC. Embryo and stem cell research in the United States: history and politics. Gene Ther 2002 Jun; 9(11):674-678.
[10]   Barack Obama Campaign Website. Available at: http://www.barackobama.com/issues/technology, 10/3/08.
[11]   Ritter H. International Legislation on Human Embryonic Stem Cell Research. Available at http://isscr.org/public/-regions/index.cfm, 3/3/ 2008.
[12]   Stem Cell Research. March 2008.
[13]   Ritter H. International Legislation on Human Embryonic Stem Cell Research. Available at www.isscr.org , 3/2008.
[14]   Parfitt T. Russian scientists voice concern over "stem-cell cosmetics". Lancet 2005 Apr 2-8; 365(9466):1219-1220.
[15]   Cyranoski D. South Korean scandal rocks stem cell community. Nat Med 2006 Jan;12(1):4.
[16]   Ethical Issues in Human Stem Cell Research. 9/1999.
[17]   Guidelines for the Clinical Translation of Stem Cells. December 3, 2008.
[18]   Trials of War Criminals before the Nuernberg Military Tribunals under Control Council Law No. 10. 1949;15 NMT 1-12.
[19]   Jones J. Bad Blood: The Tuskegee syphilis experiment. New York: Free Press; 1981.
[20]   The Belmont Report: Ethical Principles and Guidelines for the Protection of Human Subjects of Research. 4/18/1979.
[21]   Protection of Human Subjects. 2005;Title 45, Part 46, Code of Federal Regulations.
[22]   Kipnis K. Vulnerability in Research Subjects: A bioethical taxonomy. Ethical and Policy Issues Involving Human Research Participants. Online Ethics Center for Engineering and Research. Available at http://www.onlineethics.org/cms/8087.aspx , 4/15/2010.
[23]   Levine C, Faden R, Grady C, *et al*. The limitations of "vulnerability" as a protection for human research participants. Am J Bioeth 2004 Summer;4(3):44-49.
[24]   International Ethical Guidelines for Biomedical Research Involving Human Subjects 2002.
[25]   Ethical Principles for Medical Research Involving Human Subjects. 10/22/2008.
[26]   Berg J. Informed Consent: Legal Theory and Clinical Practice Oxford: Oxford University Press; 2001: 14-36.
[27]   Streiffer R. Informed consent and federal funding for stem cell research. Hastings Cent Rep. 2008 May-Jun;38(3):40-47.
[28]   Flory J, Emanuel E. Interventions to improve research participants' understanding in informed consent for research: a systematic review. JAMA 2004 Oct 6;292(13):1593-1601.
[29]   Emanuel EJ, Currie XE, Herman A, Project Phidisa. Undue inducement in clinical research in developing countries: is it a worry? Lancet 2005 Jul 23-29;366(9482):336-340.
[30]   Lo B, Chou V, Cedars MI, *et al*. Informed consent in human oocyte, embryo, and embryonic stem cell research. Fertil Steril 2004 Sep;82(3):559-563.
[31]   The Ethics Committee Of The American Society For Reproductive,Medicine. Financial compensation of oocyte donors. Fertil Steril 2007 Aug;88(2):305-309.
[32]   FitzPatrick W. Surplus embryos, nonreproductive cloning, and the intend/foresee distinction. Hastings Cent Rep. 2003 May-Jun;33(3):29-36.

[33] Hoffman DI, Zellman GL, Fair CC, *et al.* Cryopreserved embryos in the United States and their availability for research. Fertil Steril 2003 May;79(5):1063-1069.

[34] Chandra A, Martinez GM, Mosher WD, *et al.* Fertility, family planning, and reproductive health of U.S. women: data from the 2002 National Survey of Family Growth. Vital Health Stat 23 2005 Dec;(25):1-160.

[35] Grieco E, Cassidy R. Overview of Race and Hispanic Origin: Census 2000 Brief. 2000.

[36] Pouton CW, Haynes JM. Embryonic stem cells as a source of models for drug discovery. Nat Rev Drug Discov 2007 Aug;6(8):605-616.

[37] Materson BJ, Reda DJ, Cushman WC, *et al.* Single-drug therapy for hypertension in men. A comparison of six antihypertensive agents with placebo. The Department of Veterans Affairs Cooperative Study Group on Antihypertensive Agents. N Engl J Med 1993 Apr 1;328(13):914-921.

[38] Burchard EG, Avila PC, Nazario S, *et al.* Lower bronchodilator responsiveness in Puerto Rican than in Mexican subjects with asthma. Am J Respir Crit Care Med 2004 Feb 1;169(3):386-392.

[39] Choudhry S, Ung N, Avila PC, *et al.* Pharmacogenetic differences in response to albuterol between Puerto Ricans and Mexicans with asthma. Am J Respir Crit Care Med 2005 Mar 15;171(6):563-570.

CHAPTER 2

Stem Cells and their Contribution to Tissue Repair

Carmen Rios, Elisa Garbayo, Lourdes A. Gomez, Kevin Curtis, Gianluca D'Ippolito and Paul C. Schiller*

Departments of Medicine and Biochemistry & Molecular Biology, University of Miami Miller School of Medicine and Geriatric Research, Education, and Clinical Center and Research Service, Veterans Affairs Medical Center, Miami, Florida, USA

Abstract: Mammalian stem cells can be obtained mostly at all developmental stages and from numerous anatomical sites. Human adult stem cells are perhaps the most clinically relevant. Due to their broader clinical use, extensive research, and a rather more comprehensive understanding of their physiology, bone marrow-derived cells appear as the first choice for applications in regenerative medicine. Models for addressing fundamental aspects of stem cell biology and behavior have been developed in numerous species including C. elegans, drosophila, rodents, and humans. Extensive research around the world has dramatically increased our understanding of the fundamental aspects of stem cell biology and their applications for the treatment of human and animal diseases. Numerous environmental and trophic factors have been identified to play central roles in regulating the self-renewal, proliferation, migration, differentiation, senescence, and death of stem cells, their derived progeny, and the final differentiated cells that perform all tissue and organ functions. Multipotent mesenchymal stromal cells, derived primarily from the bone marrow, have been examined extensively for their capacity to repair damaged tissues. Besides direct differentiation of the stem cells to the desired mature cell type, other indirect mechanisms have been identified to play important roles in the overall repair of the injured tissue. These included production of paracrine factors, modulation of the host inflammatory response, host cell survival, and recruitment and activation of host tissue stem cells.

STEM CELLS: EMBRYONIC AND POST-NATAL

All stem cells—independently of their source—have three general properties: they are capable of dividing and self-renewing for extended periods (the stem cell's ability to replenish their undifferentiated state while undergoing normal, mitotic cell division); they are unspecialized with respect to function; and they can give rise to one or more functionally specialized cell types. As a consequence they should be capable of functionally reconstituting a given tissue *in vivo*. Cells derived from many different sources have been shown to fulfill those criteria, including embryonic stem cells (ESCs) and post-natal stem cells isolated from various tissues.

Post-natal stem cells have been isolated at term from umbilical cord blood (UCB) [1], amniotic fluid [2], placental tissue [3], and numerous tissues of young and old individuals. The later stem cell populations are generally referred to as adult stem cells. Adult stem cells are found in many tissues and in general can only give rise to differentiated cell types from the tissue of origin, thus they are considered multipotent. Some of these include neural stem cells (NSCs) which can undergo self-renewing cell divisions and give rise to neurons, astrocytes and oligodendrocytes, the three main types of nerve cells in the adult brain [4]. Other stem cells like spermatogonial, corneal and endothelial stem cells fulfill also the criteria of a stem cell, except that they differentiate only into a single type of differentiated cell. In contrast, ESCs can give rise to cells from the three somatic germ layers (ectoderm, mesoderm and endoderm) as well as to germ cells [5,6] and are considered pluripotent.

ESCs are derived from pluripotent cells in the inner cell mass of the blastocyst. These cells become lineage restricted *in vivo* at day 7–10 of human development and day 4 of mouse (except in diapause). At this point they commit to a germline or somatic cell fate and subsequently to more tissue specific cells [7]. The presumably unlimited self-renewal capacity of ESCs has to be maintained *in vitro* by specific culture conditions that allow them to self-renew and prevent them from differentiating. Interestingly, it has been recently demonstrated that unlimited self-renewal capacity and pluripotency can be conferred to differentiated cells by the introduction of three or four transcription factors [8-10]. While fibroblasts derived from human ESCs or from human fetus can be reprogrammed to generate induced pluripotent stem (iPS) cells by the   introduction of genes encoding for Oct-4, Sox-2, Klf4 and

---

Address Correspondence to this Author Paul C. Schiller: Geriatric Research, Education, and Clinical Center and Research Service, Veterans Affairs Medical Center, Miami, Florida, USA; Email: PSchille@med.miami.edu

cMyc, the efficiency of reprogramming of neonatal and adult derived fibroblasts as well as adult derived marrow stromal cells was significantly lower, and required in addition transduction with telomerase (hTeRT) and SV40 large T antigen [11]. Although iPS cells represent an interesting and useful model for developmental studies, their clinical use is limited by the requirement that several genes be introduced into somatic cells, thus all the concerns of gene therapy would be associated with them.

Adult stem cells are able to self-renew and proliferate to different extents *in vivo* depending on the turnover rate of differentiated cells which is required for maintaining tissue homeostasis. In tissues, such as in the epithelium of skin, gut and the hematopoietic system, where very large numbers of differentiated progeny need to be generated on a daily basis self-renew and proliferate extensively throughout the life if the individual. In other tissues with a low rate of differentiated progeny turnover, such as the CNS, or where proliferation of terminally differentiated cells contributes to maintain tissue homeostasis such as in the liver, tissue specific stem cells serve as a reserve for cellular replacement or repair in case of minor or major injury, respectively. Nevertheless, in most mammalian tissues there is a decline in the ability to replace mature cells with age.

We will focus our discussion primarily on the properties of adult stem cells, mainly those not covered in other chapters of this book. We will discuss aspects of the self-renewal and differentiation capacity of stem cells from the perspective of tissue and organ repair, highlighting key aspects of stem cells derived from the bone marrow (BM).

ADULT STEM CELLS

Stem cells are responsible for tissue formation during embryonic development as well as repair and maintenance throughout the organism's life. In order to achieve such feats, stem cells have developed a critical balancing act between differentiation and non-differentiation; between proliferation and non-proliferation. Stem cells are exposed to constant signals within their microenvironment that must be accurately identified and processed. The response to these signals may be latent or may progress the cell to the next stage of maturity, all at the discretion of the cell itself. How this process is controlled is the subject of great interest to stem cell researchers. A better understanding of the molecular mechanisms that mediate each turn in the life of the stem cell is gradually being achieved.

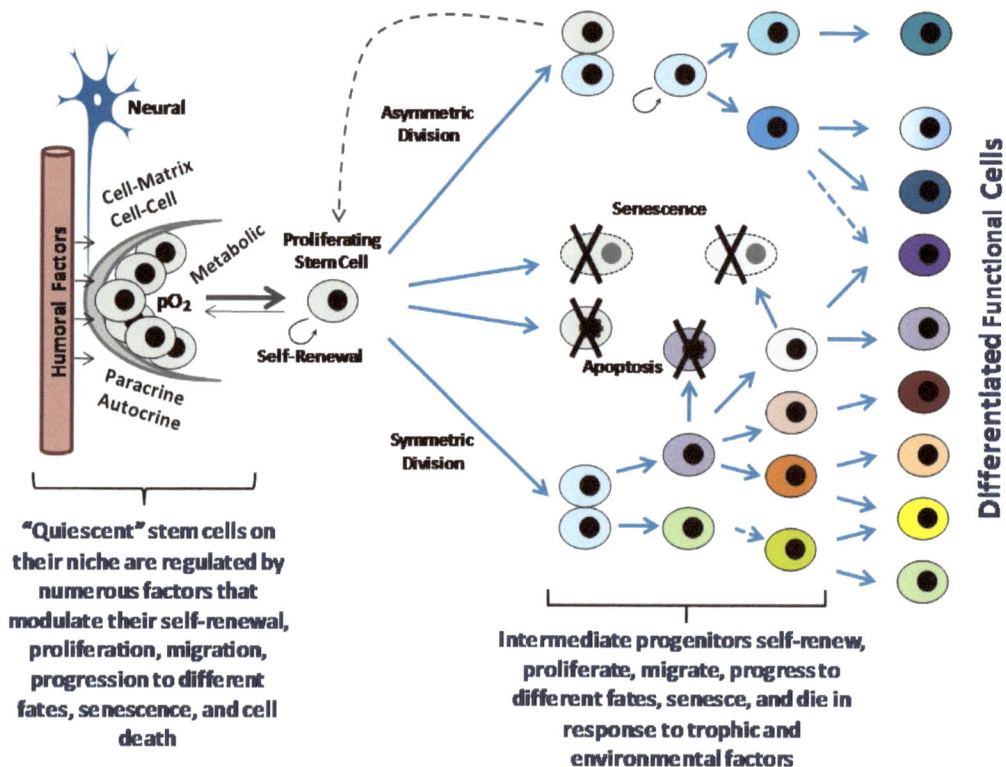

Figure 1: Adult stem cell fate determination. The most developmentally primitive stem cells are thought to localize to specific anatomical sites, or "niches," where their self-renewal is carefully regulated throughout the organisms life. As they leave the

niche stem cells give rise to intermediate progenitors, which continue to differentiate to terminally differentiated functional cells in response to an increasingly complex set of trophic and environmental factors.

One fundamental characteristic of stem cells is their ability to undergo asymmetric division – the production of daughter cells in which one retains its stem cell identity while the other engages into a differentiation program. Asymmetric cell division is a conserved mechanism for partitioning genetic information generating daughter cells (progenitors) with unlimited proliferation potential [12]. During differentiation, these progenitor cells give rise to definitive somatic cells. Both stem and progenitor cells are kept on reserve in most tissues of the organism, providing a source of constant replacement of cells lost due to cellular damage or death (Fig. **1**).

HEMATOPOIETIC STEM CELLS

It is generally accepted that the reserve of stem cells exists within a specialized microenvironment called a "niche" [13]. The niche is believed to be lined with more-differentiated cells to create a source of nourishment and protection to the stem cell population within [14]. The niche also serves as a line of communication between the stem cells and areas of need within the organism, such as a damaged artery requiring repair. The importance of the microenvironment for stem cell function was first determined after a mutation in the gene encoding membrane-bound stem cell factor (SCF; also known as KIT ligand) was revealed to cause changes in the hematopoietic stem cell (HSC) niche leading to failure of bone-marrow HSC maintenance *in vivo* [15]. However, details on the structure and localization, as well as the molecular and cellular basis for niche activity, remain complex and unclear. Current research is underway that delves into the concept of a stem cell niche with promising supporting data on the molecules and cell types that are involved after transplantation into lethally irradiated recipients [16].

Hematopoietic stem cells (HSCs) are responsible for producing all mature red and white blood cells and represent the best characterized adult stem cell population. The most primitive HSC, also termed the long-term repopulating HSC (LTR-HSC), is a relatively quiescent cell during steady state hematopoiesis and undergoes expansion and differentiation in its niche within the bone marrow. HSCs self renewal capabilities allow them to achieve a balance between differentiation and non-differentiation while ensuring an adequate population size for the lifetime of the organism [17]. The daily replenishment of blood cells is achieved to a large extent by divisions and subsequent discrete differentiation steps of cells that are immediate descendants of the most primitive LTR-HSC, termed short term repopulating HSC (STR-HSC), a slightly more committed hematopoietic progenitor cells (HPC).

Within the bone marrow, signals are received that may be either transient or dominant triggering a sequence of events that decide the cell's fate as it migrates out of the niche. The co-mingling of the HSCs with a complex network of vasculature in the bone marrow allows for easy uptake into the blood stream, transporting the cells throughout the organism.

MULTIPOTENT MESENCHYMAL STROMAL CELLS

The bone marrow niche for HSCs, is thought to be made up of stromal cells, which support the HSCs while maintaining their stem cell characteristics either through direct contact with the HSCs and or by contact with soluble factors within the niche that signal for quiescence, maintenance or expansion. Further understanding of the cellular and chemical architecture within the niche is vital in understanding stem cell behavior [18]. Human Multipotent Mesenchymal Stromal Cells (hMSCs) make up a non-hematopoietic, heterogeneous population of uncommitted and lineage-committed adult stem cells that have the ability to adhere to plastic, express the surface antigens CD73, CD90, and CD105, and are able of differentiating into osteoblasts, adipocytes, and chondrocytes [19,20]. Thus, these 2 types of marrow stem cells may share a common niche or may have similar niches that regulate their self-renewal, proliferation, differentiation, senescence or cell death. hMSCs cells were first described by A.J. Friedenstein as fibroblast-like cells residing in the bone marrow of vertebrate animals, including humans [21]. Adult stem cells assure lifelong regeneration of adult tissues (e.g. blood cells, bone, fat, cartilage, vasculature, muscle, etc.). If the rejuvenating effect of self renewal in stem cells were perfect, senescent cells (cells that have lost their ability to grow and divide) could be replaced indefinitely. In the context of aging, stem cell self renewal is important for two reasons. On the one hand, stem cells are the ideal source of regenerating aging tissue. Secondly, reactivation of stem cells, if properly controlled, could be used in treatment of degenerative diseases [22].

Recent studies have shown the multi-potentiality of hMSCs. Bone marrow used in transplantation experiments demonstrated that stromal cells can serve as long-lasting precursors for bone, cartilage, and lung [23]. Ferrari, *et al.* showed that bone marrow-derived myogenic progenitors can migrate into degenerating muscle and give rise to fully differentiated muscle fibers [24]. After isolation from the marrow, hMSCs attach to the surface of culture dishes and form colonies, and their numbers can be expanded *ex vivo* [25,26]. The population of undifferentiated hMSCs can be expanded using different culture conditions and directed to differentiate into specific phenotypic cell lineages [26,27]. The potential of hMSCs lies in their plasticity and ability to repair damaged tissue by giving rise to fully differentiated and functional cells within such tissue [24]. Interestingly, differences have been reported in number of hMSCs with *in vitro* osteogenic potential as a function of age [26]. While the number of hMSCs with osteogenic potential was high in donors less than 15 years old, a decrease was found in donors more than 40 years of age. However, the responsiveness of hMSCs to osteogenic stimulation remained intact and was unaffected by the age of the donor [26].

Human MSCs have been isolated and cultured by different labs in somewhat different conditions [28], which have led to use some different names to refer to this cell population. Methodologies have been developed to isolate, expand, and characterize these cells obtained after gradient centrifugation of human bone marrow cells [29, 30]. hMSCs are morphologically heterogeneous in culture and phenotypic differences in comparison to MSCs have been observed using flow cytometry and real time PCR [29]. hMSC-like cells have been identified in other tissues including umbilical cord blood [28], peripheral blood [31], adipose tissue [32], skeletal muscle and dermis [33].

In recent years, several groups have isolated developmentally primitive cells from BM, UCB, or fetal and adult tissues, which can be extensively cultured *in vitro* and have the ability to generate cells of multiple germinal layers, similar to the MIAMI cells. These include the multilineage adult progenitor cells (MAPCs) [34], human BM-derived multipotent stem cells (hBMSCs) [35], unrestricted somatic stem cells (USSCs) [36], fetal somatic stem cells (FSSCs) [37], amniotic fluid-derived stem (AFS) cells [2], human fetal liver multipotent progenitor cells (hFLMPCs) [38], and multipotent adult stem cells (MASCs) [39]. Some of these cell populations, including MIAMI cells, MAPC, hBMSC, AFS and MASC, may be capable to proliferate without telomere shortening. Many of them are reported to express the ES cell specific transcription factors Oct4 and Nanog. However, some of these cells are found are relatively low levels and it is not clear if they play determining roles during the normal tissue repair process.

A unique subpopulation of hMSCs have been isolated and characterized by the expression of unique distinctive markers, including those of pluripotent embryonic stem cells (Oct-4, Rex-1 and SSEA-4), distinguishing them from marrow-derived cells previously described [40]. These cells were named, marrow-isolated adult multilineage inducible (MIAMI) cells, based on their extensive proliferative capacity while maintaining telomere length and potential to generate mature cells derived from all three embryonic germ layers. MIAMI cells have been isolated as early passage cells capable of extensive expansion *in vitro* from males and females, 3 to 72 years of age, maintaining a remarkably consistent molecular profile independent of age and gender [26]. This consistent molecular profile is achieved using culture conditions that aim to mimic the niche where these cells are predicted to reside *in vivo*, which include a low oxygen tension environment. The oxygen tension (pO2) in BM ranges from 1 to 7%, which prompted an examination into the role of pO2 in regulating the capacity of MIAMI cells both to self-renew and maintain their pluripotentiality (stemness) or to progress toward osteoblastic differentiation. MIAMI cells grown under pO2 conditions (1, 3, 5, 10, and 21% oxygen) show different rates of proliferation. The proliferation rate of cells exposed to 3% oxygen increased, resulting in cell numbers more than threefold higher than those of cells exposed to air. In cells grown under osteoblastic differentiation conditions, the expression of the osteoblastic markers osteocalcin, bone sialoprotein, osterix, and Runx2 and alkaline phosphatase activity was upregulated when incubated in air; however, it was blocked at low (3%) pO2. In light of these results, a physiological scenario in which primitive MIAMI cells self-renew while localized to areas of low pO2 in the bone marrow, but tend to differentiate toward osteoblasts when they are located closer to blood vessels and exposed to higher pO2 is quite feasible. Therefore, the maintenance of developmentally primitive human cells *in vitro* at low pO2 would be more physiological and favor stemness over differentiation [26].

TISSUE-DERIVED SPECIFIC STEM CELLS

Stem cells derived from post-natal tissues are undifferentiated cells found throughout the body. As indicated, these reservoirs of specific stem cells contribute to sustain cell turnover in their respective tissues and depending of their origin, can be characterized by different properties. While the self-renewing ability of stem cells is tightly related to their ability to undergo asymmetric divisions, many stem cells can divide symmetrically, giving rise to two immature stem cell daughters or alternative to two more differentiated progenitor cells. This can take place particularly during *in vitro* expansion or when cells are responding to an injury *in vivo*. The facultative use of symmetric or asymmetric divisions by stem cells may be a key adaptation that is crucial for adult regenerative capacity [41].

The developmental origin of tissue derived stem cells is not clear, some propose that they arise during embryogenesis, usually sharing the expression of key transcription factors with cells of the embryonic rudiment that produced them and are probably in a similar developmental state [42]. It is clear to date that adult tissue contains cells that upon *in vitro* culture exhibit pluripotent capacity reminiscent to that of embryonic stem cells. Adult tissue at any age may also contain pluripotent stem cells that have the potential of differentiate into mature cells that are different to the tissue of residence of the specific stem cell and because they have migratory properties their function may not be restricted. Rather stem cell pools may serve as depositories activated at need to supply cells to different body sites [43].

EPITHELIAL STEM CELLS

Epithelia constitutes about 60% of the differentiated tissue types in the body, these cells cover the outer and inner surface of the body. Their functions are diverse and extensive, frequently involving the secretion of bioactive materials and absorption of substances, as well as preserving the integrity of the surfaces. Skin and intestine (digestive tract) are characterized by a rapid cell turnover, while the ducts of the pancreas and liver show a slower turnover under normal conditions but with special adaptations for regeneration. The stem and progenitor cells in the epithelial tissue are usually localized at a distinct anatomical niche-like site within the tissue which is distinct from where the differentiated progeny cells generally localize; i.e. in the intestine the stem cells are located in the crypt base, the transit amplifying cells constitute 2/3 of the height of the crypt, and the postmitotic differentiated cells occupy the upper part of the crypt and the villi. Almost all epithelia have this composed structural units i.e. glands of the stomach, the acini of the salivary glands, the lobules of the liver, and the nephrons of the kidney. These "structural-proliferative units" are units of self renewal, composed of one or a few stem cells. Usually epithelia are composed of different cell types, and the ability to form all of them is often considered to be a key aspect of stem cell behavior. When a damage or lesion is produced and regeneration is required, local chemicals signals must be released in tissues that can activate the dormant multipotent cells. In the epidermis an over-expression and nuclear localization of β-catenin precedes the formation of new formation of hair follicles, suggesting an involvement of Wnt pathway in the stem cell behavior [44]. Stem cells of the hair follicle are located on a specific structural niche termed the bulge. Stem cells migrating out of the bulge give rise to all of the lower hair follicle epithelial cell types [45].

HEPATIC AND PANCREATIC STEM CELLS

Liver and pancreas progenitors develop from endoderm cells in the embryonic foregut. Shortly after their specification, liver and pancreas progenitors rapidly acquire markedly different cellular functions and regenerative capacities. The liver and pancreas coordinately control body metabolism, including the modification of digested nutrients by hepatocytes in the liver and the regulation of blood glucose levels by insulin secreted from β-cells in the pancreas. Human hepatic stem cells role in liver regeneration and maintenance is not yet clear. The progenitor/oval cell compartment also known as "ductular reaction" can be activated when there is damage to the hepatocyte or cholangiocyte compartment, or when their replication is inhibited [46]. It is believed that this compartment is the stem cell niche of the liver, located in the smallest branch of bile ductules also known as the Canals of Hering, which are lined by hepatocytes and cholangiocytes. Schmelzer *et al.* published in 2007 a study that demonstrated the existence of human hepatic stem cells (hHpSC) within the canals of Hering in pediatric and adult livers [47]. Showing their capability to self-renew, to proliferate ex-vivo (>150 pd's), their pluripotency (committed biliary progenitors and hepatoblasts as well as other endodermal cell types), and the evidence that they yield mature liver tissue after transplantation.

Diabetes Mellitus is a chronic metabolic disease that affects 18.2 million people in the USA and more than 240 million worldwide. Type 1 diabetes mellitus is a chronic disease resulting from the selective autoimmune destruction of pancreatic insulin producing β-cells. Unfortunately, the exact location of the adult pancreatic stem/progenitor cells is controversial. The main treatment for years has been insulin replacement, but some patients have increased the risk for developing DM complications as nephropathy, retinopathy and neuropathy. Transplantation therapy represents a potential cure for type 1 diabetes mellitus, islet transplantation compare to whole pancreas transplantation, is minimally invasive, but is limited by availability of human pancreatic tissue, and only few patients remain insulin independent for more than a year [48,49]. MSC-like cells have been isolated from human pancreatic ductal epithelial cells, expressing cell surface antigens used to define MSCs isolated from bone marrow such as CD13, CD29, CD44, CD49b, CD54, CD90 and CD105. Pancreatic MSCs were able to differentiate into mesoderm (osteocytes, adipocytes and chondrocytes), and were also capable of deriving endoderm (hepatocytes and β-cells) [50]. Human pancreatic islet-derived mesenchymal (hPIDM) cells have been isolated *in vitro*. These cells can be expanded for 16-20 passages and differentiate into adipocytes, osteocytes and chondrocytes. Under serum removal they differentiate toward islet-like clusters (ILCs) and secrete insulin. In addition to insulin they express other endocrine pancreatic cells transcription factors including Nkx2-2 and Nkx6-1 [49]. Additional studies are necessary to optimize protocols for endocrine differentiation and generate functional β-cells that can be used for transplantation, that can improve insulin production and restore metabolic and/or glycemic control.

RENAL STEM CELLS

The kidney develops from the ureteric bud and the metanephric mesenchyme, which are mesodermal in origin. The ureteric bud forms from an outgrowth of the mesonephric duct giving rise to the ureter, renal pelvis, major and minor calyces, collecting ducts and collecting tubules. The metanephric mesenchyme forms from the caudal portion of the intermediate mass, and it surrounds the end of the ureteric bud, giving rise to all portions of the nephron, collecting tubes and renal interstitium [51]. Although cell division is infrequent in the adult kidney, it has the capacity to regenerate and repair post injury (nephrons). In our society the prevalence and incidence of chronic kidney disease is increasing at 6 to 8 % per year, in part as a consequence of the high prevalence of diabetes and obesity. This is why potential use of stem cells for regenerative medicine to treat renal diseases represents a critical goal [52]. Different cells have been localized in multiple sites in the kidney, but the basic question of whether the stem cells exist in the adult kidney still remains controversial. It remains a challenge to confirm whether the cells isolated are the same as the cells *in vivo* [53]. In recent years, approaches to the identification of renal/progenitor cells have included: the isolation based on cellular behavior, isolation based on specific markers, isolation based upon localization, with stem/progenitor features being attributed to both tubular and interstitial populations [54].

NEURAL STEM/PROGENITOR CELLS

Neural stem cells (NSC) are described as cells which (i) self renew, (ii) can undergo asymmetric cell division, and (iii) generate neurons, astrocytes and oligodendrocytes (1:5:25 ratio respectively) during development and potentially in the adult mammalian brain [4,55]. In the adult mammalian brain endogenous multipotent neural stem cell niches are limited to the forebrain subventricular zone (SVZ) lining the lateral ventricles and the subgranular layer of the dentate gyrus in primates [56] and in humans [4,57]. There are other putative neural stem cell niches in the cortex [58], olfactory bulb [59,60]. Although much is known about the brain during embryonic development, it is still unclear as to the role of NSC's during the life of the adult brain.

Human fetal brain (FBr) tissue is the main source of NSC's used for *in-vitro* study, and have a specific subset of cell surface markers: CD133$^+$, 5E12$^+$, CD34$^-$, CD45$^-$, CD24$^{-/lo}$ [61] as well as express specific genes involved in the maintenant of NPC: Sox2, E(Spl), Hes, Here genes (for a recent review see: Stigloher *et al.* [62]). Fetal brain derived

NSC's (FBr-NSC) have the potential to undergo long-term culture as neurospheres and still maintain the ability to undergo engraftment, proliferation, migration and neural differentiation upon transplantation into the brain of immunosuppressed rats [63] and neonatal mice [61]. A recent breakthrough study also showed the ability of human NSCs to migrate along the nigrostriatal pathway to degenerated tissue in a non-human primate model of Parkinson's disease (MPTP) [64]. It is unclear as to the mechanism of NSC migration in Bjugstad's study, but the inflammatory response has been shown to induce the migration of human umbilical cord blood cells in a stroke model leading to the hypothesis that localized inflammation in the brain leads to the migration of NSC. Mendoza-Torreblanca *et al.* also demonstrated that the implantation of a barrier along the rostral migratory stream in adult rats interrupted the migration of neuroepithelial progenitor cells (NPCs) from the SVZ, inducing the accumulation of periglomerular neurons [65]. This study further supports (i) the idea of an active neural precursor/stem cell niche residing in the adult mammalian brain, and (ii) that the location of the niche might determine the identity of neurons produced.

It is unknown if inflammation-induced NSC migration occurs during periods of damage/inflammation in the adult mammalian brain. It is unlikely since aging leads to a decrease in neurogenesis in rats [66] and non-human primates greater than 20 years old, but not in aged mice [67]. This would suggest that during age related neural degeneration, there are fewer self-renewing NSCs present to undergo inflammation induced migration, leading to a decrease in CNS repair, increased inflammatory response, and the onset of age-induced cognitive dysfunction. It may be that in young individuals, there is a limited capacity only for self-renewal of NSCs important in general neurogenesis observed during learning and memory [68], and not for neural repair due to brain damage or degeneration as seen in aged individuals. Due to the overall decrease in age-related tissue repair, specifically concerning the central and peripheral nervous system, the ability to extract, expand ex-vivo, and transplant NSCs which migrate to the region of damage and undergo neurogenesis would be advantageous to treating nervous system damage.

NEURAL STEM CELLS IN REGENERATIVE MEDICINE

Due to the decrease in endogenous NSC's ability to repair CNS damage during the lifetime of the human adult brain, it is hopefully that ex-vivo expanded NSCs may be used for providing therapy for diseases and CNS damage which efficacious therapy has not yet been developed. Neural stem cells derived from human fetal brain, post-mortem human brain (striatum, hippocampus SVZ, cortex, olfactory neuroepithelium retina) [69] or trans-germinally differentiated from other adult stem cell sources may provide a source for ex-vivo expanded NSCs used for cell therapy based transplantation. Not only age related degenerative diseases such as Parkinson's disease (PD), but also stroke induced cerebral ischemia, head trauma, spinal cord injury, peripheral nerve damage, and the targeting of gliomas for gene therapy are a few examples under consideration for NSC therapy.

Parkinson's disease results in the degeneration of dopamine producing substantia nigra neurons, leading to a deficiency in dopamine. Classically PD has been treated using the pharmacologic agent l-dopa to treat the symptoms of PD during the initial years of treatment. However, progressively severe side effects during prolonged treatment indicate the need for alternative therapies. An advantage of using cell-therapy in this case is due to the fact that PD is characterized by the degeneration of a limited number of neurons localized specifically to the striatum [70]. This would allow for the targeted injection of NSCs expanded under optimum conditions (3%02) in the presence of bFGF/EGF and either injected undifferentiated or predifferentiated (+IL-1b, IL-11, LIF, GNDF) as dopamine producing NSCs [71]. Initial studies showed that cell-replacement therapy replacing degenerated dopaminergic neuron with FBr-NSCs ameliorated some but not all symptoms of PD [72] the mechanism of action remains unclear. In a non-human primate model of PD, FBr-NPCs injected into the striatum migrated along the nigrostriatal pathway to the substantia nigra [64], which shows the migratory potential of NSCs toward the area in need of repair. Burnstein et al also showed that embryonic cortex NPCs pretreated with NT-4 increased the number of neurons after transplantation into the substantia nigra of a rat model of PD after 12 weeks [73]. Initial clinical trials used human fetus ventral mesencephalic graphs transplanted into patients with PD. The use of embryonic derived tissue or NPCs not only raises ethical questions but their use has also led to dyskinesias in some of the patients [74].

NSCs also have the potential to be used as seed cells for peripheral nerve repair. NSCs derived from newborn guinea pigs (<24hrs) were injected into chitosan conduits supplemented with a collagen protein sponge and showed promise in repairing the excised bucal branches of the facial nerve in adult rabbits [75].

Transplantation of NSCs migrate toward tumors in animal models of brain tumors (gliomas) [76-78]. The tumor homing ability of NPCs is also being used in combination with gene therapy in order use NPCs as vehicles for gene delivery. Yang et al used NPCs which overexpressed Il-12 in a rat glioma model in order to target a tumor specific Il-12 mediated immune response [79]. Another elegant study conducted by Aboody et al 2006 used NPCs expressing cytosine deaminase to convert an administered pro-drug (5-flourocytosine) into its active chemotherapeutic form which decreased a melanoma tumor size by about 40% in mice (Aboody et al 2006). It is still unclear as the mechanism of migration/homing toward tumors. One theory concludes that VEGF and SDF-1 may be responsible for the observed NPC-tumor homing [80].

FUNCTIONAL ACTIVITIES OF MSCs: PARACRINE EFFECTS AND IMMUNOMODULATION

Paracrine Effects

MSCs initially attracted interest for their ability to differentiate into multiple cellular phenotypes. This characteristic made MSCs ideal for use in tissue engineering therapies. However, recent evidences of functional improvement with limited engraftment indicated that stem cells do not repair tissues solely by their stem cell-like ability to differentiate [81]. In this regard, current observations have focused attention on the paracrine effect of MSCs. Since MSCs secrete large quantities of cytokines, chemokines and growth factors that are both immunomodulatory and trophic, the stem cell beneficial effect may be mediated, at least in part, by complex paracrine actions. In general, only 1% to 5% of the donor stem cells engraft and survive after transplantation and frequently, the functional improvement in the organ occurs within days or even hours after injury excluding cell differentiation as a cause. Importantly, *in vitro* and *in vivo* studies have shown that much of the functional improvement and attenuation of injury afforded by stem cells can be replicated by cell-free, conditioned media derived from stem cells [82].

Although the mechanistic basis for MSC-mediated paracrine effects remain unclear and the particular growth factors contributing to these reparative effects needs to be defined, several mechanisms have been proposed. Recently Crisostomo and co-workers reviewed the most important ones elucidated so far [82].

Stimulation of angiogenesis: MSCs transplanted into injured tissue stimulate angiogenesis that may improve regional blood flow [83]. The particular growth factors that may contribute to this neovascular effect most likely include vascular endothelial growth factor (VEGF), a potent promoter of angiogenesis, hepatocyte growth factor (HGF), an angiogenic and anti-apoptotic cytokine, and basic fibroblast growth factor (FGF2) which has been shown to be intimately involved with endothelial cell proliferation and may be a more potent angiogenic factor than VEGF (Fig. **2**).

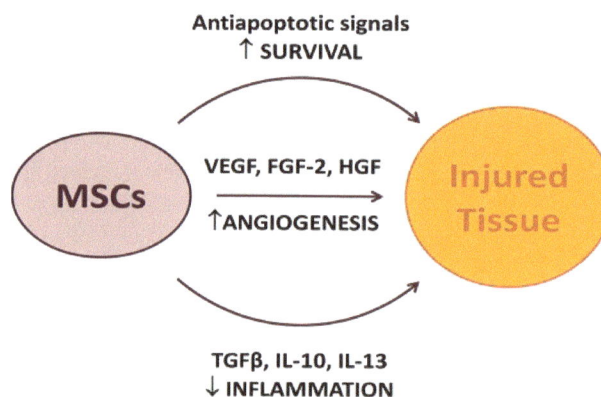

Figure 2: Alternative mechanisms of tissue repair mediated by mesenchymal stromal cells. Besides differentiated to the desired cell phenotype, MSCs can modulate pro-survival, pro-angiogenic, and anti-inflammatory pathways, as well as recruit other progenitor cells to repair the injured tissue.

Decrease of inflammation: The anti-inflammatory effects of MSCs have generated a great deal of interest. MSCs administration may affect the secretion of pro-inflammatory cytokines and chemokines attenuating local inflammation and facilitating injured tissue regeneration. MSCs may modulate allogeneic immune cell responses from a pro-inflammatory toward an anti-inflammatory environment by interacting with dendritic cells, T lymphocytes and natural killer cells [84]. Transforming growth factor beta (TGF-β) appears to be involved in the suppression of inflammation mediated by MSCs. MSCs have also been shown to release insulin like growth factor 1 (IGF-1) a survival growth factor that offers protection against apoptosis (Fig. **2**).

MSCs transplantation inhibits fibrosis and has a beneficial effect in remodelling the extracellular matrix, which prevents deterioration in organ function. In a model of global heart failure, adrenomedullin (ADM) was the antifibrotic factor that may, at least partially, mediate the antifibrotic effect of MSCs [85].

Exogenous MSCs transplantation may activate resident stem cells and mobilize circulating progenitor cells. In this regard, recent evidence corroborates the existence of organ-resident stem cells in an increasing number of organs, such as liver, gut, heart, skin and brain. HGH and IGF-1 may be the soluble factors implicated in this effect. These resident stem cells may possess growth factor receptors that can be activated to induce their migration and proliferations and to promote both the restoration of dead tissue and the improved function in damaged tissue [82]. Stem cell paracrine effects have been observed in HSCs and MSCs. However, MSC have advantages over HSC populating, including availability from small aspirates of donor bone marrow, ease of expansion in an *in vitro* cell culture, simple isolation via plastic adherence, and an innate ability to evade rejection [86].

Although MSCs were first proposed in regenerative medicine on the basis of their ability to differentiate into multiple cellular phenotypes, their therapeutic effect can result from other characteristics, such as their anti-proliferative and anti-inflammatory properties [87]. Importantly, advances in the understanding of the mechanism by which adult stem cells produce growth factors may optimize their beneficial paracrine and autocrine effects. Further investigations are needed to address the potency of intrinsic paracrine factors released by stem cells as well as the optimal localization, timing, delivery and stem cell type to be transplanted allowing earlier and more effective clinical therapies.

Immunomodulation

It is now accepted that human MSCs do not express the hematopoietic markers CD34, CD14 and CD45, while they are positive for CD44, CD71, CD73, CD90 and CD105 [88]. *In vitro* hMSCs constitutively express low surface densities of MHC class I molecules and are negative for MHC class II as well as for co-stimulatory molecules such as CD80, CD86 and CD40 [89]. In addition they express different adhesion molecules including several integrins [89]. MSC can also produce a variety of growth factors, cytokines, chemokines and proteases that are likely to play a role either in their immunomodulatory or in their migratory function. MSC are profoundly influenced by microenvironmental factors and by cell-to-cell interactions. Importantly, MSC seem to migrate preferentially to sites of injury, preferentially attracted by chemotactic signals release by injured cells, suggesting that they can sense the local microenvironment where they promote functional recovery [90]. They also respond to some inflammatory cytokines such as interleukin (IL) IL-1β, IL-17, and IFN-γ [89].

Immunosuppressive Properties of MSCs

The immunomodulatory properties of MSCs are not yet fully understood. Large number of studies reported that the immunosuppressive activities of stem cells are mediated by the secretion of immunomodulatory factors that turn off the T-cell surveillance and the chronic inflammatory processes [91] in collaboration with contact-dependent mechanism mediated by adhesion molecules [87]. It is likely that none of these molecules has an exclusive role and the immunoregulation is mediated by several molecules. Examples of molecules that are thought to collaborate in the immunosuppression effect of stem cells are inducible nitric oxide synthase (iNOS), heme oxygenase (HO), prostaglandin E2 (PGE2) an enzymatic product of arachidonic acid metabolism and the indoleamine 2,3-dioxygenase (IDO) a tryptophan-degrading enzyme which metabolizes tryptophan to kynurenine. Caplan and co-workers recently reported that the molecule IL-2 also appears to be involved in the immunomodulatory properties of MSCs [91]. Other soluble factors that suppress T-cell are members of the transforming growth factor superfamily, hepatic growth factors, IL-6, IL-10 and soluble human leukocyte antigen (HLA)-G5 which have important implications in transplantation biology.

The Effects of MSCs on Immune Cells

MSCs have immunomodulatory properties that are among the most fascinating aspects of their biology. MSCs can interact with cells of both the innate and adaptative immune system by interaction with T- and B-cells, dendritic cells (DC) and natural killer (NK) cells (Fig. **3**).

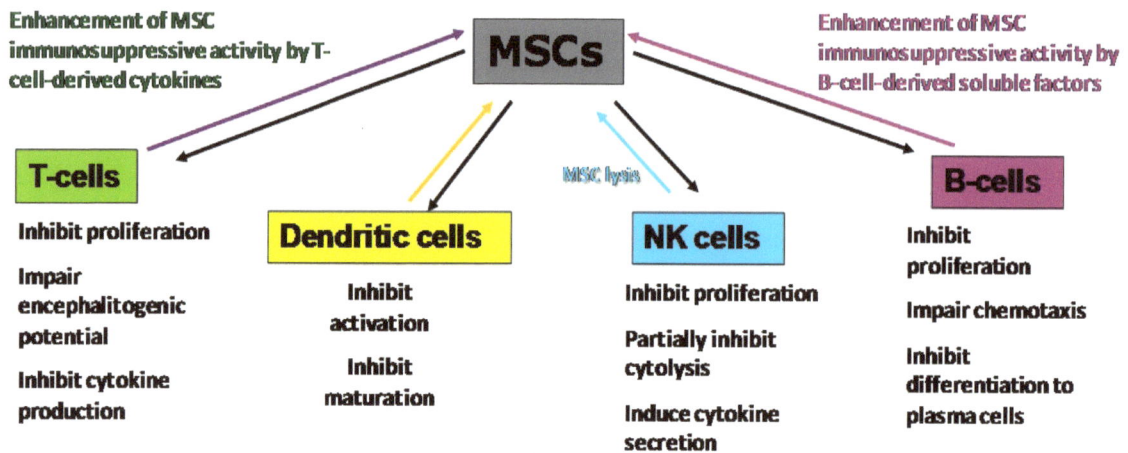

Figure 3: Interactions between MSCs and cells of the innate and adaptive immune systems.

MSCs inhibit proliferation of T cells *in vitro* and *in vivo*. However, despite the general consensus about MSC capacity to inhibit T lymphocytes proliferation, little is known regarding the responsible mechanism. Uccelli and co-workers stated that a possible explanation could be the inhibition of cell division by preventing cell to entry into the S phase of the cycle and consequent arrest in the G0/G1 phase associated with inhibition of cyclin D2 expression [89]. The same cell division inhibition was shown for B lymphocytes, NK cells and DC. The inhibition of T-cell proliferation is likely to be mediated by direct cell-cell contact and by soluble factors secretion. TGF-β1, PGE-2, HLA-G and IDO represent soluble molecules that have been proposed to inhibit T-cell proliferation. Moreover, MSCs affect several other functions of T-cells including cytokine secretion and cytotoxicity. The proliferation and activation of B-cells which are specialized for antibody production affecting antibody secretion are also regulated by MSCs. These effects seem to depend on part to the physical contact between MSCs and B cells and in part by the release of soluble factors [89].

MSCs could inhibit the differentiation of monocytes into dendritic cells by downregulation both the surface expression of CD11c, CD83 and major histocompatibility complex (MHC) class II. MSCs could also inhibit the dendritic cell maturation. MSCs can also alter the cytokine secretion profile of dendritic cells. In this sense, stem cells up-regulate the secretion of regulatory cytokines such as IL-10 and down-regulate the secretion of pro-inflammatory cytokines such as IFN-γ, IL-12 and tumor necrosis factor-α [92].

Finally, MSCs also regulate immune response through interacting with NK cells. NK cells are major effectors of the innate immune system that play a role in the elimination of cells infected by virus and malignant cells. Several authors have reported that stem cells were able to inhibit NK cell proliferation, cytokine production and cytotoxic activity. This effect was mediated by cell-cell contact and by the production of soluble factors such as IL-2, IL-15 and IFN-γ [93]. Taken together the published studies on NK cell-MSC interactions reiterate the concept that the final outcome of the interaction between MSCs and other type of cells *in vivo* will be primarily dictated by the microenvironment [89].

MSCs Clinical Translation

The potential clinical applications of MSCs are diverse. Available data suggest that MSCs exhibit two key features important for their clinical use. First, MSCs seem to be able to "freeze" immune competent cells through inhibition of cell division. Second, they support the recruitment of local precursor cells and provide trophic factors supporting the survival and repair of injured cells [90]. By virtue of their limited immunogenicity mainly based on the lack in expression of MHC class II, MSCs are particularly attractive candidates for the treatment of immune-mediated disorders including organ transplantation and autoimmune diseases such as type 1 diabetes, multiple sclerosis, therapy-resistant rheumatoid arthritis, lupus, bronchial asthma, idiopathic pulmonary fibrosis or Crohn´s disease.

However, both their condition of immunoprivileged and their immunosuppressive function have recently been challenged when analyzed under particular experimental conditions suggesting that MSCs are not as immunoprivileged as once thought [92]. Current data also suggest that the immunological outcome after *in vivo* administration of MSCs is not completely predictable because of the profound influence of microenvironmental factors that dictate the final effect of MSCs on target cells. Moreover, some practical questions including patient selection, infusion method, cells source, dose and schedule of infusion will require standardization. Finally, although few adverse effects have been reported after *in vivo* MSC administration, there are some aspects such as their potential tumorogenicity, the differentiation into undesired tissue, and long-term safety need to be addressed in order to provide safe therapies.

REFERENCES

[1]   Weiss ML, Troyer DL. Stem cells in the umbilical cord. Stem Cell Rev 2006; 2:155-162.

[2]   De Coppi P, Bartsch G, Jr., Siddiqui MM, *et al.* Isolation of amniotic stem cell lines with potential for therapy. Nat Biotechnol 2007; 25:100-106.

[3]   Matikainen T, Laine J. Placenta--an alternative source of stem cells. Toxicol Appl Pharmacol 200; 207:544549.

[4]   Gage FH. Mammalian neural stem cells. Science 2000; 287:1433-1438.

[5]   Thomson JA, Itskovitz-Eldor J, Shapiro SS, *et al.* Embryonic stem cell lines derived from human blastocysts. Science 1998; 282:1145-1147.

[6]   Martin GR. Isolation of a pluripotent cell line from early mouse embryos cultured in medium conditioned by teratocarcinoma stem cells. Proc Natl Acad Sci USA 1981; 78:7634-7638.

[7]   Rossant J. Stem cells and early lineage development. Cell 2008; 132:527-531.

[8]   Wernig M, Meissner A, Foreman R, *et al. In vitro* reprogramming of fibroblasts into a pluripotent ES-cell-like state. Nature 2007; 448:318-324.

[9]   Okita K, Ichisaka T, Yamanaka S. Generation of germline-competent induced pluripotent stem cells. Nature 2007; 448:313-317.

[10]   Yu J, Vodyanik MA, Smuga-Otto K, *et al.* Induced pluripotent stem cell lines derived from human somatic cells. Science 2007; 318:1917-1920.

[11]   Park IH, Zhao R, West JA, *et al.* Reprogramming of human somatic cells to pluripotency with defined factors. Nature 2008; 451:141-146.

[12]   Roegiers F, Jan YN. Asymmetric cell division. Curr Opin Cell Biol 2004; 16:195-205.

[13]   Schofield R. The relationship between the spleen colony-forming cell and the haemopoietic stem cell. Blood Cells 1978; 4:7-25.

[14]   Calvi LM, Adams GB, Weibrecht KW, *et al.* Osteoblastic cells regulate the haematopoietic stem cell niche. Nature 2003; 425:841-846.

[15]   Barker JE. Early transplantation to a normal microenvironment prevents the development of Steel hematopoietic stem cell defects. Exp Hematol 1997; 25:542-547.

[16]   Wilson A, Trumpp A. Bone-marrow haematopoietic-stem-cell niches. Nat Rev Immunol 2006; 6:93-106.

[17]   Oakley EJ, Van Zant G. Unraveling the complex regulation of stem cells: implications for aging and cancer. Leukemia 2007; 21:612-621.

[18]   Wagner W, Horn P, Bork S, *et al.* Aging of hematopoietic stem cells is regulated by the stem cell niche. Exp Gerontol 2008; 43:974-980.

[19]   Colter DC, Sekiya I, Prockop DJ. Identification of a subpopulation of rapidly self-renewing and multipotential adult stem cells in colonies of human marrow stromal cells. Proc Natl Acad Sci USA 2001; 98:7841-7845.

[20]   Dominici M, Le Blanc K, Mueller I, *et al.* Minimal criteria for defining multipotent mesenchymal stromal cells. The International Society for Cellular Therapy position statement. Cytotherapy 2006; 8:315-317.

[21]   Friedenstein AJ, Chailakhjan RK, Lalykina KS. The development of fibroblast colonies in monolayer cultures of guinea-pig bone marrow and spleen cells. Cell Tissue Kinet 1970; 3:393-403.

[22]   Ho AD, Wagner W, Mahlknecht U. Stem cells and ageing. The potential of stem cells to overcome age-related deteriorations of the body in regenerative medicine. EMBO Rep 2005; 6 Spec No: S35-38.

[23]   Pereira RF, Halford KW, O'Hara MD, *et al.* Cultured adherent cells from marrow can serve as long-lasting precursor cells for bone, cartilage, and lung in irradiated mice. Proc Natl Acad Sci USA 1995; 92:4857-4861.

[24]   Ferrari G, Cusella-De Angelis G, Coletta M, *et al.* Muscle regeneration by bone marrow-derived myogenic progenitors. Science 1998; 279:1528-1530.

[25]   Jaiswal N, Haynesworth SE, Caplan AI, *et al.* Osteogenic differentiation of purified, culture-expanded human mesenchymal stem cells *in vitro.* J Cell Biochem 1997; 64:295-312.

[26]   D'Ippolito G, Schiller PC, Ricordi C, *et al.* Age-related osteogenic potential of mesenchymal stromal stem cells from human vertebral bone marrow. J Bone Miner Res 1999; 14:1115-1122.

[27]   Bruder SP, Jaiswal N, Haynesworth SE. Growth kinetics, self-renewal, and the osteogenic potential of purified human mesenchymal stem cells during extensive subcultivation and following cryopreservation. J Cell Biochem 1997; 64:278-294.

[28]   Minguell JJ, Erices A, Conget P. Mesenchymal stem cells. Exp Biol Med (Maywood) 2001; 226:507-520.

[29]   Majumdar MK, Thiede MA, Mosca JD, Moorman M, Gerson SL. Phenotypic and functional comparison of cultures of marrow-derived mesenchymal stem cells (MSCs) and stromal cells. J Cell Physiol 1998; 176:57-66.

[30]   Haynesworth SE, Goshima J, Goldberg VM, *et al.* Characterization of cells with osteogenic potential from human marrow. Bone 1992; 13:81-88.

[31]   Huss R. Isolation of primary and immortalized CD34-hematopoietic and mesenchymal stem cells from various sources. Stem Cells 2000; 18:1-9.

[32]   Zuk PA, Zhu M, Mizuno H, *et al.* Multilineage cells from human adipose tissue: implications for cell-based therapies. Tissue Eng 2001; 7:211-228.

[33]   Young HE, Duplaa C, Katz R, *et al.* Adult-derived stem cells and their potential for use in tissue repair and molecular medicine. J Cell Mol Med 2005; 9:753-769.

[34]   Jiang Y, Jahagirdar BN, Reinhardt RL, *et al.* Pluripotency of mesenchymal stem cells derived from adult marrow. Nature 2002; 418:41-49.

[35]   Yoon YS, Wecker A, Heyd L, *et al.* Clonally expanded novel multipotent stem cells from human bone marrow regenerate myocardium after myocardial infarction. J Clin Invest 2005; 115:326-338.

[36]   Kogler G, Sensken S, Airey JA, *et al.* A new human somatic stem cell from placental cord blood with intrinsic pluripotent differentiation potential. J Exp Med 2004; 200:123-135.

[37]   Kues WA, Petersen B, Mysegades W, *et al.* Isolation of murine and porcine fetal stem cells from somatic tissue. Biol Reprod 2005; 72:1020-1028.

[38]   Dan YY, Riehle KJ, Lazaro C, *et al.* Isolation of multipotent progenitor cells from human fetal liver capable of differentiating into liver and mesenchymal lineages. Proc Natl Acad Sci U S A 2006; 103:9912-9917.

[39]   Beltrami AP, Cesselli D, Bergamin N, *et al.* Multipotent cells can be generated *in vitro* from several adult human organs (heart, liver, and bone marrow). Blood 2007; 110:3438-3446.

[40]   D'Ippolito G, Diabira S, Howard GA, *et al.* Marrow-isolated adult multilineage inducible (MIAMI) cells, a unique population of postnatal young and old human cells with extensive expansion and differentiation potential. J Cell Sci 2004; 117:2971-2981.

[41]   Morrison SJ, Kimble J. Asymmetric and symmetric stem-cell divisions in development and cancer. Nature 2006; 441:1068-1074.

[42]   Slack JM. Origin of stem cells in organogenesis. Science 2008; 322:1498-1501.

[43]   Zipori D. The stem state: plasticity is essential, whereas self-renewal and hierarchy are optional. Stem Cells 2005; 23:719-726.

[44]   Slack JM. Stem cells in epithelial tissues. Science 2000; 287:1431-1433.

[45]   Cotsarelis G. Epithelial stem cells: a folliculocentric view. J Invest Dermatol 2006; 126:1459-1468.

[46]   Kitisin K, Shetty K, Mishra L, *et al.* Hepatocellular stem cells. Cancer Biomark 2007; 3:251-262.

[47]   Schmelzer E, Zhang L, Bruce A, *et al.* Human hepatic stem cells from fetal and postnatal donors. J Exp Med 2007; 204:1973-1987.

[48]   Baeyens L, Bouwens L. Can beta-cells be derived from exocrine pancreas? Diabetes Obes Metab 2008; 10 Suppl 4:170-178.

[49]   Gallo R, Gambelli F, Gava B, *et al.* Generation and expansion of multipotent mesenchymal progenitor cells from cultured human pancreatic islets. Cell Death Differ 2007; 14:1860-1871.

[50]   Seeberger KL, Dufour JM, Shapiro AM, *et al.* Expansion of mesenchymal stem cells from human pancreatic ductal epithelium. Lab Invest 2006; 86:141-153.

[51]   Herzlinger D, Koseki C, Mikawa T, *et al.* Metanephric mesenchyme contains multipotent stem cells whose fate is restricted after induction. Development 1992; 114:565-572.

[52]   Sagrinati C, Netti GS, Mazzinghi B, *et al.* Isolation and characterization of multipotent progenitor cells from the Bowman's capsule of adult human kidneys. J Am Soc Nephrol 2006; 17:2443-2456.

[53]   Gupta S, Verfaillie C, Chmielewski D, *et al.* Isolation and characterization of kidney-derived stem cells. J Am Soc Nephrol 2006; 17:3028-3040.

[54]   Hopkins C, Li J, Rae F, Little MH. Stem cell options for kidney disease. J Pathol 2009; 217:265-281.

[55]   Zhao M, Momma S, Delfani K, Carlen M, *et al.* Evidence for neurogenesis in the adult mammalian substantia nigra. Proc Natl Acad Sci U S A 2003; 100:7925-7930.

[56]   Gould E, Reeves AJ, Fallah M, *et al.* Hippocampal neurogenesis in adult Old World primates. Proc Natl Acad Sci U S A 1999; 96:5263-5267.

[57]   Eriksson PS, Perfilieva E, Bjork-Eriksson T, et al. Neurogenesis in the adult human hippocampus. Nat Med 1998; 4:1313-1317.

[58]   Arsenijevic Y, Villemure JG, Brunet JF, *et al.* Isolation of multipotent neural precursors residing in the cortex of the adult human brain. Exp Neurol 2001; 170:48-62.

[59]   Liu Z, Martin LJ. Olfactory bulb core is a rich source of neural progenitor and stem cells in adult rodent and human. J Comp Neurol 2003; 459:368-391.

[60]   Pagano SF, Impagnatiello F, Girelli M, *et al.* Isolation and characterization of neural stem cells from the adult human olfactory bulb. Stem Cells 2000; 18:295-300.

[61]   Uchida N, Buck DW, He D, *et al.* Direct isolation of human central nervous system stem cells. Proc Natl Acad Sci U S A 2000; 97:1472014725.

[62]   Stigloher C, Chapouton P, Adolf B, *et al.* Identification of neural progenitor pools by E (Spl) factors in the embryonic and adult brain. Brain Res Bull 2008; 75:266-273.

[63]   Fricker RA, Carpenter MK, Winkler C, *et al.* Site-specific migration and neuronal differentiation of human neural progenitor cells after transplantation in the adult rat brain. J Neurosci 1999; 19:5990-6005.

[64]   Bjugstad KB, Teng YD, Redmond DE, Jr., *et al.* Human neural stem cells migrate along the nigrostriatal pathway in a primate model of Parkinson's disease. Exp Neurol 2008; 211:362-369.

[65]   Mendoza-Torreblanca JG, Martinez-Martinez E, Tapia-Rodriguez M, *et al.* The rostral migratory stream is a neurogenic niche that predominantly engenders periglomerular cells: *in vivo* evidence in the adult rat brain. Neurosci Res 2008; 60:289-299.

[66]   Olariu A, Cleaver KM, Cameron HA. Decreased neurogenesis in aged rats results from loss of granule cell precursors without lengthening of the cell cycle. J Comp Neurol 2007; 501:659-667.

[67]   Aizawa H, Goto M, Sato T, *et al.* Temporally regulated asymmetric neurogenesis causes left-right difference in the zebrafish habenular structures. Dev Cell 2007; 12:87-98.

[68]   Drapeau E, Montaron MF, Aguerre S, *et al.* Learning-induced survival of new neurons depends on the cognitive status of aged rats. J Neurosci 2007; 27:6037-6044.

[69]   Feldmann RE, Jr., Mattern R. The human brain and its neural stem cells postmortem: from dead brains to live therapy. Int J Legal Med 2006; 120:201-211.

[70]   Dunnett SB, Bjorklund A. Prospects for new restorative and neuroprotective treatments in Parkinson's disease. Nature 1999; 399:A32-39.

[71]   Storch A, Paul G, Csete M, *et al.* Long-term proliferation and dopaminergic differentiation of human mesencephalic neural precursor cells. Exp Neurol 2001; 170:317-325.

[72]   Freed CR, Greene PE, Breeze RE, *et al.* Transplantation of embryonic dopamine neurons for severe Parkinson's disease. N Engl J Med 2001; 344:710-719.

[73]   Burnstein RM, Foltynie T, He X, *et al.* Differentiation and migration of long term expanded human neural progenitors in a partial lesion model of Parkinson's disease. Int J Biochem Cell Biol 2004; 36:702-713.

[74]   Wenning GK, Odin P, Morrish P, *et al.* Short- and long-term survival and function of unilateral intrastriatal dopaminergic grafts in Parkinson's disease. Ann Neurol 1997; 42:95-107.

[75]   Guo BF, Dong MM. Application of neural stem cells in tissue-engineered artificial nerve. Otolaryngol Head Neck Surg 2009; 140:159-164.

[76]   Shah K, Bureau E, Kim DE, *et al.* Glioma therapy and real-time imaging of neural precursor cell migration and tumor regression. Ann Neurol 2005; 57:34-41.

[77]   Glass R, Synowitz M, Kronenberg G, *et al.* Glioblastoma-induced attraction of endogenous neural precursor cells is associated with improved survival. J Neurosci 2005; 25:2637-2646.

[78]   Furnari FB, Fenton T, Bachoo RM, *et al.* Malignant astrocytic glioma: genetics, biology, and paths to treatment. Genes Dev 2007; 21:2683-2710.

[79]   Yang SY, Liu H, Zhang JN. Gene therapy of rat malignant gliomas using neural stem cells expressing IL-12. DNA Cell Biol 2004; 23:381-389.

[80]   Dwain I, Xiangpeng Y, Zeng Z, *et al.* Neural stem cells--a promising potential therapy for brain tumors. Curr Stem Cell Res Ther 2006; 1:79-84.

[81]   Prockop DJ. "Stemness" does not explain the repair of many tissues by mesenchymal stem/multipotent stromal cells (MSCs). Clin Pharmacol Ther 2007; 82:241-243.

[82]   Crisostomo PR, Markel TA, Wang Y, *et al.* Surgically relevant aspects of stem cell paracrine effects. Surgery 2008; 143:577-581.

[83]   Houchen CW, George RJ, Sturmoski MA, *et al.* FGF-2 enhances intestinal stem cell survival and its expression is induced after radiation injury. Am J Physiol 1999; 276:G249-258.

[84]   Aggarwal S, Pittenger MF. Human mesenchymal stem cells modulate allogeneic immune cell responses. Blood 2005; 105:1815-1822.

[85]   Li L, Zhang S, Zhang Y, *et al.* Paracrine action mediates the antifibrotic effect of transplanted mesenchymal stem cells in a rat model of global heart failure. Mol Biol Rep 2009; 36:725-731.

[86]   Prockop DJ. Marrow stromal cells as stem cells for nonhematopoietic tissues. Science 1997; 276:71-74.

[87]   Uccelli A, Moretta L, Pistoia V. Mesenchymal stem cells in health and disease. Nat Rev Immunol 2008; 8:726-736.

[88]   Uccelli A, Mancardi G, Chiesa S. Is there a role for mesenchymal stem cells in autoimmune diseases? Autoimmunity 2008; 41:592-595.

[89]   Uccelli A, Moretta L, Pistoia V. Immunoregulatory function of mesenchymal stem cells. Eur J Immunol 2006; 36:2566-2573.

[90]   Uccelli A, Pistoia V, Moretta L. Mesenchymal stem cells: a new strategy for immunosuppression? Trends Immunol 2007; 28:219-226.

[91]   Caplan AI. Why are MSCs therapeutic? New data: new insight. J Pathol 2009; 217:318-324.

[92]   Abdi R, Fiorina P, Adra CN, *et al.* Immunomodulation by mesenchymal stem cells: a potential therapeutic strategy for type 1 diabetes. Diabetes 2008; 57:1759-1767.

[93]   Larghero J, Vija L, Lecourt S, *et al.* Mesenchymal stem cells and immunomodulation: Toward new immunosuppressive strategies for the treatment of autoimmune diseases? Rev Med Interne 2009; 30:287-299.

CHAPTER 3

The Role of Microenvironment Stromal Cells in Regenerative Medicine

Ian McNiece* and Joshua Hare

Interdisciplinary Stem Cell Institute, University of Miami, Miami, FL, USA

Abstract: Regenerative medicines offer the potential for treatment and possibly cure of debilitating diseases including heart disease, diabetes, Parkinson's disease and liver failure. Approaches using stem cells from various sources are in pre clinical and clinical testing. The goal of these studies is to deliver cellular products capable of replacing damaged tissue and/or cells. However, the balance between cellular proliferation and differentiation is a carefully controlled process involving a range of growth factors and cytokines produced in large part by tissue stromal cells. These stromal cells make up the tissue microenvironment and appear to be essential for normal homeostasis. We hypothesize that tissue damage in many instances involves damage to the microenvironment resulting in a lack of signals through growth factor networks necessary to maintain survival and proliferation of tissue specific stem cells and progenitor cells. Therefore, optimal repair of disease tissue must account for the damage to the stromal environment. We propose that optimal cellular therapies for regenerative medicine will require combination cellular products consisting of a stromal cell population to reconstitute the microenvironment and to support the survival, proliferation and differentiation of the tissue specific stem cells or progenitor cells.

INTRODUCTION

The homeostasis of cellular content is an ongoing process in most tissue, representing a balance between cell death and new cell production. One of the best studied systems in the body is the hematopoietic system which requires ongoing blood cell production due to blood cell turnover. The bone marrow (BM) is the principal site for blood cell formation in humans. In normal adults the body produces about 2.5 billion red blood cells (RBC), 2.5 billion platelets and 10 billion granulocytes per kilogram of body weight per day [1]. The production of mature blood cells is a continual process that is the result of proliferation and differentiation of stem cells, committed progenitor cells and differentiated cells. Within these three stages, extensive expansion of cell numbers occurs through cell division. A single stem cell has been proposed to be capable of more than 50 cell divisions or doublings and has the capacity to generate up to 10^{15} cells, or sufficient cells for up to 60 years [2]. The proliferation and differentiation of cells is controlled by a group of proteins called hematopoietic growth factors (HGFs). The GFs and other cytokines are produced in part by stromal cells of the BM microenvironment. In addition, hematopoietic stem cells (HSC) reside in the BM in close proximity to stromal cells which provide the "stem cell niche". Deficiencies in the microenvironment at a cellular or molecular level result in abnormal cell production resulting in anemia, leukemia or embryonic lethality [3].

To date there is little data on the presence of stromal cells in tissues such as the heart, liver, lungs etc. However, recent studies have demonstrated the existence of tissue specific stem cells. We have proposed that stromal cells make up a "BM like" stem cell niche in tissues, such as the heart, and in this manuscript we discuss the implications for regenerative medicine.

THE BONE MARROW MICROENVIRONMENT

The BM from a wide range of mammalian species contains precursor cells that generate adherent colonies of stromal cells *in vitro*. The BM stroma represents the non-hematopoietic connective tissue elements that provide a system of structural support for developing hematopoietic cells. The complex cellular composition of marrow stromal tissue comprises a heterogenous population of cells including reticular cells, adipocytes, osteogenic cells near bone surfaces, vascular endothelial cells, smooth muscle cells in vessel walls, and macrophages [4-7].

*Address Correspondence to this Author Ian K. McNiece:** University of Miami, 1120 NW 14th St, room 1113, Miami, FL, USA; E-mail: imcniece@med.miami.edu

The concept that adult hematopoiesis occurs in a stromal microenvironment within the BM was first proposed by Dexter and colleagues, leading to the establishment of the long-term BM culture (LTMC). These studies demonstrated that an adherent stromal-like culture could support maintenance of hematopoietic stem cells (HSC) [8]. Mesenchymal stem cells (MSC) represent the major stromal cell population in the BM.

Mesenchymal Stem Cells (MSC)

MSCs were recognized by Friedenstein who isolated cells from guinea pig bone marrow which were adherent in culture and which differentiated into bone [9]. Surface antigens have been reported for identification and phenotyping of human MSCs [10-12]. Although MSCs are rare, representing approximately 0.01% of the bone marrow mononuclear cell fraction, they have attractive features for therapy, including the ability to expand many log-fold *in vitro*, and unique immune characteristics allowing their use as an allogeneic graft. They are typically isolated based upon adherence to standard tissue culture flasks. Low density BM mononuclear cells (MNCs) are placed into culture in basal media plus FCS (typically 20%) and after 2 to 3 days adherent cells can be visualized on the surface of the flask. The non adherent cells are removed at this time and fresh media added until a confluent adherent layer forms. The MSC are harvested by treatment with trypsin and further passaged expanding the number of MSC. A number of different cell populations have been isolated using different culture conditions however, the morphology of these cells is very similar. Phenotypical characterization of MSC has been performed by many groups and a standard criterion has been proposed by the International Society of Cellular Therapy (ISCT) [13]. The minimal criteria proposed to define human MSC by the Mesenchymal and Tissue Stem Cell Committee of the ISCT consists of the following: 1) the MSC must be plastic-adherent when maintained in standard culture conditions; 2) MSC must express CD105, CD73 and CD90, and lack expression of CD45, CD34, CD14 or CD11b, CD79 alpha or CD19 and HLA-DR surface molecules; and 3) MSC must differentiate into osteoblasts, adipocytes and chondrocytes *in vitro* [13].

A standard *in vitro* assay for MSC is the colony-forming unit fibroblast (CFU-F) assay [14]. BM MNCs are plated at low density and colonies of fibroblasts develop attached on the surface of the culture dish. Based upon the results of this assay, the frequency of MSC precursor cells is one in 10^4 to 10^5 BM MNC. The frequency is highly variable between individuals and the number of MSC has been shown to be decreased in older people. Other studies have demonstrated that MSC precursors can be isolated based upon surface antigen expression. Antibodies to CD271 and Stro-1 have been used to enrich MSC precursors. CD271, also known as low affinity nerve growth factor receptor (LNGFR) or p75NTR belongs to the low affinity neurotrophin receptor and the tumor necrosis factor receptor superfamily. Selection of CD271+ cells from human BM enriches CFU-F and MSC are preferentially selected in the CD271+ fraction compared to the CD271- fraction [10, 11]. Similarly, isolation of Stro-1+ cells from BM MNC results in enrichment of CFU-F in the Stro-1+ fraction compared to the Stro-1- fraction [12].

Immunologic Properties of MSCs

MSCs are ideal candidates for allogeneic transplantation because they show minimal MHC class II and ICAM expression and lack B-7 costimulatory molecules necessary for T-cell mediated immune responses [15-17]. Indeed MSCs do not stimulate a proliferative response from alloreactive T-cells even when the MSCs have differentiated into other lineages or are exposed to proinflammatory cytokines [17]. As previously reviewed [18], MSCs have significant immunomodulatory effects, inhibiting T-cell proliferation [19], prolonging skin allograft survival [20], and decreasing graft-versus-host disease (GVHD) [21]. Recently human MSCs were shown to alter the cytokine secretion profile of dendritic cells, T cells, and natural killer cells *in vitro*, inhibiting secretion of proinflammatory cytokines (e.g. TNF-a, IFN-γ) and increasing expression of suppressive cytokines (e.g.IL-10), possibly via a prostaglandin E2 mediated pathway [22]. In vivo studies of the fate of MSCs have shown that, when transplanted into fetal sheep, human MSCs engraft, undergo site-specific differentiation into various cell types, including myocytes and cardiomyocytes and persist in multiple tissues for as long as 13 months after transplantation in non-immunosuppressed immunocompetent hosts [23]. Further, *in vivo* studies using rodents, dogs, goats, and baboons demonstrate that allogeneic MSCs can be engrafted into these species without stimulating systemic alloantibody production or eliciting a proliferative response from recipient lymphocytes [24-27]. These properties present MSC as a promising source of allogeneic cells for tissue repair.

The Stem Cell Niche

The control of proliferation and differentiation of a number of types of stem cells (SC) occurs in the micro environmental niche or the stem cell niche. Hematopoietic stem cells (HSC) have been studied in detail and shown to reside in the bone marrow in association with stromal cells which make up the hematopoietic micro environment [28]. The stroma consists of several cell populations including mesenchymal stem cells (MSC), fibroblasts and adventicular reticulocytes [29]. HSC exist in a quiescent state in close relationship with the stromal cells in the bone marrow. These stromal cells produce a number of cytokines and growth factors that are either secreted or expressed as membrane bound proteins and these cytokines and growth factors control the differentiation and proliferation of the HSC. *In vitro*, MSC have been shown to support the proliferation and differentiation of HSC, generating committed hematopoietic progenitor cells over a six week period [8]. If the microenvironment is compromised, such as in patients who receive multiple rounds of high dose chemotherapy regimens, normal homeostasis is disrupted and deficiencies in blood cells occur.

Stromal Cells in Cardiac Tissue

The extracellular matrix (ECM) of cardiac tissue provides elasticity and mechanical strength. The cardiac ECM is composed of a number of cells including cardiac fibroblasts, mesenchymal cells, fibronectin and other matrix proteins [30-32]. We have isolated several stromal cell populations from human fetal heart which are positive for CD105, CD90 and CD73 but negative for CD34 and CD45, which is consistent with the phenotype of BM derived MSC [McNiece I, unpublished data]. Given the homeostatic role of MSC in regulation of HSC it is highly likely that cardiac stromal cells play a regulatory role in the control of proliferation and differentiation of cardiac stem and progenitor cells (CSC and CPC). This role could be performed through the secretion of a range of growth factors and cytokines.

MI results in ischemic damage which results in cell death of not only cardiomyocytes but also fibroblasts and most likely stromal cells. Even with migration of viable CSCs and CPCs to the ischemic tissue, the lack of stromal elements would result in the failure of the CSCs and CPCs to proliferate and differentiate, hence failure of remodeling. Along with the recent identification of cardiac stem cells in heart tissue, this offers insights into the biology of ischemic heart damage. Patients with an MI have ischemic tissue which fails to regenerate and we propose that this is in part due to destruction of cardiac stromal cells.

MSC derived from BM cells have been evaluated for cardiac regenerative therapy [33] and as presented above, offer advantages over other sources of stem cells because of their availability, immunologic properties, and record of safety and efficacy. Studies of MSC engraftment in rodent and swine models of myocardial infarction demonstrate: 1) functional benefit in post-myocardial infarction (MI) recovery with administration 2) evidence of neoangiogenesis at the site of the infarct 3) decrease in collagen deposition in the region of the scar 4) some evidence of cells expressing contractile and sarcomeric proteins but lacking true sarcomeric functional organization. Administration of autologous or allogeneic human MSCs to cardiovascular patients has been performed in several clinical studies to date, all in the post-myocardial infarction (MI) setting. The MSC have been administered via the intracoronary route (IC), via peripheral intravenous (IV) injection or direct injection into the cardiac tissue with surgery.

Based upon these data we propose that optimal repair of ischemic tissue requires regeneration of both stromal elements and cardiomyocytes. Delivery of MSC to the ischemic tissue can regenerate the stroma and delivery of cardiac stem/progenitor cells can regenerate cardiomyocytes. We further propose that the combination cellular therapy is necessary for optimal repair as delivery of cardiac stem/progenitor cells will result in minimal repair due to the lack of a niche and the absence of appropriate growth factors and cytokines for these cells to proliferate and differentiate.

IN VITRO APPLICATIONS OF STROMAL CELLS

The delivery of stem cells to damaged tissue, such as the heart, has demonstrated promising results. However, the capacity for stem cells to differentiate into functional mature cells may be limited in some clinical settings. An example may be the need to deliver functional islet cells in patients with diabetes. Also the clinical application may have limitations on the potential of stem cells – an example is the use of cord blood (CB) products as a source of hematopoietic cells for cancer patients undergoing high dose chemotherapy. The time to recovery of neutrophils and platelets is critical for the optimal outcome and the literature demonstrates that hematopoietic progenitor cells provide faster recovery than HSC. Therefore a number of Investigators have explored *ex vivo* culture conditions to differentiate HSC into progenitor cells increase the dose of progenitor cells available [34]. The use of growth factors to drive differentiation has been less than optimal however; we have described culture conditions that utilize stromal cells for co culture with CB cells. This demonstrates an approach to use the potential of stromal cells to manipulate stem cells *in vitro* to generate a cellular product for clinical use.

Ex Vivo Expansion of Cord Blood Cells on MSC

A number of approaches have been explored for *ex vivo* expansion of CB products from liquid culture in bags to bioreactors. A number of groups have demonstrated that selection of CD34+ cells or CD133+ cells was necessary for optimal expansion. In 1997 we reported that culture of CB mono nuclear cells (MNC) in a HGF cocktail of stem cell factor (SCF) plus granulocyte colony stimulating factor (G-CSF) and thrombopoietin (Tpo) resulted in only a 1.4 fold expansion of total cells, 0.8 fold in mature progenitor cells (GM-CFC) and 0.3 fold in erythroid progenitors (BFU-E) [35]. In contrast, CD34+ selected CB cells resulted in 113 fold expansions of total cells, 73 fold expansion of GM-CFC and 49 fold expansion of BFU-E. Based upon these results we initiated expansion cultures in clinical trials with CD34-selected CB cells. Processing of clinical products has led us to two conclusions:

a) Although we can expand significantly the total nucleated cells (TNC) and committed progenitor cells from CD34+ cells we rarely reached pre selection TNC numbers.

b) The performance of clinical trials using CB grafts in the unrelated setting requires the use of frozen CB products. Selection of frozen CB products results in significant losses of CD34+ cells (50% or greater loss of CD34+ cells) and often results in low purities [36]. With a 50% recovery of CD34+ cells after selection we now require at least a 400 fold cell expansion to obtain equivalent TNC as we started with. Again from our experience with clinical studies the purity of the CD34-selected product impacted the level of expansion achieved. Therefore the use of CD34 selected products has rarely resulted in increased cell doses of *ex vivo* expanded cells compared to the starting unmanipulated product. Therefore, we have evaluated methods for expanding CB products without an initial CD34- or CD133-selection.

Based upon the ability of MSC to support hematopoietic cells, we have developed a co culture system which is capable of expanding CB MNC by culturing the CB MNC on confluent MSC layers [36]. The literature contains many reports of the ability of MSC to support the growth of hematopoietic cells. It has been demonstrated that MSC produce a number of HGFs and adhesion molecules that may stimulate growth of hematopoietic cells. Our data reproducibly demonstrated a 10 to 20 fold expansion of TNC with 18 fold expansion of GM-CFC and 16 to 37 fold expansions of CD34+ cells.

We have evaluated the potential of *ex vivo* expansion of frozen CB products using the co culture on MSC [McNiece and colleagues, unpublished data]. CB products were thawed and washed, resulting in a median of 3.3 $x10^8$ TNC (range 1.4 to 3.6 $x10^8$, n=5). For a 50 kg recipient, these CB products would provide only 0.73 $x10^7$ TNC/kg with zero of 5 products reaching the minimal target dose of 1 $x10^7$ TNC. Each product was expanded by culturing the MNC fraction from each product on preformed layers of MSC. A median of 9 fold expansion of TNC was obtained with a range of 6.5 to 24 fold. The median TNC post expansion was 21.6 $x10^8$ (range 11 to 79 $x10^8$ TNC). A median expansion of mature progenitor cells (GM-CFC) of 46 fold was also obtained in the co culture. For a 50 kg recipient, the expanded CB product would be equivalent to 4.3 $x10^7$ TNC/kg (range 2.2 to 16 $x10^7$), with all 5 expanded products reaching the minimal target of $1x10^7$ TNC/kg. In fact all expanded products contained more the 1 $x10^7$ TNC/kg based upon a 100 kg recipient.

A clinical trial to evaluate the potential of *ex vivo* expanded cells generated using this co culture approach, is currently being conducted at MD Anderson by Dr E.J. Shapll.

SUMMARY

Stem cells have the potential to repair damaged tissue in a number of organs and tissues of the body, however, these cells require an appropriate niche for survival and proliferation. Inflammation associated with cell death and damage results in further damage to cells and the microenvironment. We propose that Combination Cell Therapy will be necessary for optimal tissue repair. MSC are a unique cell population that exhibit immune properties that minimize graft rejection or immune activation. The use of MSC to reestablish the stem cell niche will be critical in several diseases to ensure that stem cells used for regenerative approaches have an appropriate niche. In particular we are focused on using Combination Cell Therapy for heart disease using MSC to repair the microenvironment of ischemic tissue and cardiac stem cells for regeneration of cardiomyocytes. We plan to move forward with large animal studies combining MSC with c-kit+ cardiac stem cells in animals with an MI to move towards clinical trials.

REFERENCES

[1]   Williams WJ, Beutler E, Erslev AJ, Lichtman MA, Eds. Hematology. 4th ed. McGraw-Hill Inc: New York 1990.

[2]   Kay HEM. How many cell-generations? Lancet 1995; August 28: 418-419

[3]   Mintz B, Russell ES. Gene induced embryological modifications of primordial germ cells in the mouse. J Exp Zool 1957; 134:207-237.

[4]   Weiss L. The hematopoietic microenvironment of the bone marrow: an ultrastructural study of the stroma in rats. Anatom Rec 1976; 186: 161.

[5]   Westen H, Bainton DF. Association of alkaline phosphatase-positive reticulum cells in bone marrow with granulocyte precursors. J Exp Med 1979; 150: 919.

[6]   Lichtman MA. The ultrastructure of the hematopoietic microenvironment of the marrow: a review. Exp Hematol 1981; 9: 391.

[7]   Bianco P, Riminucci M. The bone marrow stroma in vivo: ontogeny, structure, cellular composition and changes in disease. In: Beresford JN, Owens ME, Eds. Marrow stromal cell culture. Handbooks in Practival Animal Cell Biology. Cambrdge, UK: Cambridge University Press, 1998; p. 1025.

[8]   Dexter TM. Stromal cell associated haemopoiesis. J Cell Physiol Suppl 1982; 1: 87.

[9]   Friedenstein AJ. Precursor cells of mechanocyte. Int Rev Cytol 1976; 47: 327.

[10]   Quirici N, Soligo D, Bossolasco P, *et al*. Isolation of bone marrow mesenchymal stem cells by anti- nerve growth factor receptor antibodies. Exp Hematol 2002; 30(7): 783.

[11]   Jones E, English A, Kinsey SE, *et al*. Optimization of a flow cytometry-based protocol for detection and phenotypic characterization of multipotent mesenchymal stromal cells from human bone marrow. Cytometry B Clin Cytom 2006; 70: 391-399.

[12]   Zannettino A, Paton S, Kortesidis A, *et al*. Human multipotential mesenchymal/stromal stem cell are derived from a discrete subpopulation of STRO-1^{bright}/CD34-/CD45-/glycophorin-A- bone marrow cells. Haematogica 2007; 92(12): 1707.

[13]   Dominici M, Le Blanc K, Mueller I, *et al*. Minimal criteria for defining multipotent mesenchymal stromal cell. The International Society of Cellular Therapy position statement. Cytotherapy 2006; 8(4): 315.

[14]   Freidenstein AJ, Gorskaja JF, Kilagina NN. Fibroblast precursors in normal and irradiated hematopoietic organs. Exp Hematol 1976; 4(5): 267-274.

[15]   Le Blanc K, Tammik C, Rosendahl K, *et al*. HLA expression expression and immunologic properties of differentiated and undifferentiated mesenchymal stem cells. Exp Hematol 2003; 31(10): 890-896.

[16]   Klyushnenkova E, Shustova V, Mosca J, *et al*. Human mesenchymal stem cells induce unresponsiveness in preactivated but not naïve alloantigen specific T cells. Exp Hematol 1999; 27: abstract 122.

[17]   Klyushnenkova E, Mosa JD, Zernetkina V, *et al*. T cell responses to allogeneic human mesenchymal stem cells: immunogenicity, tolerance, and suppression. J Biomed Sci 2005; 12(1): 47-57.

[18]   Le Blanc K, Ringden O. Immunobiology of human mesenchymal stem cells and future use in hematopoietic stem cell transplantation. Biol Blood Marrow Transplant 2005; 11(5): 321-334.

[19]   Le Blanc K, Rasmusson I, Gotherstrom C, *et al*. Mesenchymal stem cells inhibit the expression of CD25 (interleukin-2 receptor) and CD38 on phytohaemagglutinin-activated lymphocytes. Scand J Immunol 2004; 60(3): 307-315.

[20]   Bartholomew A, Sturgeon C, Siatskas M, *et al*. Mesenchymal stem cells suppress lymphocyte proliferation *in vitro* and prolong skin graft survival in vivo. Exp Hematol 2002; 30(1): 42-48.

[21]   Lazarus HM, Koc ON, Devine SM, *et al.* Cotransplantation of HLA-identical sibling culture-expanded mesenchymal stem cells and hematopoietic stem cells in hematologic malignancy patients. Biol Blood Marrow Transplant 2005; 11(5): 389-398.

[22]   Aggarwal S, Pittenger MF. Human mesenchymal stem cells modulate allogeneic immune cell responses. Blood 2005; 105(4): 1815-1822.

[23]   Lietchy KW, MacKenzie TC, Shaaban AF, *et al.* Human mesenchymal stem cells engraft and demonstrate site-specific differentiation after in utero transplantation in sheep. Nat Med 2000; 6(11): 1282-1286.

[24]   Grinnemo KH, Mansson A, Dellgren G, *et al.* Xenoreactivity and engraftment of human mesenchymal stem cells transplanted into infracted rat myocardium. J Thorac Cardiovasc Surg 2004; 127(5): 1293-1300.

[25]   Arinzeh TL, Peter SL, Archambault MP, *et al.* Allogeneic mesenchymal stem cells regenerate bone in a critical-sized canine segmental defect. J Bone Joint Surg Am 2003; 85-A(10): 1927-1935.

[26]   Murphy JM, Fink DJ, Hunziker EB, Barry FP. Stem cells therapy in a caprine model of osteoarthritis. Arthritis Rheum 2003; 48(12): 3464-3474.

[27]   Mahmud N, Pang W, Cobbs C, *et al.* Studies on the route of administration and role of conditioning with radiation on unrelated allogeneic mismatched mesenchymal stem cell engraftment in a nonhuman primate model. Exp Hematol 2004; 32(5): 494-501.

[28]   Haylock DN, Nilsson SK. Stem cell regulation by the hematopoietic stem cell niche. Cell Cycle 2008; 4(10): 1353-1355.

[29]   Weiss L. The hematopoietic microenvironment of the bone marrow: an ultrastructural study of the stroma in rats. Anatom Rec 1976; 186: 161.

[30]   Decker C, Greggs R, Duggan K, *et al.* Adhesive multiplicity in the interaction of embryonic fibroblasts and myoblasts with extracellular matrices. J Cell Biol 1984; 99: 1398.

[31]   Choy M, Oltjen SL, Otani YS, *et al.* Fibroblast growth factor-2 stimulates embryonic cardiac mesenchymal cell proliferation. Dev Dyn 1996; 206: 193.

[32]   Baudino TA, Carver W, Giles W, Borg TK. Cardiac fibroblasts: friend or foe? Am J Physiol Heart Circ Physiol 2006; 291: H1015.

[33]   Mazhari R, Hare JM. Mechanisms of action of mesenchymal stem cells in cardiac repair: potential influences on the cardiac stem cell niche. Nat Clin Pract Cardiovasc Med 2007; 4 suppl 1: S21-26.

[34]   McNiece I, Briddell R. *Ex vivo* expansion of hematopoietic progenitor cells and mature cells. Exp. Hematol. 2001; 29(1): 3-11.

[35]   Briddell R, Kern BP, Zilm KL, *et al.* Purification of CD34+ cells is essential for optimal *ex vivo* expansion of umbilical cord blood cells. J. Hematotherapy 1997; 6: 145-150.

[36]   McNiece I, Harrington J, Turney J, *et al.* *Ex vivo* expansion of cord blood mononuclear cells on mesenchymal stem cells (MSC). Cytotherapy 2004; 6(4): 311-317.

Send Orders for Reprints to reprints@benthamscience.net

Stem Cell and Regenerative Medicine, 2010, 29-39

CHAPTER 4

The Role of Mechanical Forces on Stem Cell Growth and Differentiation

Daniel Pelaez[1, 2], Jason R. Fritz[1] and Herman S. Cheung[1, 2,]*

[1]Department of Biomedical Engineering, College of Engineering, University of Miami, 1251 Memorial Drive, Coral Gables, FL 33146, USA and [2]Geriatrics Research, Education and Clinical Center, Miami VA Healthcare System, 1201 NW 16 Street, Miami, FL 33125, USA

Abstract: The application of biomimetic mechanical forces for stem cell differentiation is a technique that has been on the rise in recent years. Bioreactors are being designed and constructed in order to accurately direct these forces onto stem cells in both 2D and 3D configurations. Currently, the most widely investigated mechanical forces are compressive forces and tensile strain, while a small number of researchers are making use of more complex systems of forces such as torsion, shearing and, still more complex, hemodynamic forces. The effects of these forces on mesenchymal stem cells, adipose derived stem cells, and embryonic stem cells are the most commonly explored combinations in functional tissue engineering. Fortunately, recent breakthroughs in the area of adult dental stem cells have brought viable alternatives to the use of these three cell types to the forefront of stem cell research. Yet for certain target cell types, the application of mechanical force alone is not the optimal stimulus for the induction of differentiation programs, which then requires the addition of a chemical stimulus as well. Elucidation of the optimal recipes and how these protocols affect the cells is the ultimate goal of current tissue engineering endeavors. This chapter will summarize the most current findings in functional tissue engineering, explain the importance of engineering in medical research, and describe the ways tissue engineers are attempting to understand what biochemical changes are occurring in the stem cells during the application of mechanical stress.

INTRODUCTION

Functional tissue engineering (FTE) has become a paradigm which was coined and defined in 2003 [1]. This paradigm has many key concepts including the determination of in vivo force pattern exposure of repair tissues [2] and adequate cell source selection. The type and magnitude of these forces has been extensively modeled for some systems in the human body. For functional tissue engineering purposes, these models are used in the design of bioreactors, which recreate the physiological environment of a specific tissues [3].

In part, FTE relies only on the application of a mechanical force to differentiate the stem cells into a desired cell type. However, it has been demonstrated that this may require the combination of biological agents and mechanical forces to attain a desired cellular phenotype [4]. Yet a complete picture of all the necessary guiding stimuli will only occur when the individual mechanotransduction pathways elicited for each desired cell type or tissue has been fully constructed. Members of these pathways will undoubtedly include various cytokines manufactured by the cells themselves and/or moieties of the mitogen-activated protein kinase (MAPK) family.

Mechanotransduction, which falls into the category of mechanobiology, refers to the biochemical cascade which occurs during the application of different modes of physical stress to stem and progenitor cell populations [5]. It has been shown that the application of different mechanical loads can regulate the self-renewal and guide the differentiation of stem cells, but the actual mechanisms through which this is achieved intra-cellularly remain largely unknown [6]. Once these mechanisms are better understood, engineers will have the ability to design and build more appropriate bioreactors [5], which are specially designed cell culture apparatuses designed to impart a mechanical force on the cells in question while maintaining the appropriate conditions for cell survival (generally 5% CO_2 levels and a humidified atmosphere).

MAPKs convert mechanical signals into biological responses and are responsible for cellular growth, differentiation, and response to stresses. The mechanical impulses applied to the cells generally have an impact on

---

*Address Correspondence to this Author Herman S. Cheung: Research Service, Miami VA Healthcare System, 1201 NW 16th Street, Miami, FL 33125, USA; E-mail: hcheung@med.miami.edu

one or more of the three major MAPK pathways: p38 MAPK, p42/44 MAPK and c-Jun N-terminal kinase (JNK). These three proteins are activated through ATP-dependent phosphorylation and have the ability to translocate to the nucleus or bind to various cytoplasmic substrates, including cytokines.

Cell selection is also a crucial element of FTE. The cell type chosen must be highly renewable and have the ability to differentiate into the desired cell type. Most of the tissues in the body that are under constant mechanical strain, for example, are members of the mesodermal germ layer. Taking all this into consideration, it is not all too surprising to see that the primary cell source for these bioreactor systems is mesenchymal stem cells (MSCs). These cells have the ability to differentiate into all the cell types of the mesodermal germ layer [7] and generally do not advocate an immune response from transplant recipients [8,9], making them an ideal candidate for tissue engineering. Furthermore, adipose-derived stem cells (ASCs) are a very commonly accepted alternative to MSCs and have been utilized in several FTE projects. Recent discoveries have shown considerable similarities in the transcriptome of MSCs and ASCs during differentiation into the mesodermal germ layer [10]. Lastly, the use of embryonic stem cells (ESCs), especially human ESCs (hESCs), is not as widely investigated, but are used nonetheless. ESC use in research is still important due to their plasticity and ability to differentiate into all three germ layers. However, their use is not as widespread due to the common contamination with exogenous animal proteins as a result of the culturing techniques used on them, and their potential for teratoma formation once implanted.

This chapter will discuss the need for the inclusion of engineering principles in biotechnology, the way those principles are being translated into reality and the results of some of these efforts to do so. These results will be presented for the application of the major physical forces currently being utilized in the quest to attain engineered tissues.

THE IMPORTANCE OF APPLICATIONS OF ENGINEERING PRINCIPLES

What sets biomedical and, more specifically, tissue engineering apart from all the other life sciences is quite simply the engineering. This may sound oversimplified, but this concept is what seems to be pushing biomedical engineering to the forefront of current medical technology. For instance, the crux of this chapter is to discuss the application of mechanical and biomimetic forces to stem cells to induce differentiation to a desired lineage. It now becomes the engineer's responsibility to ensure the forces applied are imparted on the cells and scaffolds just as they would be during repair and regeneration in the human body.

For instance, it is now well accepted the microenvironment of the stem cell can have an influence on its differentiation and phenotypic expression [11]. It requires an understanding of biological systems combined with the engineering ability to properly recreate those physical and biochemical signals in a laboratory setting, to accurately design bioreactor systems that accurately mimic the in-vivo environment. These complex designs have been implemented in such projects as the engineering of articular cartilage [12,13], bone [14], ligaments [15], cardiac muscle [16] and vascular smooth muscle cells (VSMCs) [17,18]. Furthermore, some reactors, like microfluidic reactors, are built solely for the purpose of bettering cell culture outcomes for cells that have proven hard to culture, such as hESCs [19]. These have also been validated with other cell types [20].

Additionally, some researchers have gone so far as to begin modeling cellular behavior itself, including their physical and biological properties. One group has mathematically modeled the proliferation and differentiation of human MSCs (hMSCs) in a porous biopolymer based on oxygen consumption from previously acquired experimental data [21]. Another group investigated the actual mechanical property differences between hMSCs and fully differentiated osteoblasts [22]. Their findings show there is a difference between the Young's modulus and an even greater difference in the membrane tether of the cells. These differences are attributed mostly to the differential actin cytoskeleton organization within the cells. This data will be helpful in future tissue engineering endeavors such as the design and implementation of superior bioreactors and may serve as motivation for other investigators to perform similar testing on several other cell types.

COMPRESSIVE FORCES

Compressive forces can be applied to cells and cellular constructs in a number of different and unique ways. One obvious example is simply placing a large force on the cells and allowing it to act on the cells for different periods of time. Additionally, there are more complex systems being employed for the application of compressive forces. One such system involves the use of a bioreactor to subject the cells and the constructs they are seeded on, to hydrostatic pressure in both static and intermittent configurations. Furthermore, there are even more complex bioreactors, which impart compressive forces in a dynamic unconfined arrangement with the purpose of simulating tissues under a periodic, yet continuous stress (such as the force experienced by the cartilage in the knee as a person walks). For some of these experiments, stem cells need to be encased in a variety of synthetic and natural 3D matrix scaffolds that range from synthetic hydrogels to natural polymers like fibrin depending on the parameters of each study.

In the least complex method for applying a compressive force to stem cells, different amounts of lead weights were applied to a monolayer of C2C12 cells for a defined time course. This investigation discovered that these cells differentiate into a mixed population of osteogenic and chondrogenic cell constituents as evidenced by the increase of expression of Runx2 and Osterix, common osteogenic genetic markers, as well as (sex determining region Y)-box 5 (SOX-5) and SOX-9, which are markers of chondrogenic differentiation [23]. This study also went on to illustrate the involvement of p38 MAPK during the differentiation of C2C12 cells, but made no mention of the other two MAPK pathways and did not determine which cell type (osteogenic or chondrogenic) utilized the p38 MAPK pathway as a part of its differentiation program. One discovery, which is noteworthy, was made during the application of centrifugal or gravitational force to a culture of human MSCs in a technique commonly known as pellet culture. Human MSCs in this environment synchronized their cell cycle in the G0/G1 phase after 7 days in the pellet culture system [24]. This predictable behavior can be a very helpful tool for later experiments in which the cell cycle is important to the subject under investigation. This study also went on to show retention of the cells in pellet culture for 21 days resulted in a decrease in expression of cluster of differentiation 105 (CD105), a response indicative of cellular differentiation. Signs of phenotypic changes further supported the initiation of differentiation after 21 days of pellet culture from a MSC lineage to a chondrogenic lineage.

Work done with cyclic hydrostatic pressure (sometimes called intermittent hydrostatic pressure) and hMSCs has met with some success, but is still in the early stages of development. This is evident from two studies performed at Stanford University in which it took upwards of 10 days for the hMSCs to express chondrogenic markers when subjected to this form of mechanical stress. The first study done in 2006 which utilized pelletized hMSCs in an osteogenic medium required 14 days of compression before the expression of chondrogenic markers was detected [25]. The second, from 2008, used hMSCs seeded on collagen scaffolds in a very similar osteogenic media as in the 2006 study and required 10 days of compression before the appearance of chondrogenic markers [26]. These Stanford studies suggest it is possible to overcome the effects of media additives if the mechanical force is applied for a sufficient length of time, but do not offer much more. The most compelling evidence of the inefficiency of this system comes from work done by Finger et al, which utilized a media with no additives. The expression of chondrogenic markers required 4 days of compressive stress to be achieved, yet the cells quickly lost this genotype after 9 days of compression for unknown reasons [27]. These conditions are very similar to conditions described for some of the dynamic unconfined compression experiments, which will be discussed shortly

However, the application of cyclic hydrostatic pressure may have a positive impact in the differentiation of hMSCs toward an osteogenic lineage. One very promising study demonstrates that the application of cyclic hydrostatic pressure significantly increases the expression of osteogenic markers, osteocalcin and osteopontin, in the presence of osteogenic media over those of the unloaded constructs in the same osteogenic media [28]. This study goes on to show osteogenesis is suppressed in the presence of U0126, a potent selective inhibitor of p42/44 MAPK, in both compressed and non-compressed cellular constructs.

Dynamic unconfined compressive forces have mostly been utilized for the initiation of chondrogenesis of cells in manufactured cellular constructs. One such study encapsulated mesenchymal progenitors from human ESCs in a poly (ethylene glycol)-diacrylate (PEGDA) hydrogel both with and without functionalization of the scaffold with transforming growth factor (TGF)-β1. Here it was shown the necessity of TGF-β1 for the mesenchymal progenitors to differentiate into articular cartilage. This was demonstrated by the expression of chondrogenic markers SOX-9, aggrecan and collagen II after 2-3 weeks of daily compression [29]. In the gel constructs that were not functionalized, dynamic compression had the inverse effect and suppressed these chondrogenic markers after 7 days of static culture and only 1 hour of dynamic compression.

More efficient processes have been developed that employ dynamic unconfined stress as part of the differentiation protocol, including the compression of human MSCs in alginate scaffolds, which produced signs of chondrogenic differentiation after 8 days of daily compression [30]. This study also illustrated the complex interactions between the several epigenetic factors involved in the differentiation of stem cells when TGF-β3, a known inducer of chondrogenesis in hMSCs, was added to the media yet its effects were shown to not be additive to the chondrogenic response. Additional studies have shown even greater efficiency in the differentiation of hMSCs toward a chondrogenic lineage in fibrin gel scaffolds after only two days (8 total hours) of dynamic unconfined compression stimulation [13]. A very similar study which encased rabbit MSCs (rMSCs) in an alginate scaffold and achieved dynamic compression with the use of an electromagnet also showed signs of differentiation along a chondrogenic lineage after very short compression periods of 10 minutes per day for 3, 5, and 7 days in the absence of any exogenous TGF-β supplementation [31].

Based off of mechanical stimulation alone, the experiments performed in our laboratory show the potential for dynamic compressive loading to induce chondrogenic differentiation of hMSCs. One study using rMSCs seeded in an agarose construct confirmed the findings made by Park et al. in which chondrogenesis could be achieved in the absence of serum and exogenous TGF-β supplementation in our custom built bioreactor [32]. Here it was also shown that the electromagnetic field employed by Park *et al* is immaterial to the results of the experiment and that the induction of chondrogenesis depends only on the application of the compressive deformation. A follow-up study went on to demonstrate the increase in the expression of both TGF-β receptors as well as the involvement of p42/44 MAPK due to the increase in the expression of c-Fos [33], which is a known downstream target of p42/44 MAPK [34]. Ongoing studies are making at an attempt at uncovering the mechanotransduction pathway of dynamic unconfined compression as it applies to the chondrogenesis of stem cells.

TENSILE STRAIN

Tension in any form is one of the two major forces employed to assist and guide the differentiation of stem cells to a committed cell type. In this section, we will discuss the most popular techniques involving tensile force along with some of the instruments being utilized in these processes.

Equiaxial Strain

Although this form of dynamic deformation is sometimes referred to as uniaxial stretching, this is a misnomer. Uniaxial, or longitudinal, strain occurs when the deformation is directed along a single axis in the construct. On the other hand, equiaxial strain is defined as a circumferential deformation that is equal in magnitude along all axes. This is most commonly achieved by a deformation (either up or down) of the central region of a circular, circumferentially bound elastic scaffold. In such a case, cells in the centrally deformed region would experience radial tensile loading in all possible directions.

When analyzed closely, we can infer that most studies into the effects of mechanical stresses on stem and progenitor cell populations rely on the implementation of the form of mechanical force that the differentiated tissues should eventually encounter in vivo to guide the differentiation phenomena. Under the proper conditions, mechanical forces are capable of guiding cell orientation and structured matrix deposition, thus theoretically improving mechanical properties of the final tissues. This is a crucial aspect in highly structured tissues such as muscle, cartilage and bone where matrix alignment allows for the compensation and generation of directed force.

Consequently, tensile strain is most commonly applied force in the achievement of myogenic lineages for the cardiovascular system (composed of smooth and cardiac muscle). One very notable and extensive study was performed on mouse ESCs (mESCs) with the goal of understanding the chemical cascade involved in their differentiation along a cardiomyogenic and angiogenic lineages [16]. Schmelter et al. utilized flexible bottomed culture plates along with the Flexcell tension plus® system to apply equiaxial strain to their cells. They performed their experiments in the absence of any cardiopoietic inducing moieties, either synthetic or natural, with cyclic tensile strain as their only added stimulus. The group describes a direct correlation between the amount of applied force and the number of beating foci seen after 7-9 days of culture. The study also proposes the reactive oxygen species (ROS) pathway as the major intracellular pathway guiding the differentiation of the cells into both cardiomyocytes and vascular cells. They conclude this by both direct measurement of the ROS post-stress application and the lack of differentiation observed under ROS inhibition. Subsequently, in an effort to elucidate the MAPK involved in tensile loading-induced cardiomyogenic differentiation, Schmelter *et al* also discovered that under the same strain conditions, cardiomyogenesis could be diverted to angiogenesis by the addition of a specific inhibitor to the p38 MAPK, SB203580. This observation followed data suggesting that p38, p42/44 and JNK were all activated by the application of tensile load and elucidates the importance of all three MAPK cascades in the cardiomyogenic and angiogenic processes.

The insights provided by the Schmelter et al. study provide encouraging evidence for the use of tensile strain in the achievement of functional tissue engineered grafts for regenerative therapies. The ability of tensile force to initiate the agiogenic program in stem and progenitor cells is being exploited by several researchers focused on the creation of new blood vessels for afflicted patients. A very elegant study demonstrated the effects this type of mechanical force can have on hMSCs [17]. Their attempts at constructing a functional blood vessel in-vitro analyzed many of the variables to which cells in this environment are exposed, including mechanical force, extracellular matrix (ECM) proteins, soluble factors and other growth factors. Differentiation of the cells to smooth muscle cells (SMCs) was assisted by the addition of TGF-β1 and tensile loading on fibronectin coated plates. Not surprisingly, the group observed that these same factors had an inhibitory effect on the proliferation rates of the undifferentiated hMSCs. Conversely, the conditions that enhanced the proliferation of the undifferentiated cells, platelet-derived growth factor BB (PDGF-BB) and Vitamin C along with mechanical strain appeared to inhibit the differentiation of the hMSCs. The dual and contradictory effect that mechanical force exerts upon the cells is often seen in other bioreactor systems and will be discussed later in this chapter.

One unlikely candidate for the use of this form of stress would be in the assistance of osteogenesis. Stretching the cells does not constitute a biomimetic approach to osteogenesis as these cells are not commonly placed under tensile loads. Yet some researchers have tried to utilize this method in the generation of bone cells. One such attempt was made on calcifying vascular cells (CVCs), with equiaxial mechanical strain in the presence of β-glycerophosphate (a known osteogenic promoter) supplemented medium. This effort was successful, and showed signs the application of mechanical stretching would accelerate the rate of alkaline phosphatase (ALP) expression over that of simple media supplementation [35]. This group's previous application of the same protocol was not as successful when applied to hMSCs. A known osteogenic-inducing media [36] was used both with and without the application of cyclic stretching. Unfortunately, the use of mechanical force in this system was of no benefit and bordered on being a hindrance to the osteogenic differentiation of hMSCs [37]. No change in ALP activity was seen at any of the time points as a consequence of mechanical strain application. Mechanical force also inhibited the growth of the hMSCs in culture; data which was later reproduced in a very similar system [17].

This mechanical system has also brought about a glimmer of light in the immense challenge that is the adequate culturing of hESCs. Most all cell culture of hESCs involves the use of mouse embryonic fibroblast (MEF) cells as a feeder layer for the hESCs to grow on. However, it has been noted that the application of equiaxial force to hESCs cultured on flexible plates coated with Matrigel (a basement membrane matrix) has maintained the pluripotency of the hESCs and has not interfered with the proliferation of the cells [38]. This may seem to solve some of the problems of foreign protein contamination and introduction of animal disease, which have plagued the use of hESCs in clinical settings. However, the use of media conditioned with MEF cells and exogenous basic fibroblast growth factor (bFGF) is still required.

Uniaxial Stretching

Uniaxial stretching implies that the stretch applied to the cells is directed only in one direction. This is also sometimes referred to as longitudinal stretching, but for the purposes of this chapter, uniaxial will be the term used to describe this type of dynamic deformation.

Unlike equiaxial stretching, uniaxial stretching can be carried out by a variety of different means. Some involve the use of commercially available bioreactor systems like the Flexcell Tissue Train® system, while other researchers have opted for the fabrication of machines of their own design which fit their specific design parameters [39]. Here we will examine the utilization of these instruments for the differentiation of stem cells to a defined lineage.

Again, as described above, VSMCs are under a constant state of cyclic mechanical strain and the application of this force to stem cells in the pursuit of differentiating them is a very logical choice. This is supported by the evidence which has been uncovered for the past twenty years suggesting that mechanical strain maintains VSMC phenotype in vivo [18]. As promising as this evidence is, the impact this mechanical force has on stem cells is still poorly understood. In a custom-built bioreactor, Kurpinski et al. [39], subjected hMSCs to uniaxial strain in normal growth medium with no additional supplements. Cells were either stretched on a regular membrane or on a membrane with parallel microgrooves to force the cells to align in a specific direction with respect to the applied stress. It was shown that the direction of the cellular alignment versus the axis of stretching has an impact on the differentiation of the cells as observed by the differences in SMC genetic markers like calponin 1 [40]. Interestingly, Kurpinski *et al* noted a decrease in cartilage matrix proteins providing the hypothesis that mechanical stretching might suppress the phenotype of load-bearing tissues to favor a tensile-bearing phenotype. Additionally, attempts have been made to obtain VSMCs from other stem cells sources, including human ASCs (hASCs). Unfortunately, unlike with the hMSCs, cyclic uniaxial strain was observed to inhibit the proliferation of the hASCs. However, these cells still aligned perpendicular to the axis of strain, suggesting this phenomenon is independent of the type of cell used. Along with proliferation, expression of VSMC markers, including α-smooth muscle actin (α-SMA) and calponin 1, were decreased as a result of stretching alone. These studies taken together, suggest that supplementation may be required to drive stem cells to terminal differentiation as VSMCs.

In the realm of osteogenic differentiation, uniaxial stretching has also been applied to both hMSCs and hASCs. The results are very promising when using hMSCs and the Flexcell Tissue Train culture system. It has been shown that cyclic strain alone in this apparatus, in unsupplemented media, has the ability to maintain the viability of the hMSCs [41], increase the expression of bone morphogenic protein-2 (BMP-2) [42] and trigger the transcription of known cellular differentiation factors interleukin-6 (IL-6) and interleukin-8 (IL-8) mRNA [43]. When applied to hASCs in the presence and absence of osteogenic supplements, cyclic stretching had an additive effect in the increase of the number of cells committed to an osteogenic lineage [44]. This data hints at the possibility that molecular pathways involved in the mechanical and chemical differentiation methods are independent of each other. Furthermore, another study utilizing their own custom built bioreactor for the application of uniaxial stretching, applied the same stress under very similar culture conditions and showed evidence of upregulated osteogenic differentiation from both hMSCs and hASCs [45]. These data reflect the importance of a suitable cell source selection for the creation of effective regenerative therapies and suggest both hMSCs and hASCs as possible candidates for bone and myocyte regeneration.

Finally, one very important and breakthrough study was performed to compare the differing effects of uniaxial versus equiaxial stretching in the differentiation of hMSCs into SMCs [46]. What was most important about this study has less to do with the fact they achieved their goal of differentiation with uniaxial stretching, but more to do with how the markers of SMCs, including α-SMA and collagen I were down-regulated with the application of equiaxial stretching. This was one of the first studies to show that the form and pattern of presentation of mechanical forces to undifferentiated cells plays an important role in determining the final lineage commitment of the cells.

TORSION, SHEAR STRESS AND HEMODYNAMIC FORCES

Torsion, shear stress and hemodynamic forces are some of the lesser-explored, highly complex types of mechanical stimulation being applied to stem cells in current research endeavors. Although they may not be widely investigated, they are still very important developing areas of research and will be discussed here.

Torsion

The application of torsion to stem cells is reserved mostly for the engineering of tendons and ligaments. Evidence has shown the application of this type of mechanical strain, in the absence of ligament inducing cytokines, can direct hMSCs to a ligament-like lineage as determined by the increase of expression of collagen I, collagen III, and tenascin-C, while lacking chondrogenic or osteogenic genetic markers [15,47]. Cells in the stimulated constructs were elongated and aligned themselves in a helical pattern along a vertical axis while un-stimulated constructs contained cells, which were morphologically spherical and showed no indication of reorganization.

Even in the wake of these successes, further improvements have been made to these bioreactors, including constant media perfusion to keep nutrient concentrations at intended levels, while exposing the cellular construct to conditions which are closely relevant to the anterior cruciate ligament [48]. Also, the addition of precision computer control to be certain the reactor is operating at the optimal biomimetic level is quickly advancing research performed in this area [49].

One novel study worthy of mention has taken the next step in FTE by implanting their construct into an animal model. Butler et al. used a torsion bioreactor for the preconditioning of rMSCs in either a collagen gel or collagen sponge prior to implantation into rabbit patellar tendon defects. These preconditioned constructs improved the structural and material properties of the repaired tendons over and above the non-preconditioned constructs of either scaffold [2]. It is exciting to see what will come from these new developments in the near future.

Shear Stress

Shear stress is a force one would believe would be most prevalent in the circulatory system. However, the forces exhibited in the circulatory system are much more complex and will be mentioned shortly. This fact does not displace the utility of this kind of mechanical force for uses in other tissue engineering protocols.

One such protocol analyzed the difference between the application of a constant high or low shear stress to hESCs in a microfluidic chamber using a continuous flow of fresh, unsupplemented medium and without the use of a feeder layer of mouse fibroblasts [19]. The application of the two different shear stress levels led to significantly different outcomes. Under the high shear stress conditions and a low cell density, the hESCs differentiated into SMCs as evidenced by an increase in the expression of α-SMA. On the other hand, under low shear stress and a high cell seeding density, the flow of the fresh media seemed to only remove loosely adhered cells and allowed the hESCs to retain their "stem-ness". These results are a massive step forward in the future of hESC culturing techniques.

In an attempt to engineer a functional blood vessel, hESCs, which were pre-differentiated to an endothelial cell (EC) lineage were placed into a parallel plate flow chamber and perfused with a constant flow of endothelial differentiating inducing medium. Even if the application of mechanical force is a secondary effect of the fluid flow, it is still noteworthy to mention the mechanical force directed the cells to reorganize their cytoskeleton to align with the direction of flow [50]. This observation will be useful in further attempts at the engineering of vessel grafts and could assist in the design of reactors for the differentiation of stem cells into ECs.

The application of low levels of shear stress was also used in an attempt to engineer bone tissue from hMSCs. Collagen constructs were seeded with hMSCs, placed into a low shear stress bioreactor and perfused with osteogenic media for 5 weeks [14]. Although there is an application of shear stress to the cells, it is most likely the appearance of mineralization and increased ALP activity is due to the supplements added to the medium and has little to do with the application of mechanical stress. In addition, this system also shows alignment of the cells to the direction of fluid flow.

Hemodynamic Force

As mentioned previously, hemodynamic forces are a complex combination of several types of mechanical stresses including, but not limited to, pulsatile shear stress and cyclic radial stretch. In order to apply all these mechanical stimuli in concert in vitro, hMSCs were seeded onto the inside of a flexible silicone tube with mechanical properties similar to natural vessels and attached to a pulsatile pump [51]. The application of hemodynamic forces caused the hMSCs to begin to differentiate and take on the morphology of ECs including alignment with the direction of flow (as described in previous experiments). Yet the cells lacked expression of EC genetic markers making the study somewhat inconclusive. It is possible the differentiation of hMSCs into ECs cannot be done without the addition of medium supplements [3], but more studies will have to be performed to rationalize this hypothesis.

Nevertheless, other research performed utilizing hemodynamic forces have already paved to way for the engineering of vascular grafts. It has been observed these mechanical forces can increase the confluence of ECs and their organization within a graft [52]. In addition, this type of conditioning of the graft can lead to a lower occurrence of in vivo graft thrombosis and neointimal hyperplasia [53,54].

Furthermore, a different kind of bioreactor can also be classified as a system for the application of hemodynamic forces. Tissue engineered heart valves (TEHVs) are another up and coming branch of cardiovascular tissue engineering, which is taking advantage of biomimetic preconditioning. Engelmayr et al. have constructed a novel bioreactor that applies flexion, tension, and shear stress to their constructs seeded with sheep MSCs. The group discovered that the application of the three forces simultaneously for three weeks, significantly increased the collagen content and effective stiffness values (which was not very different than values measured for vascular smooth muscle cells) of the constructs over those which were exposed to only one or no mechanical force [55]. In addition, this group has gone on to validate and quantifying all parameters of the forces being imparted on the cells in the bioreactor by the addition of computer control [56].

CONCLUSIONS AND FUTURE DIRECTIONS

Mechanobiology and mechanotransduction are two of the most important topics being researched today by tissue engineers. It has been pointed out that mechanobiology and its applications to FTE should be the focus of future tissue engineering conferences [4].

The full extent of the mechanobiological events involved in the differentiation of stem cells will not be known until the underlying mechanisms for differentiation of each stem cell into the desired target cell type is elucidated. Though it may not have been explicitly enumerated in each study reported in the previous sections, many of them have investigated the role that the different MAPK pathways play during the mechanical stimulation of the cells. It is becoming increasingly apparent that the reaction to external stimuli and the involvement of these powerful molecules during mechanical stimulation of stem cells must be more closely examined. In addition, profiling the up- and down-regulation of cytokines during the mechanical stimulation process will help fill in the gaps in knowledge currently hindering the applicability of functional tissue engineering techniques.

Until now, the most notable information gathered shows certain cellular lineages favor one kind of mechanical deformation over others; more specifically, the adaptation to the force that the cells would normally experience in vivo is the most effective when it comes to in vitro differentiation. This is quite obvious from the experiments that have been performed in the absence of serum and exogenous cytokine supplementation resulting in differentiated cells. In short, chondrocytes develop from dynamic compression, cardiac muscle and VSMCs from cyclic stretching, ligament from torsion and alignment of vascular cells due to hemodynamic forces. Moreover, it should not be overlooked that the usefulness of bioreactors is not limited to the production of biomimetic forces; they can also be built to mimic other conditions in the body, such as the transport of nutrients to and waste away from the cells.

Until recent history, most studies on FTE employed a small group of stem cells including ESCs and adult stem cells, including MSCs and ASCs. Yet more recent investigations have begun to involve recently discovered adult stem cells in their work and in particular, stem cells from dental tissue. While the research done on these stem cells is in its infancy, the cells are being harvested from human exfoliated deciduous teeth (SHED), dental pulp stem cells (DPSC), and periodontal ligament stem cells (PDL). SHED cells are taken from donors 7-9 years of age, DPSCs are harvested from extracted third molars from donors 17-30 years old, and PDL cells are scraped from the root of extracted molars from donors of various ages. These new dental stem cells have been shown to express Stro-1, a surface marker of MSCs, and have the ability to differentiate toward the osteogenic, chondrogenic, and adipogenic lineages [57-59]. Furthermore, when DPSCs are co-cultured with rat cardiomyocytes, the cells differentiate into cardiomyocytes, adding greater potential to these cells [60]. In addition, many agree the most important characteristic of MSCs has been their immunomodulatory effects, allowing for allogenic transplantation. It has just recently been shown that PDL and SHED cells also possess this ability, which opens the door for these cells to be used as viable alternatives in all the mechanical differentiation modalities discussed here [61].

The more that is understood about the interactions of these biochemical and mechanical effectors, as well as their effects on different types of stem and progenitor cell populations will eventually lead to a multitude of stable, well developed, functional tissue engineering grafts for regenerative therapies.

REFERENCES

[1]   Guilak F, Butler DL, Goldstein SA, *et al*. Functional Tissue Engineering.Springer: NY 2004.

[2]   Butler DL, Juncosa-Melvin N, Boivin GP, *et al*. Functional tissue engineering for tendon repair: A multidisciplinary strategy using mesenchymal stem cells, bioscaffolds, and mechanical stimulation. J Orthop Res 2008; 26: 1-9.

[3]   Burdick JA, Vunjak-Novakovic G. Review: Engineered Microenvironments for Controlled Stem Cell Differentiation. Tissue Eng 2008; Part A.

[4]   Freed LE, Guilak F, Guo XE, *et al*. Advanced tools for tissue engineering: scaffolds, bioreactors, and signaling. Tissue Eng 2006; 12: 3285-3305.

[5]   Haudenschild AK, Hsieh AH, Kapila S, Lotz JC. Pressure and distortion regulate human mesenchymal stem cell gene expression. Ann Biomed Eng 2009; 37: 492-502.

[6]   Wang JH, Thampatty BP. Mechanobiology of adult and stem cells. Int Rev Cell Mol Biol 2008; 271: 301-346.

[7]   Pittenger MF, Mackay AM, Beck SC, *et al*. Multilineage potential of adult human mesenchymal stem cells. Science 1999; 284: 143-147.

[8]   Amado LC, Saliaris AP, Schuleri KH, *et al*. Cardiac repair with intramyocardial injection of allogeneic mesenchymal stem cells after myocardial infarction. Proc Natl Acad Sci USA 2005; 102: 11474-11479.

[9]   Grudeva-Popova JG. Cellular therapy--the possible future of regenerative medicine. Folia Med (Plovdiv) 2005; 47, 5-10.

[10]   Liu TM, Martina M, Hutmacher DW, Hui JH, Lee EH, Lim B. Identification of common pathways mediating differentiation of bone marrow- and adipose tissue-derived human mesenchymal stem cells into three mesenchymal lineages. Stem Cells 2007; 25: 750-760.

[11]   Estes BT, Gimble JM, Guilak F. Mechanical signals as regulators of stem cell fate. Curr Top Dev Biol 2004; 60: 91-126.

[12]   Hung CT, Mauck RL, Wang CC, *et al*. A paradigm for functional tissue engineering of articular cartilage via applied physiologic deformational loading. Ann Biomed Eng 2004; 32: 35-49.

[13]   Pelaez D, Huang CY, Cheung HS. Cyclic Compression Maintains Viability and Induces Chondrogenesis of Human Mesenchymal Stem Cells in Fibrin Gel Scaffolds. Stem Cells Dev. 2008; 93-102

[14]   Meinel L, Karageorgiou V, Fajardo R, *et al*. Bone tissue engineering using human mesenchymal stem cells: effects of scaffold material and medium flow. Ann Biomed Eng 2004; 32: 112-122.

[15]   Altman GH, Horan RL, Martin I, *et al*. Cell differentiation by mechanical stress. FASEB J 2002; 16: 270-272.

[16]   Schmelter M, Ateghang B, Helmig S, *et al*. Embryonic stem cells utilize reactive oxygen species as transducers of mechanical strain-induced cardiovascular differentiation. FASEB J 2006; 20: 1182-1184.

[17]   Gong Z, Niklason LE. Small-diameter human vessel wall engineered from bone marrow-derived mesenchymal stem cells (hMSCs). FASEB J 2008; 22: 1635-1648.

[18]   Kurpinski K, Park J, Thakar RG, Li S. Regulation of vascular smooth muscle cells and mesenchymal stem cells by mechanical strain. Mol Cell Biomech 2006; 3: 21-34.

[19]   Cimetta E, Figallo E, Cannizzaro C, *et al*. Micro-bioreactor arrays for controlling cellular environments: design principles for human embryonic stem cell applications. Methods 2009; 47: 81-89.

[20]   Korin N, Bransky A, Khoury M, *et al*. Design of well and groove microchannel bioreactors for cell culture. Biotechnol Bioeng 2009; 102: 1222-1230.

[21]   Lemon G, Waters SL, Rose FR, King JR. Mathematical modelling of human mesenchymal stem cell proliferation and differentiation inside artificial porous scaffolds. J Theor Biol 2007; 249: 543-553.

[22]   Titushkin I, Cho M. Modulation of cellular mechanics during osteogenic differentiation of human mesenchymal stem cells. Biophys J 2007; 93: 3693-3702.

[23]   Yanagisawa M, Suzuki N, Mitsui N, *et al*. Effects of compressive force on the differentiation of pluripotent mesenchymal cells. Life Sci 2007; 81: 405-412.

[24]   Yang JW, De IN, Huselstein C, *et al*. Evaluation of human MSCs cell cycle, viability and differentiation in micromass culture. Biorheology 2006; 43: 489-496.

[25]   Miyanishi K, Trindade MC, Lindsey DP, *et al*. Dose- and time-dependent effects of cyclic hydrostatic pressure on transforming growth factor-beta3-induced chondrogenesis by adult human mesenchymal stem cells in vitro. Tissue Eng 2006; 12: 2253-2262.

[26]   Wagner DR, Lindsey DP, Li KW, *et al*. Hydrostatic pressure enhances chondrogenic differentiation of human bone marrow stromal cells in osteochondrogenic medium. Ann Biomed Eng 2008; 36: 813-820.

[27]   Finger AR, Sargent CY, Dulaney KO, *et al.* Differential effects on messenger ribonucleic acid expression by bone marrow-derived human mesenchymal stem cells seeded in agarose constructs due to ramped and steady applications of cyclic hydrostatic pressure. Tissue Eng 2007; 13: 1151-1158.

[28]   Kim SH, Choi YR, Park MS, *et al.* ERK 1/2 activation in enhanced osteogenesis of human mesenchymal stem cells in poly(lactic-glycolic acid) by cyclic hydrostatic pressure. J Biomed Mater Res A 2007; 80: 826-836.

[29]   Terraciano V, Hwang N, Moroni L, *et al.* Differential response of adult and embryonic mesenchymal progenitor cells to mechanical compression in hydrogels. Stem Cells 2007; 25: 2730-2738.

[30]   Campbell JJ, Lee DA, Bader DL. Dynamic compressive strain influences chondrogenic gene expression in human mesenchymal stem cells. Biorheology 2006; 43: 455-470.

[31]   Park SH, Sim WY, Park SW, *et al.* An electromagnetic compressive force by cell exciter stimulates chondrogenic differentiation of bone marrow-derived mesenchymal stem cells. Tissue Eng 2006; 12: 3107-3117.

[32]   Huang CY, Hagar KL, Frost LE, *et al.* Effects of cyclic compressive loading on chondrogenesis of rabbit bone-marrow derived mesenchymal stem cells. Stem Cells 2004; 22: 313-323.

[33]   Huang CY, Reuben PM, Cheung HS. Temporal expression patterns and corresponding protein inductions of early responsive genes in rabbit bone marrow-derived mesenchymal stem cells under cyclic compressive loading. Stem Cells 2005; 23: 1113-1121.

[34]   Karin M. The regulation of AP-1 activity by mitogen-activated protein kinases. J Biol Chem 1995; 270: 16483-16486.

[35]   Simmons CA, Nikolovski J, Thornton AJ, *et al.* Mechanical stimulation and mitogen-activated protein kinase signaling independently regulate osteogenic differentiation and mineralization by calcifying vascular cells. J Biomech 2004; 37: 1531-1541.

[36]   Jaiswal RK, Jaiswal N, Bruder SP, *et al.* Adult human mesenchymal stem cell differentiation to the osteogenic or adipogenic lineage is regulated by mitogen-activated protein kinase. J Biol Chem 2000; 275: 9645-9652.

[37]   Simmons CA, Matlis S, Thornton AJ, *et al.* Cyclic strain enhances matrix mineralization by adult human mesenchymal stem cells via the extracellular signal-regulated kinase (ERK1/2) signaling pathway. J Biomech 2003; 36: 1087-1096.

[38]   Saha S, Ji L, de Pablo JJ, Palecek SP. Inhibition of human embryonic stem cell differentiation by mechanical strain. J Cell Physiol 2006; 206: 126-137.

[39]   Kurpinski K, Li S. Mechanical stimulation of stem cells using cyclic uniaxial strain. J Vis Exp 2007; 242.

[40]   Kurpinski K, Chu J, Hashi C, Li S. Anisotropic mechanosensing by mesenchymal stem cells. Proc Natl Acad Sci USA 2006; 103: 16095-16100.

[41]   Sumanasinghe RD, Osborne JA, Loboa EG. Mesenchymal stem cell-seeded collagen matrices for bone repair: effects of cyclic tensile strain, cell density, and media conditions on matrix contraction in vitro. J Biomed Mater Res A 2009; 88: 778-786.

[42]   Sumanasinghe RD, Bernacki SH, Loboa EG. Osteogenic differentiation of human mesenchymal stem cells in collagen matrices: effect of uniaxial cyclic tensile strain on bone morphogenetic protein (BMP-2) mRNA expression. Tissue Eng 2006; 12: 3459-3465.

[43]   Sumanasinghe RD, Pfeiler TW, Monteiro-Riviere NA, Loboa EG. Expression of proinflammatory cytokines by human mesenchymal stem cells in response to cyclic tensile strain. J Cell Physiol 2009; 219: 77-83.

[44]   Wall ME, Rachlin A, Otey CA, *et al.* Human adipose-derived adult stem cells upregulate palladin during osteogenesis and in response to cyclic tensile strain. Am J Physiol Cell Physiol 2007; 293: C1532-C1538.

[45]   Van GM, Diederichs S, Roeker S, *et al.* Mechanical Strain Using 2D and 3D Bioreactors Induces Osteogenesis: Implications for Bone Tissue Engineering. Adv Biochem Eng Biotechnol 2008.

[46]   Park JS, Chu JS, Cheng C, *et al.* Differential effects of equiaxial and uniaxial strain on mesenchymal stem cells. Biotechnol Bioeng 2004; 88: 359-368.

[47]   Goh JC, Ouyang HW, Teoh SH, *et al.* Tissue-engineering approach to the repair and regeneration of tendons and ligaments. Tissue Eng 2003; 9 Suppl 1: S31-S44.

[48]   Altman GH, Lu HH, Horan RL, *et al.* Advanced bioreactor with controlled application of multi-dimensional strain for tissue engineering. J Biomech Eng 2002; 124: 742-749.

[49]   Kahn CJ, Vaquette C, Rahouadj R, Wang X. A novel bioreactor for ligament tissue engineering. Biomed Mater Eng 2008; 18: 283-287.

[50]   Metallo CM, Vodyanik MA, de Pablo JJ, *et al.* The response of human embryonic stem cell-derived endothelial cells to shear stress. Biotechnol Bioeng 2008; 100: 830-837.

[51]   O'Cearbhaill ED, Punchard MA, Murphy M, Barry FP, *et al.* Response of mesenchymal stem cells to the biomechanical environment of the endothelium on a flexible tubular silicone substrate. Biomaterials 2008; 29: 1610-1619.

[52]   Hoerstrup SP, Zund G, Sodian R, *et al.* Tissue engineering of small caliber vascular grafts. Eur J Cardiothorac Surg 2001; 20: 164-169.

[53] Dardik A, Liu A, Ballermann BJ. Chronic in vitro shear stress stimulates endothelial cell retention on prosthetic vascular grafts and reduces subsequent in vivo neointimal thickness. J Vasc Surg 1999; 29: 157-167.

[54] Shirota T, He H, Yasui H, *et al*. Human endothelial progenitor cell-seeded hybrid graft: proliferative and antithrombogenic potentials in vitro and fabrication processing. Tissue Eng 2003; 9: 127-136.

[55] Engelmayr GC Jr, Sales VL, Mayer JE Jr, Sacks MS. Cyclic flexure and laminar flow synergistically accelerate mesenchymal stem cell-mediated engineered tissue formation: Implications for engineered heart valve tissues. Biomaterials 2006; 27: 6083-6095.

[56] Engelmayr GC Jr, Hildebrand DK, Sutherland FW, *et al*. A novel bioreactor for the dynamic flexural stimulation of tissue engineered heart valve biomaterials. Biomaterials 2003; 24: 2523-2532.

[57] Gay IC, Chen S, MacDougall M. Isolation and characterization of multipotent human periodontal ligament stem cells. Orthod Craniofac Res 2007; 10: 149-160.

[58] Koyama N, Okubo Y, Nakao K, *et al*. Evaluation of pluripotency in human dental pulp cells. J Oral Maxillofac Surg 2009; 67: 501-506.

[59] Singhatanadgit W, Donos N, Olsen I. Isolation and characterisation of stem cell clones from adult human ligament. Tissue Eng Part A 2009.

[60] Arminan A, Gandia C, Bartual C, *et al*. Cardiac differentiation is driven by NKX2.5 and GATA4 nuclear translocation in tissue specific mesenchymal stem cells. Stem Cells Dev 2008.

[61] Wada N, Menicanin D, Shi S, *et al*. Immunomodulatory properties of human periodontal ligament stem cells. J Cell Physiol 2009; 667-676

CHAPTER 5

Functional Cartilage Tissue Engineering with Adult Stem Cells: Current Status and Future Directions

Alice H. Huang[1,2], Clark T. Hung[3], and Robert L. Mauck[1,2,]*

[1]McKay Orthopaedic Research Laboratory, Department of Orthopaedic Surgery, University of Pennsylvania. Philadelphia, PA 19104, USA; [2]Department of Bioengineering, University of Pennsylvania, Philadelphia, PA 19104, USA and [3]Cellular Engineering Laboratory, Department of Biomedical Engineering, Columbia University, New York, NY, 10027, USA

Abstract: Adult mesenchymal stem cells (MSCs) hold great promise for engineering replacements for damaged or degraded articular cartilage. This promise has long been contemplated, and its arrival has recently been marked by the implantation of engineered human trachea using autologous adult stem cells [1]. While tracheal cartilage is not the same as the articulating cartilage lining the ends of load bearing joints, the demonstration of *in vivo* efficacy provides a major step forward clinically. However, not all progress with MSC-based cartilage has been successful and considerable challenges remain in the realization of these constructs for load-bearing applications. Thus the intent of this chapter is to define the functional metrics required for engineering articular cartilage, and to situate the current state of MSC-based constructs within this framework. In doing so, we briefly define the components and function of the native tissue, and review the progress made to date using differentiated cartilage cells (chondrocytes) for cartilage tissue engineering. This discussion includes methods of formation, biochemical formulations for enhancing *in vitro* development, as well as progress made towards using mechanical forces to further direct maturation. We next overview the origins and applications of adult multi-potential stem cells, and discuss how routes towards cartilage tissue engineering with stem cells match (or fail to match) those approaches that were successful using differentiated cells. In particular, we describe new requirements for cartilage formation with MSCs, and outline several research areas that may inform this new direction in cartilage tissue engineering.

INTRODUCTION

It is well appreciated that articular cartilage is a unique tissue whose function is predicated on a precise balance of extracellular matrix (ECM) components and cells. Together, these components produce and maintain structure and mechanical function over a lifetime of use. Disruption of the articulating cartilages, either through trauma or progressive degenerative diseases such as osteoarthrititis (OA), engenders pain and loss of function to millions in the US, and hundreds of millions worldwide. The antecedents of OA have yet to be fully elucidated, but certain mechanical, genetic, and lifestyle risk factors have been identified [2]. Pathologies associated with OA arise both within the articulating cartilage layers (fissuring, loss of matrix properties, progressive vascularization and eburnation), as well as within the subchondral bone supporting the cartilage layer. Many of the same features that enable cartilage function (a dense ECM, a lack of vascularity) also appear to impede normal healing responses in the tissue, and predispose a loss in functional capacity once the careful regulatory mechanisms that maintain the tissue become imbalanced.

This lack of endogenous repair necessitates methods for repair to restore joint function, the most common of which is total joint replacement. This replacement of bone and soft tissue with metal and plastic components represents the most significant advance in orthopaedic medicine over the last several decades; joint replacement has restored function to millions of patients who otherwise would be incapable of carrying out the functions of daily life. Indeed, with the aging of the US population, as well as increases in lifespan, total joint replacement

---

*Address Correspondence to this Author Robert L. Mauck: Assistant Professor of Orthopaedic Surgery and Bioengineering, McKay Orthopaedic Research Laboratory, Department of Orthopaedic Surgery, University of Pennsylvania, 36th Street and Hamilton Walk, Philadelphia, PA 19104, USA; Tel: (215) 898-3294; Fax: (215) 573-2133; E-mail: lemauck@mail.med.upenn.edu

procedures are only becoming more common. A recent study suggested that the number of total knee replacements would increase by >600% by 2030, reaching as many as 3.5 million procedures performed per year in the US alone [3]. Despite the successes of joint replacement in restoring function, the lifetime of implanted prosthetic components range between 10-15 years, and surgical methods are limited to only one revision procedure (in which a failing implant is replaced with a new component). Given the prevalence of this disease, the number of replacements performed annually, and the limited alternatives available, solutions to OA are increasingly in demand.

To address this pressing clinical need, the field of tissue engineering has focused on biologic reconstruction of articulating joints. Tissue engineering is loosely defined as the combination of cells and biocompatible materials to generate new, living, biologic tissues for implantation. A tenet of this approach is that biologic substitution is superior to material implantation as a biologic substitute by definition can remodel and sustain itself through normal cellular processes, much like the normal functioning tissue. Early successes in the production of cartilage and bone from cells cultured *ex vivo* as replacement tissue have suggested that tissue engineering may be a viable approach that can eliminate or forestall the need for joint replacement. Even in the absence of full functionality with engineered biologics, provision of an additional decade of joint health via a biologic substitute (prior to joint replacement) would immeasurably improve patient health, particularly as life expectancies continue to improve in the aged population.

To improve the function and utility of engineered materials, several major challenges must be addressed to enable translation of early research to clinically useful therapies in cartilage tissue engineering. First and foremost, methods to improve the function and maturation of engineered cartilage constructs themselves must be optimized. This chapter details progress made to date in these efforts, and highlights mechanisms by which engineered constructs have been produced with near-native tissue properties. An additional consideration in this research area is the most appropriate cell source on which to focus efforts. Autologous chondrocytes (cartilage forming cells) may not be the ideal cell source for repair methodologies given their limited supply, age, and diseased status with OA. One opportunity for overcoming such concerns is the use of multi-potential autologous mesenchymal stem cells (MSCs). These cells are easily obtained from bone marrow and other tissues (such as adipose) [4], are expandable in culture [5], and may be grown in sufficient numbers to populate engineered scaffolds. These cells also have a proven capacity to adopt phenotypes that reproduce many features of primary bone and cartilage cells, and so are particularly suitable for engineering bone and cartilage replacements. While promising, recent work has clearly demonstrated that cartilage formed by MSCs is of different quality and stability in comparison with cartilage formed by primary cells. Moreover, methods of optimization that have been successful with primary chondrocytes are not directly translatable to optimization of engineered cartilage formed from MSCs. These differences may be related to a different developmental state and/or inherent potential of a newly differentiated cell in comparison to a cell that has undergone a full differentiation process. These issues will be addressed in this chapter by defining the state of the art in cartilage tissue engineering with adult mesenchymal stem cells, and outlining several new research areas that may further their optimization and clinical application.

ARTICULAR CARTILAGE PROPERTIES AND ENGINEERING BENCHMARKS

To fully appreciate the challenge of articular cartilage tissue engineering, an in-depth appreciation of the structure, composition, and function of the native tissue is required. The following sections briefly describe the main structural and mechanical features of cartilage that are critical to its functional role, as well as the events that underlie its formation, maturation, and maintenance through a lifetime of use.

Adult Articular Cartilage: Composition, Mechanical Properties, and Physiologic Loading

As the load bearing material of diarthrodial joints, articular cartilage lines the bony surfaces and functions to transmit the high stresses that originate with motion through an elegant transition from soft to hard tissue, Fig. **1**. Articular cartilage consists of both a solid matrix [6-8] and a fluid phase [9, 10]. The solid matrix is composed of a dense network of type II collagen fibrils enmeshed in a solution of charged, aggregated proteoglycans (PGs: aggrecan core protein plus glycosaminoglycan (GAG) side chains). Collagen content ranges from 5-30% by wet weight and PG content from 2-10% [11, 12], with the remainder of the tissue made up of water. Collagen forms a cross-linked co-polymeric network composed of collagens II, IX and XI [13], and acts to immobilize proteoglycans within the ECM [14]. In developing articular cartilage, the proportions of collagens are roughly ≥10% IX, ≥10% XI, ≥80% II, falling to ~1% IX, ~3% XI, ≥90% II in adult cartilage [15]. Mutations in collagen types II, IX and XI genes have been associated with the onset of cartilage degeneration and osteoarthritis-like features [16, 17]. Trifunctional hydroxypyridinium cross-links stabilize these collagen components and contribute to the tensile properties of the tissue. In chondrocyte-based tissue-engineered constructs, collagen content and pyridinium crosslinks are markedly reduced relative to native tissue, although the fractions of collagen types II and IX are comparable [18]. Chondrocytes make up less than 10% of the tissue [19] and produce ECM to balance continual degradation and remodeling by MMPs (collagenases and aggrecanases) [20-23]. The composition, architecture, and remodeling of cartilage are uniquely adapted to function over a lifetime of repetitive use.

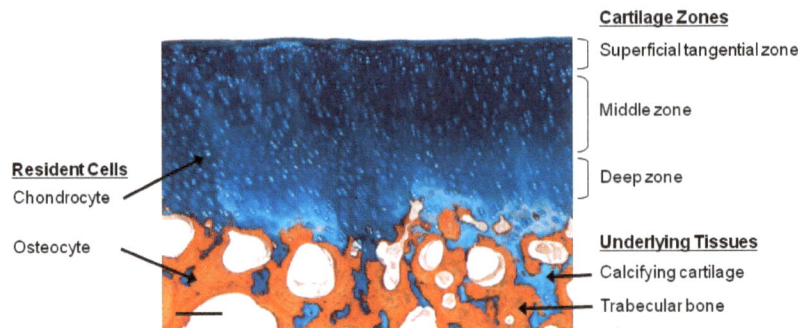

Figure 1: Articular cartilage histology showing zonal dependence and integration with underlying bone. Ovine tissue sample stained for proteoglyan (alcian blue) and collagen (picrosirius red). Scalebar: 200 μm.

A normally active adult takes 1-2 million steps per year [24] and the resulting forces acting on cartilage range from 2.5 to 4.9 times the body weight [25-27]. Loading is cyclical/intermittent [26, 28] and stresses at the cartilage surface can range from 2-10 MPa [29-35]. The dense PG-rich collagenous matrix of cartilage resists this loading environment with its high equilibrium compression modulus of 0.2-1.4 MPa [36-41] and even higher tensile modulus of 1-30 MPa [42-46] in the plane of the tissue. The organization and prevailing direction of collagen fibers (the split line direction) is of particular importance for the tensile properties, which are highest at the surface and in the split line direction [46-50]. Split lines have a different organization in loaded and unloaded regions of joints [51] that is similar between patients, consistent with the idea that use defines structural organization [52]. With this dense specialized matrix, cyclical compressive loading at physiologic frequencies (0.1-2 Hz) causes the interstitial fluid pressure to increase [53], resulting in a higher dynamic modulus than equilibrium modulus [54]. This is enhanced by the disparity between the tensile and compressive moduli [55-60]. In addition to these factors, the dynamic compressive modulus is also dependent on the collagen content and tensile properties of the tissue [54, 59, 61]. Treatment with collagenase results in marked reduction of the dynamic compressive modulus of cartilage explants [62-64]. With contact loading, the enhanced fluid pressurization at the point of contact supports >90% of applied stress, shielding the solid matrix from excess deformation [57, 65]. Remarkably, with its high contact stresses, cartilage thickness *in vivo* changes by <6-20% with use [25, 66-68]. This mechanical interplay between the solid and fluid components of cartilage has been defined by sophisticated biphasic and poroelastic models [60, 69, 70]. It is precisely this combination of tensile and compressive properties, promoting fluid pressurization, which enables cartilage mechanical function and must be recapitulated in any successful repair.

Articular Cartilage: Formation and Maturation

While the current understanding of articular cartilage structure and function is fairly extensive, the mechanism by which cartilage develops these properties is less clear. It is also unclear how articular chondrocytes acquire and maintain their characteristic phenotype during embryogenesis. A better understanding of these developmental processes is important from a tissue engineering standpoint as it would allow researchers to more effectively engineer replacement tissues with a stable phenotype. The first appearance of a cartilage-like tissue (dense organization of PG and type II collagen) is in the limb bud [71]. Limb bud cells aggregate and undergo chondrogenesis under a complex array of morphogenetic and transcription factors, and other signaling cues [71].

While this material is 'cartilage', it is transient in nature, and much of it is eventually replaced through endochondral ossification [72-74] and forms the long bones of the skeleton. Articular chondrocytes however, escape hypertrophy and ossification, and acquire permanent phenotypic traits that allow them to maintain and remodel cartilage throughout a lifetime of use. The origin of these cells and the factors directing the development of their unique phenotype are only beginning to be elucidated.

The formation of articular joints (a process known as cavitation) begins with the interruption of the cartilage template (the anlagen) within the limb bud by a specialized layer called the interzone. This specialization is directed by a host of molecular factors, including GDF-5, Wnt-4, ERG and PTHrP. Wnt-4 is a soluble factor expressed early in the developing joint, and may be an important molecule in determination of the interzone site. GDF-5 is a member of the BMP family and appears to play many roles during joint development, including cavitation and joint patterning. PTHrP is expressed in cartilage cells from the embryonic stage through adulthood, and may maintain the articular cartilage phenotype [75, 76]. While the precise sequence of events has yet to be definitively mapped, at least a portion of the interzone appears to be populated by invading cells from the anlagen periphery [77, 78]. Cells within the interzone differentiate into all of the fibrous joint structures, and occupy at least the superficial and middle zones of the eventual permanent articular cartilage. In addition to biological factors, mechanical forces are essential for articular joint formation [79, 80]. For example, inhibitors of muscle contraction *in ovo* lead to incomplete joint formation and decreased properties [81-83]. Many signaling factors, including PTHrP [84], are themselves modulated by mechanical factors, suggesting that the promotion and maintenance of the chondrocyte phenotype is a highly regulated process in development.

After birth, articular cartilage undergoes dramatic maturational changes that results in an adult tissue with unique load-bearing capacity. Collagen fiber organization within the tissue is transformed from an isotropic arrangement to a mature configuration with superficial fibers arranged into split lines parallel to the surface [85]. Compared to the initial anlagen formation, less is known about the cells in the articulating cartilage, and the signaling events that define their maturation. Unlike cells within other skeletal structures, articulating cartilage cells never undergo hypertrophy. Pacifici and co-workers recently reviewed the extant literature on these articular chondrocytes, and concluded that articular cells that retain a permanent cartilage phenotype are distinguishable from the transient chondrocytes that form the initial anlagen and growth plate [86]. While these different cell types likely share some signaling mechanisms, it is not yet clear whether these factors act in the same fashion. Nevertheless, what is clear is that the maturation of cartilage results in dramatic increases in tissue mechanics (particularly tensile properties) [87-89]. In mice, MMPs-2,-3, and -9 are absent at birth and peak 2 weeks later, suggesting an intense early ECM remodeling [90, 91]. In the cow, mechanical and biochemical properties increase rapidly in juvenile compared to fetal cartilages [12, 92], with increases in tensile properties correlated to increases in collagen content and cross-linking. At the same time, tissue cellularity decreases markedly, from 120 million cells/mL in fetal calf tissue to 50 million cells/mL in adult tissues [93]. When embryonic and juvenile bovine cartilage explants are removed from the joint environment, tensile properties decrease [94]. While one cannot overstate the importance of biologic factors in the *in situ* milieu, these findings also suggest that the demands placed on cartilage, coincident with use, help define organization and properties (e.g., collagen split lines), allowing the tissue to achieve its mature load bearing capacity. Thus, a developmental cascade of events, from formation in the embryo through maturation in the adult, results in the unique properties of the native tissue – incorporation of this understanding, and application of these principles may aid in the generation of functional engineered cartilage constructs.

CARTILAGE TISSUE ENGINEERING WITH CHONDROCYTES

As cartilage healing is limited, there exists a growing demand for cell-based strategies for cartilage repair. A now standard tissue engineering approach consists of a chondrocytic cell type encapsulated in or seeded on a three-dimensional (3D) biomaterial support. Chondrocytes are a well-characterized and useful cell type for these applications, as they readily produce a cartilage-like matrix composed of proteoglycans and collagens *in vitro* in a number of supportive media and material conditions.

Materials for Cartilage Tissue Engineering

A number of materials have been employed in cartilage tissue engineering, including porous scaffolds (foams and fibrous meshes) fabricated from poly(α-hydroxy esters) including poly(glycolic acid), poly(lactic acid), and their copolymers [95-99]. Foams and meshes based on natural materials (Type I, II collagen, PG/collagen composites) support cartilage growth as well [100, 101]. Chondrocytes cultured on these porous scaffolds form ECM and increased mechanics with culture. However, uniform seeding throughout the scaffold expanse is a challenge; cells flatten and line the pore spaces, collagen contents remain lower than native tissue, and directionality of formed matrix has not been achieved. Alternatively, hydrogels are attractive biomaterials for cartilage regeneration and many natural (e.g., collagen and alginate) and synthetic polymers (e.g., Pluronics) have been investigated. Specific examples in the literature include alginate [102-104], agarose [105, 106], fibrin [107, 108], type I and II collagen [109, 110], peptide gels [111], and poly(ethylene glycol) (PEG) [112-114], to list but a few. This focus on hydrogels is motivated by the observation that in hydrogel culture, chondrocytes can be well dispersed and cells may assume their natural round shape and phenotype. This shape is particularly important, as it has long been demonstrated that de-differentiated chondrocytes can regain their cartilage ECM producing capacity when seeded in even simple hydrogels [115]. Furthermore, these gels efficiently entrap the cartilage-like ECM produced by the cells [115-117], and can rapidly assemble a neo-cartilage matrix with functional properties. Combinations of gels and fibrous structures might be particularly valuable, as demonstrated in work by Moutos and co-workers developing a cell-laden gel-infused fiber scaffold using advanced weaving technologies [118].

Recent focus has also turned to highly functionalized hydrogels, including photopolymerizable networks that can be optimally modified to elicit specific cell responses *in vivo* and *in vitro*. Elisseeff *et al.* [119] first used a transdermally polymerized hydrogel formed from dimethacrylated poly(ethylene oxide) and semi-interpenetrating linear poly(ethylene oxide) chains. This work illustrated both the ability to photoencapsulate viable chondrocytes in a hydrogel network with light transmitted through dermal tissue and the production of neocartilage with both PG and collagen present. Bryant and Anseth later showed that photocrosslinked scaffolds could be fabricated that span the thickness of native cartilage found *in vivo* while maintaining PG production [113]. More recently, chemically and photocrosslinked natural materials such as elastin like protein (ELP) and hyaluronic acid (HA) have been employed in the formation of chondrocyte-seeded hydrogels [120-123]. A number of investigators have examined how changes in hydrogel properties (e.g., crosslinking density) influence the synthesis and distribution of collagen and PGs by encapsulated chondrocytes [124-126]. This work generally showed that higher crosslinking densities limit matrix distribution. To hasten matrix distribution, dynamic hydrogels have been developed that either incorporate degradable linkages or have enzymatic treatment methods applied to cell-seeded constructs during maturation. For example, we have applied agarase (which degrades agarose) to remove the remnants of this gel from the neo-tissue [127]. Others have engineered the hydrogel itself via the inclusion of hydrolytically degradable linkages in synthetic PEG gels; findings from this work show a markedly greater level of collagen deposition and distribution by chondrocytes seeded within [128]. Other gels have been designed with MMP-cleavable linkages and backbones, such that remodeling of a synthetic matrix can occur by natural, cell-mediated mechanisms [129]. For example, an MMP-sensitive PEG based gel developed by Lutolf [130] was used to encapsulate bovine chondrocytes [131]. This study showed a greater distribution of formed matrix in gels with MMP-sensitive linkages, as well as greater expression of aggrecan and type II collagen. From this body of work it is clear that a cell encapsulating material can be appropriately designed to promote maximum levels of matrix formation, as well as eventually be removed to further ECM distribution throughout the construct.

Functional Cartilage Tissue Engineering

Simply supporting matrix formation is sufficient for enabling cartilage-like tissue formation, but absent other cues, this tissue does not typically develop into a tissue construct with native tissue properties. Articular cartilage exists in a mechanically challenging environment, and this environment is critical in the development of mechanical properties, as the dynamic environment guides new tissue formation. Drawing on this concept, the primary goal of functional tissue engineering is to recapitulate critical structural and mechanical benchmarks necessary to restore function in the joint [132]. This approach incorporates our understanding of the mechanical signals that arise in the tissue microenvironment [133], and then uses these signals to inform *in vitro* culture conditions to better direct tissue growth and modulate cell behavior. To that end, bioreactors that provide an appropriate mechanical environment for constructs are an important element in tissue engineering. Constructs can be cultured in the presence of mechanical signals, including hydrostatic pressurization (e.g., [134]), fluid flow (e.g., [135]), or direct mechanical stimulation through mechanical compression (e.g., [105, 106, 136, 137]). Since mechanical stimulation plays a crucial role in the native environment of cartilage, mechanical preconditioning may be an especially suitable strategy for engineering cartilage [136]. Studies in hydrogels have shown that biosynthesis of collagen and proteoglycans are up-regulated with compressive loading [138] and are modulated by amplitude, frequency and loading duration [139, 140]. In chondrocyte-based constructs, long-term application of dynamic compression enhances both the mechanical properties and biochemical content of loaded gels [137]. To date, however, the collagen content of engineered constructs remain well below native values; failure of constructs to achieve the dynamic compressive properties and tensile properties found in cartilage can be attributed to this lack in collagen content and organization [18].

New Media Formulations for Cartilage Tissue Engineering

In addition to mechanical loading, a number of other optimization strategies have been employed to improve engineered cartilage formation. Several studies have shown that increasing the initial cell number within the construct can lead to more rapid and/or greater cartilage-ECM formation and mechanics [99, 105, 106, 141, 142]. Increased levels of nutrient supplementation can likewise increase growth rates [106]. Specific inclusion of anabolic growth factors normally found in the maturing and mature synovial fluid (such as IGF-1, TGF-β family members, and FGF) can further improve cartilage-like tissue development in engineered constructs [143-147]. In a series of recent studies we have shown that such approaches can lead to rapid and robust growth. Specifically, transient (rather than continuous) application of TGF-β3 in a serum-free, chemically defined medium dramatically enhances the compressive properties and GAG content of chondrocyte-laden hydrogels to near-native levels [148, 149], Fig. **2**. In these studies, after removal of the growth factor, constructs undergo an explosive growth phase, and reach equilibrium compressive moduli of ~0.8 MPa and proteoglycan levels of 6-7% wet weight in less than 2 months of culture. These findings have particular implications for clinical use, as the media used for culture does not contain poorly characterized and potentially immunogenic serum elements, and induction is superior when growth factor is discontinued, as would be the case when such constructs are implanted *in vivo*. While promising, however, it should be noted that both collagen content and dynamic modulus of such constructs remains well below that of native tissue, suggesting that further optimization will be required to achieve full functionality. Towards that end, we applied dynamic loading to these constructs and showed that in the presence of TGF-β3, loading reduced the mechanical properties of chondrocyte-seeded constructs relative to free-swelling controls [148]. In contrast, sequential application of TGF-β3 followed by dynamic compression (after removal of TGF-β3) significantly enhanced mechanical properties [148], with constructs reaching a compressive moduli in excess of 1 MPa. These findings indicate that the biologic and mechanical environments are highly interactive, and that optimization of growth can be tuned to the current state of the microenvironment.

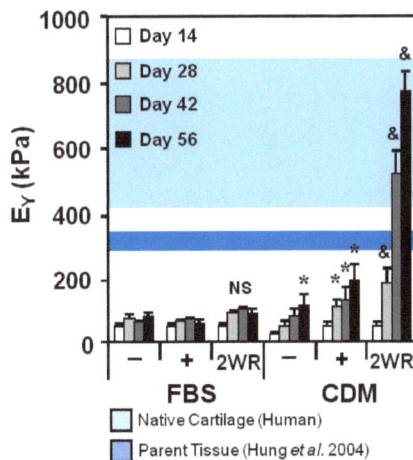

Figure 2: Equilibrium unconfined compressive modulus of chondrocyte-seeded constructs maintained in serum-containing (FBS) or chemically defined (CDM) media supplemented continuously with (+), transiently with (2WR), or in the absence of (-) 10 ng/mL TGF-β3. Data represent mean and standard deviation of 8-22 samples from two to five replicate studies. * indicates significant difference versus day 14, & indicates significant difference from all other time-matched samples, p<0.05. Modified from [149] with permission from Mary Ann Liebert, Inc.

Age Dependent Chondrocyte Differences

While much of the work outlined above has shown the promise of cartilage tissue engineering with chondrocytes, a large proportion of the studies were carried out with juvenile cells. Disparities in chondrocyte biosynthetic activity and healing response that reflect cartilage tissue age are well established (e.g., [150, 151]), with aged chondrocytes and cartilage tissue generally showing reduced biosynthetic potential relative to immature cells. Cell and tissue age also mediates the response to the biochemical and biomechanical environment. In the bovine model system, transient addition of growth factors is capable of introducing explosive development of tissue properties in primary immature chondrocyte-seeded engineered cartilage, whereas continuous application of growth factors is necessary for growth of constructs seeded with primary adult chondrocytes [152], Fig. **3**. With respect to clinical applications, the ability to successfully expand adult chondrocytes while maintaining their subsequent chondrogenic potential (i.e., ability to make cartilaginous tissue) is critical in providing sufficient cells for cartilage repair strategies. During monolayer expansion, chondrocytes exhibit a de-differentiated phenotype, where type I collagen levels are elevated and type II collagen and aggrecan decreased [153]. Expansion of chondrocytes with growth factors or in the presence of primary chondrocytes has also been successful in re-establishing the chondrogenic phenotype and matrix production capacity in passaged chondrocytes (e.g., [154, 155]). Our lab has reported that adult canine chondrocytes, primed using a growth factor expansion protocol originally reported for human chondrocytes [156], produce engineered cartilage [157] with mechanical and biochemical properties at native levels and that are 20-fold greater than primary chondrocytes (Fig. **4**). This finding is reminiscent of observations that extended passaging increases chondrogenic potential of adipose-derived stem cells [158]. A better understanding of the mechanisms by which the chondrogenic potential of adult chondrocytes is enhanced after passaging may therefore be key in providing important clues for developing successful strategies to optimize the chondrogenic potential of stem cells.

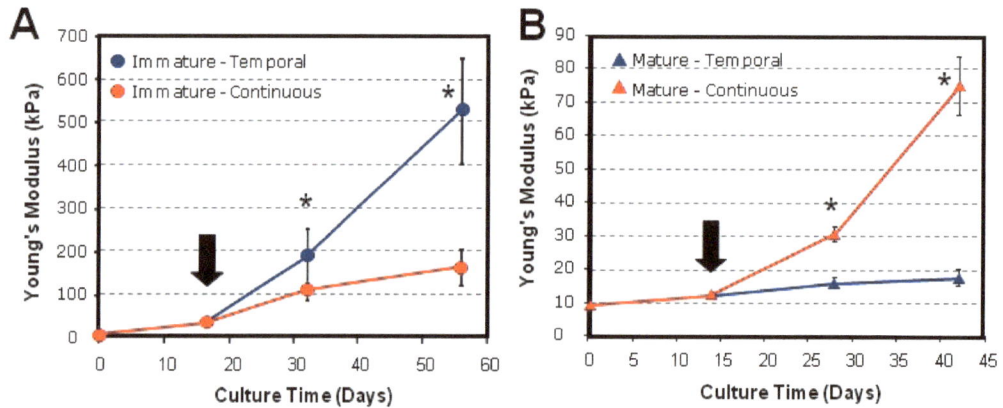

Figure 3: Compressive young's modulus of (A) immature and (B) mature chondrocyte-laden agarose constructs under continuous or temporal exposure to TGF-β3. Arrow indicates point during *in vitro* culture at which TGF-β3 was removed from the media. * indicates significant differences between groups, p<0.05, n=4-5/group. Modified from [148] and [247] with permission from Elsevier and the Orthopaedic Research Society.

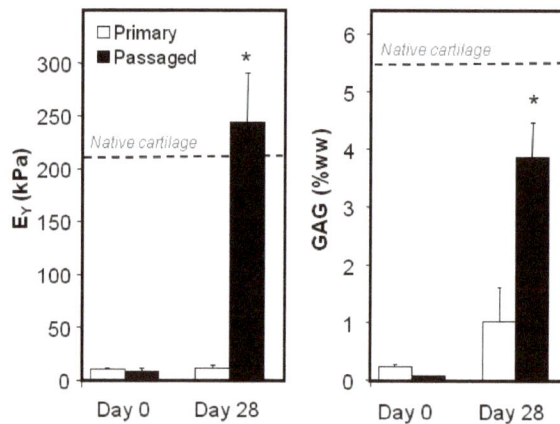

Figure 4: (A) Equilibrium compressive modulus and (B) GAG content of primary and passaged canine chondrocytes embedded in agarose. Passage in the presence of growth factor significantly enhanced matrix production and mechanical

properties. * indicates greater than all groups (p<0.05). n=4-5/group. Data modified from [248] with permission from the Orthopaedic Research Society.

CARTILAGE TISSUE ENGINEERING WITH MESENCHYMAL STEM CELLS

Mesenchymal Stem Cells: Isolation and Differentiation

Despite these successes in cartilage tissue engineering with primary cells, limitations in chondrocyte availability and donor site morbidity may preclude their use in clinical applications. Therefore, over the last decade, there has been increasing interest in mesenchymal stem cells (MSCs) as an alternative cell type for cartilage engineering. MSCs are a self-renewing and multi-potent cell type with great potential for cell-based regenerative therapies. In the original descriptions of MSC multi-potentiality, MSCs were induced toward bone, fat, and cartilage phenotypes [159, 160], and these assays remain the accepted metric for characterization of these cells. Although there is no definitive marker for MSC selection, hematopoietic surface antigens (i.e., CD45, CD34 and CD14) are not present on MSCs [159]. Because there is no single defining surface marker for MSC identification, cell selection through plastic adhesion and colony formation is widely utilized. As a result, the starting population of cells may include a heterogeneous mixture of MSCs and other cells. MSCs can be readily isolated from a wide variety of tissue sources; while bone marrow is a common source of MSCs, these cells (and cells with similar multi-lineage capacity) have been derived from adipose tissue [161], periosteum [162], synovium [163], and trabecular bone chips [164]. In standard assays of MSC chondrogenesis, cells are collected into high-density pellets to induce a rounded morphology (mimicking mesenchymal condensation in the limb bud). Indeed, in some ways, these cells possess a similar capacity as limb bud mesenchyme cells, as they can form both bone and cartilage. It should be noted that these two cell types are distinct; while limb bud cells transit through cartilage and on to an osteogenic lineage *in vitro* in micromass culture without specific additives, adult MSCs must be treated with specific biofactors to take on a cartilage phenotype. Common chondrogenic media formulations for MSCs include TGF-β superfamily members and dexamethasone presented in a chemically defined serum-free medium [159, 160, 165]. Under these conditions, MSCs synthesize a cartilage-specific ECM rich in sulfated GAGs and type II collagen and express cartilage markers, including the transcription factor sox 9 (Fig. **5**). In addition to their chondrogenic potential, there is also evidence suggesting that MSCs are nonimmunogenic or hypoimmunogenic, which may be useful for therapeutic applications [166].

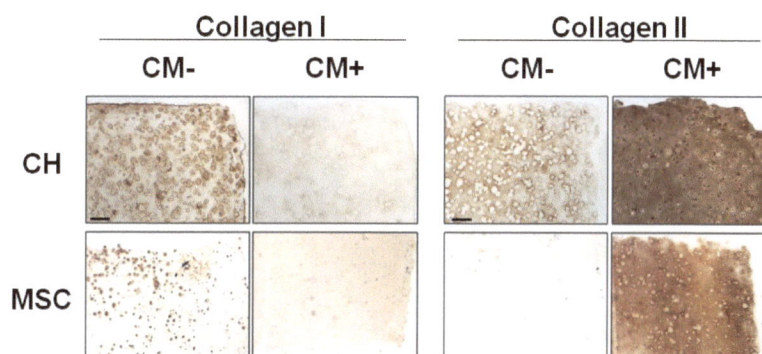

Figure 5: Immunohistochemical detection of type I and type II collagen deposition in chondrocyte (CH) - and MSC-seeded agarose constructs seeded at 10 million cells/mL after 56 days of *in vitro* culture in a chemically defined medium in the presence (CM+) or absence (CM-) of TGF-β3. Scale Bar: 100 µm. Data adapted from [197] with permission from Elsevier.

MSC Chondrogenesis in 3D Culture

Given their ability to take on a cartilage-like phenotype, MSCs have attracted intense interest for cartilage tissue engineering, and their ability to form cartilage-like tissues has been evaluated in a variety of 3D culture configurations. Indeed, in defined media conditions, it has been shown that MSCs undergo chondrogenesis in a number of biocompatible scaffolds, including fibrin [167], agarose [168, 169], HA/gelatin [168, 170], and alginate hydrogels [161, 168, 171-173], as well as in polyester foams [174] and polyester/alginate amalgams [175, 176]. MSC-biomaterial interactions may be particularly important for MSCs, both in terms of initial viability as well as subsequent chondrogenesis. For example, unlike chondrocytes, the viability of human MSCs decrease in hydrogels when not presented with the appropriate 3D adhesive niche and media formulation [177, 178]. MSCs are generally isolated based on their adhesion to tissue culture plastic, and thus precipitating the first step in phenotypic conversion may be necessary to maintain viability in this anchorage dependent population. Conversely, these same adhesive cues may both positively and negatively regulate chondrogenic differentiation; increasing densities of RGD presented in modified alginate decreased the extent of MSC chondrogenesis as measured by ECM production [179], while inclusion of a collagen mimetic peptide in a PEG background increased chondrogenesis [180]. These findings suggest that hydrogels for MSC-based cartilage TE must preserve viability while still promoting chondrogenic conversion and functional maturation.

In one recent study, we examined the potential of bovine MSCs to undergo chondrogenesis in 3D culture in three distinct hydrogels [181]. We employed agarose [182] as well as two hydrogels based on natural materials. The first, a commercially available self-assembling peptide gel (Puramatrix), possesses favorable properties for the culture of numerous cell types and supports chondrocyte-mediated ECM deposition [111, 183]. More recently, we and others have demonstrated that equine [184] and human [185] MSCs undergo chondrogenesis in this hydrogel as well. While not providing specific receptor mediated interactions (e.g., RGD signaling cascades are not activated), the gel does appear to promote cell adhesion and neurite extension [186] and may further be susceptible to proteolytic breakdown. The second biopolymer used was a photocrosslinked hyaluronan (HA)-based hydrogel. This gel supports ECM deposition by articular and auricular chondrocytes, both *in vitro* and *in vivo* [121, 122, 187]. Particularly relevant to chondrogenesis, HA expression is regulated during limb bud formation and mesenchymal cell condensation, and is a primary structural component of adult cartilage ECM [188, 189]. Chondrocytes interact with HA in the pericellular environment via CD44 receptors located on the cell surface [190, 191] and actively endocytose HA fragments [192]. Short term studies have shown that these HA gels induce greater levels of chondrogenesis in human MSCs compared to culture in PEG gels, even after controlling for viability and mechanics [193]. Results of this study showed robust cartilage formation in each of these hydrogels, with increasing mechanical properties observed with time in *in vitro* culture [181], Fig. **6**. These findings suggest great potential for MSCs in forming cartilage-like tissues *in vitro*. As with chondrocytes, continued optimization may result in even better tissue formation with variation in hydrogel material parameters; for example, polymer concentration [194] and degradation kinetics [195] appear to regulate matrix distribution in MSC-seeded HA hydrogels.

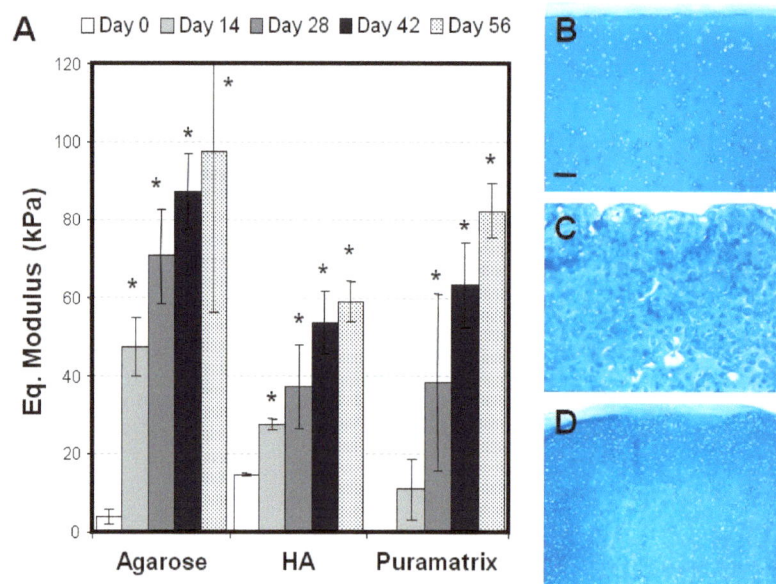

Figure 6: (A) Equilibrium compressive modulus of MSC-seeded agarose, photo-crosslinked hyaluronic acid (HA), and self-assembling Puramatrix hydrogels with *in vitro* culture in a chemically defined media containing 10 ng/mL TGF-β3. Data represent the mean and standard deviation of 3-4 samples per time point; * indicates p<0.05 versus Day 0. (B-D) Alcian blue staining demonstrates robust proteoglcyan deposition in agarose (B), HA (C) and Puramatrix (D) hydrogels on day 56. Scale Bar: 100 μm. Data adapted from [181] with permission from Mary Ann Liebert, Inc.

Cartilage Tissue Formation with MSCs: Mechanical and Molecular Evaluation

Despite the potential of MSCs to be directed toward a chondrogenic phenotype and to deposit functional matrix in 3D culture, recent studies are beginning to elucidate some limitations in MSC-based engineered cartilage, particularly relative to fully differentiated chondrocytes. Indeed most studies show MSC chondrogenesis at the molecular/histological level, but few have evaluated the resultant mechanical properties developed in these MSC-laden constructs or compared them directly to those achieved by chondrocytes. In one study using adipose derived adult stem (ADAS) cells, the mechanical properties of cell-laden agarose, alginate, and fibrous gelatin based foams were evaluated over a 4-week time course [168]. In that study, mechanical properties increased modestly with time, though primary chondrocyte controls were not examined. More recently, we acquired bovine chondrocytes and MSCs from the same donor or groups of healthy donors and evaluated their maturation with long-term culture in agarose in a pro-chondrogenic media formulation [182, 196], Fig. **7A**. Testing the equilibrium and dynamic mechanical properties of these constructs showed that while MSC-laden constructs increased in mechanical properties, they did so to a lesser extent than chondrocyte-laden constructs. In contrast, the collagen content and tensile properties of MSC-laden constructs are comparable to chondrocyte-laden constructs, though both of these properties remain well below native tissue levels [197]. A number of studies have examined the effects of varying cell seeding density on MSC chondrogenesis [198-203] and functional matrix evolution. Cell-cell contact and/or communication is a recognized factor in the initiation of chondrogenesis in pellet cultures [204], and does appear to increase molecular level conversion of MSCs to the chondrocyte phenotype. Similar to chondrocyte-laden hydrogels, increasing MSC seeding density increases matrix formation rates (on a per cell basis) at low seeding densities (1-5 million cells/mL) in collagen microspheres [202], though other work suggests a limit to these increases at higher (20-60 million cells/mL) seeding densities in agarose hydrogels [205, 206]. These findings suggest that limitations in functional properties are not due simply to too few cells, but rather underscore the differences between MSCs that have undergone chondrogenesis and fully differentiated chondrocytes. Furthermore, our recent microarray analysis of whole genome expression of these two cell types reveals a large number of genes that remain differentially regulated, even after chondrogenesis is fully developed [196], Fig. **7B**. These findings suggest that new methods must be considered to further the potential of MSCs for cartilage tissue engineering applications. Appreciation of these differences in phenotypic state, and development of enabling methods to overcome these gaps, will be essential in the functional formation of cartilage using MSCs.

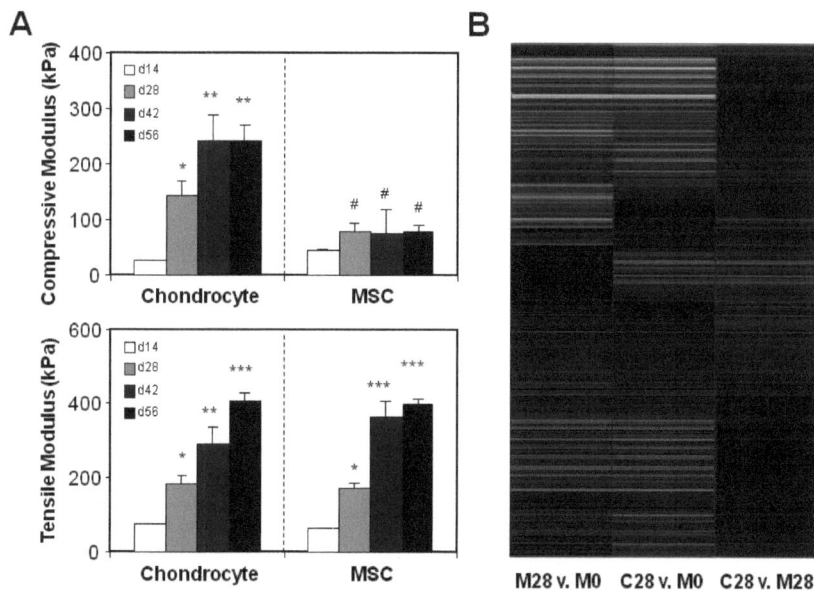

Figure 7: (A) Compressive (top) and tensile (bottom) modulus of chondrocyte- and MSC-seeded agarose gels cultured in a chemically defined media with TGF-β3 over 56 days (n=4-10 per assay). (B) Heat map generated from microarray data showing differential gene expression (green = greater, red = lower) between undifferentiated MSCs in agarose on day 0 (M0), chondrogenically differentiated MSCs in agarose on day 28 (M28) and chondrocytes in agarose on day 28 (C28). * indicates greater than lower, ** indicates greater than lower, *** indicates greater than lower, # indicates lower than same time-point versus chondrocyte group (p<0.05).

Optimization of Culture Conditions and Media Formulations for MSC Chondrogenesis

As noted above, inductive cues are critical for the initial lineage specification in MSC cultures. However, consideration must also be given to the totality of commitment to that lineage with a given set of factors, as well as the persistence of phenotype when inductive cues are altered (either *in vitro* or with *in vivo* implantation). Cells that have undergone lineage specification may not need the same set of persistent cues once a specific threshold has been achieved. These thresholds can involve duration of exposure, as well as the dose of the biofactors employed.

When considering MSC chondrogenesis, for example, induction on a molecular level can be achieved equivalently (in terms of common genes like type II collagen and aggrecan) by short exposure to a high dose of TGF-β (added for three days, followed by removal to a non-inductive media) versus a continual exposure to a lower dose of this morphogen [175]. In one study by Mehlhorn et al, human MSCs in alginate beads synthesized lower amounts of aggrecan after transient application of TGF-β3 compared to constructs cultured continuously with TGF-β3. However, the level of aggrecan accrued was still greater than that of control constructs and chondrogenic genes remained expressed, suggesting maintenance of the chondrocytic phenotype [207]. In our work, this was shown to be true on a biochemical and mechanical basis as well – comparable outcomes were found in mechanical properties, cartilage-specific matrix accumulation, and expression of cartilage markers when agarose-based 3D cultures were cultured transiently (3 weeks) or continuously with TGF-β over a 7 week time course [205]. Taken together, these studies indicate that a brief exposure to TGF-β may be sufficient to initiate and maintain a basal level of chondrogenesis in induced MSCs.

In addition to timing considerations, some thought should be given to the inductive media itself. Since the late 1990s, nearly every chondro-inductive media has employed the same set of molecules. Some parameterization has been attempted, most notably by Awad and colleagues in terms of ascorbate and dexamethasone [208] and by Estes and co-workers for combinations of TGF and BMP isoforms [209]. As our microarray data shows, however, there exists a wide gulf between full differentiation (chondrocytes) and chondrogenically induced MSCs. This should not be surprising, given the large number of biologic molecules shown to interact with initial joint formation stages as well as establishment of the 'permanent' chondrocyte phenotype. To begin to address this, we recently developed and validated a high throughput screening method to identify novel small molecule modulators of chondrogenic differentiation [210]. This method provides a facile means for screening new growth factors and their combinations, as well as to rapidly interrogate small molecule libraries for new elements that can influence this conversion process.

Mechanical Preconditioning of MSC-Based Cartilage Constructs

Enhancing biologic and small molecule induction certainly bears further examination, but other means of optimization of MSC chondrogenesis should be considered as well. As noted above, mechanical stimuli play a role in the original establishment of the joint cavity, as well as in the retention of the permanent chondrocyte phenotype as the rest of the cartilage rudiments undergo ossification. In chick limb-bud mesenchyme cells (a related but distinct cell type to MSCs) in agarose culture, compressive loading induced enhanced chondrogenesis in a manner modulated by both frequency and duration of loading [211, 212]. Based on these findings, as well as the success of functional tissue engineering approaches for chondrocyte-based tissue engineering applications, it should not be surprising that similar mechanical stimulation regimens have been attempted for MSC based constructs. Mesenchymal stem cells are sensitive to mechanical loading, with even simple loading modalities such as substrate stretch of monolayer cultures modulating cell division and osteogenic differentiation potential [213]. For chondrogenesis, hydrostatic pressurization, an indirect loading modality, has been applied to both MSC pellets and cell-seeded constructs. In these studies, cyclic hydrostatic pressure enhanced the expression of cartilaginous genes, including sox 9, collagen type II and aggrecan, as well as GAG deposition [214-216]. Indeed, repeated application of hydrostatic pressure was more beneficial for chondrogenesis compared to single applications of load [216]. These data implicate mechanical perturbation as a potentially positive modulator of MSC chondrogenesis.

To date, the effect of direct cyclic compression (and tension) on MSC chondrogenesis and the development of functional properties in engineered constructs remains unclear. In seminal work by Huang and co-workers, compressive loading of MSCs in agarose induced the expression of transcription factors known to mediate TGF-β signaling, including sox 9, AP-1 and c-Jun [217]. When MSCs were seeded in a porous hyaluronan-gelatin sponge, an initial period of repeated compressive loading was sufficient to induce the expression of chondrogenic genes relative to non-loaded controls [218]. In agarose, a single application of cyclic compression improved both collagen type II and aggrecan expression when MSC-seeded agarose gels were pre-cultured in TGF-β1 containing media for 16 days [219]. In another study, short-term loading of MSC-laden agarose cultures in the absence of TGF-β increased aggrecan promoter activity, Fig. **8** , but decreased collagen type II promoter activity [220]. Under cyclic tension (10% strain, 1Hz), the rate of GAG synthesis was enhanced in MSCs seeded on collagen-GAG scaffolds [221, 222], suggesting a positive role for cyclic tensile loading in chondrogenesis. However, when tensile stretch was applied to MSCs seeded on silicon membranes, strains of 7.5% or greater (applied at 0.17 Hz) was sufficient to induce apoptosis of seeded cells [223].

While these initial findings with dynamic loading appear promising, and certainly indicate the mechanosensitivity of MSCs in 3D culture, few studies have examined the effects of long-term loading on MSC chondrogenesis or on the development of functional properties. Several studies have demonstrated positive effects on gene expression with repeated loading, however, mechanical properties were not reported in those studies [220, 224-226]. Rather, one recent study showed that long-term mechanical compression actually impairs functional realization of MSC chondrogenesis. When loaded daily for 42 days in TGF-β containing media, the compressive modulus and GAG content of MSC-seeded agarose was considerably reduced compared to free-swelling controls [227]. From this study and similar studies from within our own group, it appears that MSC and chondrocyte response to mechanical stimulation are not identical. Moreover, these findings also suggest that a direct link between gene expression and accrual of mechanical properties does not always exist. Recent work by Terracciano and co-workers illustrated that while MSCs respond favorably to compressive loading, embryonic stem cells, in the same 3D environment and with the same mechanical loading regime, respond adversely until they have been stimulated toward the chondrogenic lineage [225]. This suggests that additional work will be necessary to determine the optimal parameters for the application of this loading modality to improve MSC-based cartilage constructs. Moreover, the molecular mechanisms underlying the different cell responses, and how these change with differentiation status, must be understood to improve these outcomes.

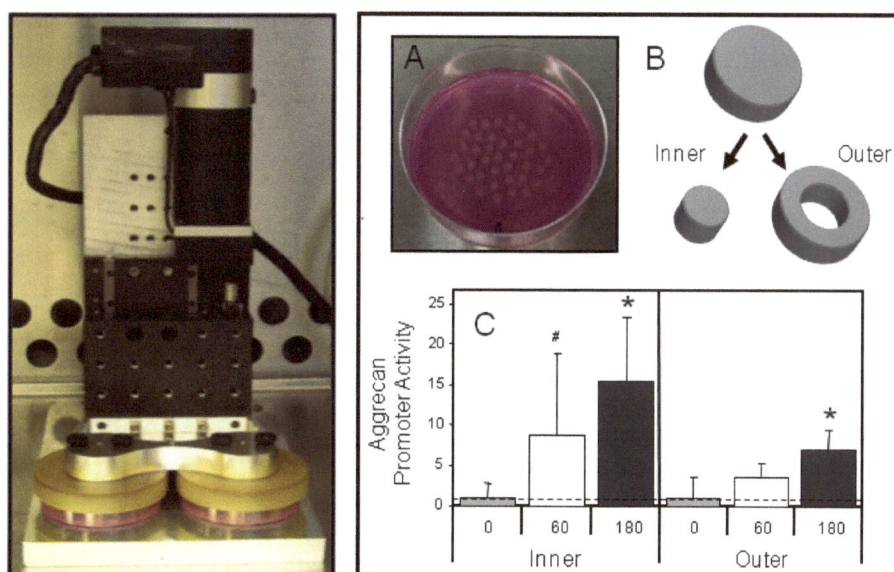

Figure 8: (A) Compression loading bioreactor for mechanical stimulation of cell-seeded hydrogel constructs. (B) MSC-seeded agarose disks in prepared mold for dynamic loading. (C) Schematic of agarose disk cored into inner and outer regions to determine region-specific gene expression responses with dynamic loading. (D) Aggrecan promoter activity in the inner and outer regions of MSC-seeded constructs after 0, 60 and 180 minutes of dynamic compressive loading. # indicates p<0.1 versus free-swelling, * indicates p<0.05 versus free swelling, n=7-8 per group. Data adapted from [220] with permission from Springer-Verlag.

Stem Cell Mechanical Properties

One opportunity for enhancing success with loading of stem cell based constructs may arise from a better understanding of stem cell mechanobiology and signaling. As physical stimuli do not appear to have the same potency on stem cells (with respect to production of tissue) as their native differentiated counterparts, it may be possible that stem cells perceive these stimuli differently. Transfer of physical forces to cells from the surrounding environment in 3D systems (e.g., cell-seeded scaffolds) may depend on the cell properties relative to the surrounding tissue matrix. To gain an appreciation of the temporal-spatial mechanical environment around cells during applied tissue loading, knowledge of cell and tissue properties as well as a proper theoretical constitutive framework are necessary [228].

Micropipette aspiration and atomic force microscopy (AFM) studies have been used to characterize stem cell viscoelastic properties [229, 230]. MSC and adipose-derived stem cells are similar in properties and different from chondrocytes [230]. It has been suggested that cell stiffness could be used as a biomarker for classification of cells capable of differentiating toward predictable lineages [231]. The ability of MSCs to survive extreme hypotonic shock without lysis, an observation that may reflect their mechanical properties, has been used in a strategy of osmotic selection to enrich the MSC population from umbilical cord blood [232]. Differences in osmotic loading behavior and calcium signaling between MSCs and chondrocytes have also been observed and may also be related to disparate cell physicochemical properties [233].

Chondrocytes and MSCs possess nuclei with viscoelastic properties [234]. The stem cell nucleus has been reported to be pliable and to stiffen significantly with terminal differentiation [235]. The latter may underlie reported differences between stem cell and differentiated cell mechanotransduction in 3D applied loading studies, as plasma membrane surface receptors bound to the surrounding tissue are mechanically coupled to the nucleus via the cytoskeleton, providing a mechanism for tissue deformation to be transmitted intracellularly [236]. Adding to this complexity, substrate (2D) stiffness that dictates cell stiffness has been found to control MSC fate [237] and may imply that cell-matrix interactions modulate cell mechanical properties. Further investigations into these cell level properties, as well as micromechanical analysis of the local matrix formed by MSCs, will be required to inform loading modalities towards enhancing MSC chondrogenesis and functional tissue formation.

In Vitro and In Vivo Stability of MSC-Based Cartilage Constructs

As a final point, while induction of phenotype is a challenge, and production of functional tissue has yet to be realized, we must also understand that MSCs are and remain multi-potential, and so retention of phenotype is a particular concern. For example, fate switching or 'transdifferentiation' has been reported in MSCs. In these studies, after the differentiated phenotype is achieved, cells sorted based on lineage-specific promoters can be de-differentiated and 'pushed' to alternative lineages [238]. Moreover, work by Pelltari and co-workers showed, for example, that MSCs that had been chondrogenically differentiated *in vitro* formed vascularized and mineralized nodules when implanted *in vivo* in a subcutaneous model [239]. While it was not clear in those studies whether all cells comprising the osteogenic nodules were from the original implant, it does suggest that chondrogenesis can be subsumed by osteogenesis in the *in vivo* environment. Similarly, Jukes and colleagues recently demonstrated that bone formation from embryonic stem cells required a cartilage intermediary state, and that bone formed on this cartilage template upon subcutaneous implantation [240]. *In vitro* assays of such phenomenon have yielded mixed results; our work in 3D MSC-seeded agarose gels suggests that simply removing TGF-β was not sufficient to alter phenotype, while other studies using chondrogenic pellets demonstrated that removal of TGF-β did induce hypertrophy and osteogenic conversion, but only when coupled with the reduction in dexamethasone concentration and the addition of thyroid hormone (T3) [241].

In addition to removal of differentiation cues, other conflict signals such as inflammatory cytokines are present in the inflamed joint environment that can adversely impact the engineered construct. For chondrocyte-based constructs, it is well appreciated that inflammatory cytokines can reduce engineered tissue properties [242]. For MSCs, these changes might operate through dedifferentiation or enhanced catabolism of matrix, with both factors likely playing a role. In one study using BMP-2 differentiated MSC pellets, IL-1 decreased the expression of sox9 (and its downstream targets collagen 2 and aggrecan) [171]. Most interestingly, that same study showed that addition of BMP-2 could partially offset the effect of IL-1, suggesting that persistent inductive cues may act to 'harden' a construct against loss of function in a conflict environment. We recently examined the effect of varying doses of IL-1β (an inflammatory cytokine) on both chondrocyte- and MSC-based engineered cartilage constructs [243]. MSC- and chondrocyte-based constructs were grown for 21 days in a chemically defined media containing TGF-β3. At this point, TGF was removed and the media further supplemented with IL-1β at graded levels for an additional 6 days. Mechanical, biochemical, and histological features of the constructs were evaluated as a function of time, revealing dramatic effects of the challenge (Fig. **9**). MSC-laden construct modulus decreased with IL-1β concentrations >2.5 ng/mL on day 6. These findings suggest that while MSC constructs produce neo-cartilage with increasing mechanical properties, they are sensitive (even more so than primary cell derived cartilage constructs) to conflicting signals that arise from an inflamed environment. While this study did not distinguish between molecular changes (de-differentiation events) or the more likely increased catabolism (matrix degradation) occurring over this short time period in the presence of conflicting signals, these issues must be addressed as MSCs move towards clinical implementation for cartilage repair *in vivo*.

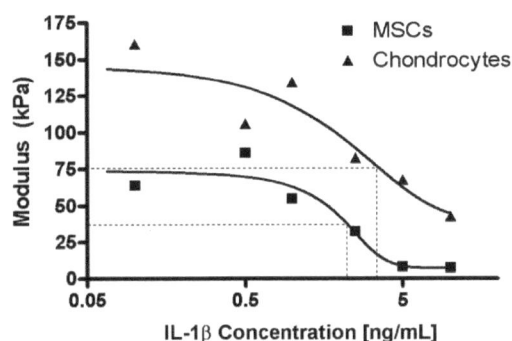

Figure 9: Engineered cartilage constructs are sensitive to inflammatory challenge. Data showing compressive modulus versus IL-1β concentration for chondrocyte- and MSC-laden constructs after 6 days of exposure. Analysis indicates that MSC-laden constructs are more sensitive to challenge than are chondrocyte laden-constructs; MSCs lose one-half of their properties at IL-1β concentrations of 2.2 ng/mL, while 4.1 ng/mL is required to elicit a similar reduction in chondrocyte based constructs. Data adapted from [243].

CONCLUSIONS AND FUTURE DIRECTIONS

The last decade has witnessed excellent progress on many fronts in the tissue engineering of chondrocyte- and MSC-based cartilage constructs for implantation. Recent reports of clinical implementation of human autologous cartilage formation by MSCs are especially promising, signaling as they do a new era in regenerative medicine using patient-derived stem cells. Restoration of cartilage in diarthrodial joints (including the hip and knee) will require engineered constructs that can sustain the intense mechanical demands encountered in those loading environments. While demanding, these environments are generally considered to be immune-privileged, and thus the use of both allogeneic and autogenic cells and tissues are possible without the need for immunosuppressive drugs. As such, it is a unique opportunity to use allogeneic cells such as chondrocytes and MSCs from other donors, allowing for the possibility of optimization and wide-spread distribution of these cell-based therapies. Despite this progress to date and inherent potential of this emerging technology, several key questions remain in the transition of MSC-based products for applications where load-bearing capacity is required (Fig. **10**).

As discussed above, it is now well established that MSCs can be induced to take on a chondrocyte-like phenotype, and that they, like chondrocytes, produce engineered tissues with increasing mechanical properties with time. However, the full assumption of the chondrocyte phenotype by MSCs has yet to be accomplished, and as a consequence, the mechanical properties of MSC-based cartilage still remains less than that of engineered cartilage formed from primary chondrocytes. A better understanding of how these cells are similar (differentiated chondrocytes and chondrogenically differentiated adult stem cells) or how they are dissimilar, both before and after differentiation are equally as important as understanding how to use these cells to generate new tissues. Of particular note, a better understanding of the most appropriate biologic and mechanical signals tuned to the differentiation status of the MSC will further these goals. Additional investigations into the differences between these two cell types (on a molecular, biochemical, and mechanical level), as well as the development of novel materials, soluble differentiation cues, and mechanical pre-conditioning regimens all hold promise in advancing this pursuit. Each of these research areas should be pursued both in isolation and in combination, and studies should span development through adult function and critically evaluate quantitative outcomes from both *in vitro* and *in vivo* systems, including large animal models of joint repair.

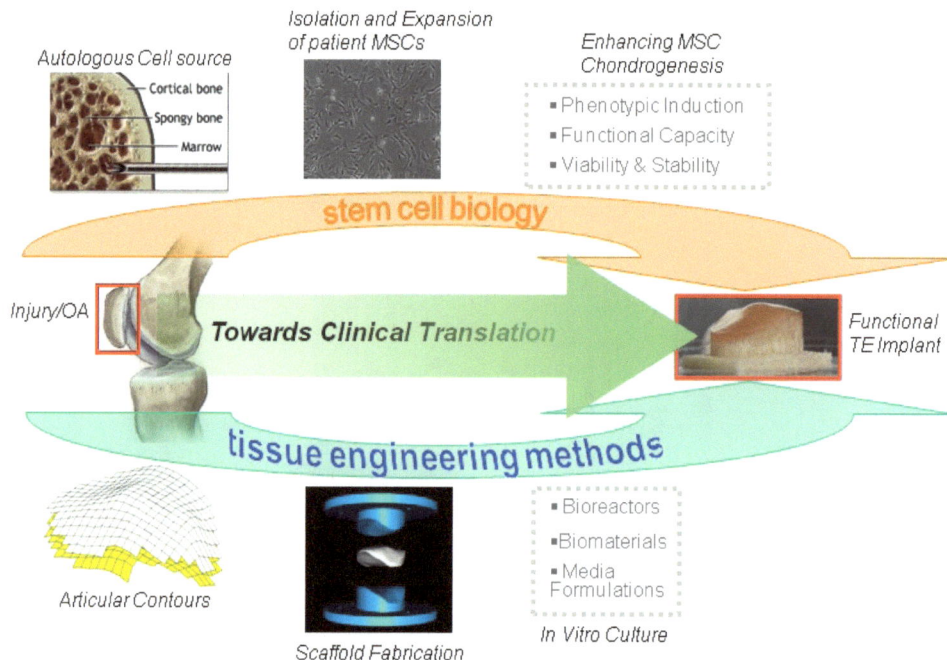

Figure 10: Schematic illustrating ideal multiple interacting paths towards the clinical implantation of a functional MSC-based engineered cartilage replacement.

Realization of the potential of MSC-based cartilage will require the combination of advanced stem cell biology and novel tissue engineering methodologies. These routes and technologies are highly interactive, with each discipline providing new insight and methods to the other. New research questions, some discussed above, some yet to be anticipated, will inform and direct the growth of this discipline. For example, scaffold technology could be harnessed to direct tissue specific lineage specification via topographic or biochemical cues that can enforce and sustain a robust differentiation status *in vivo*. These same materials may gradually modify a phenotypic status by controlled evolution of the biomaterial structure. Once implanted, MSCs may be modulated by the cells around them, as well as influence their neighboring MSCs through lineage modification, as has recently been demonstrated *in vitro* for combinations of differentiated cells and MSCs [244]. Advances in embryonic stem cells or embryonic-like stem cells (e.g., IPS cells), or MSCs derived from these sources may subsume the need for adult cells entirely [245]. Concerns of teratoma formation notwithstanding, these new cell populations hold incredible promise for engineering cartilage. Finally, these versatile cells and engineering methods may be combined to address whole joint arthroplasty, producing both functional cartilage layers and seamlessly integrated subchondral bone in patient-specific anatomic form, obviating the need for metal and plastic prosthetics [246]. This worthy goal, once achieved, will signal a new era in regenerative medicine and restore function and health to the millions worldwide who are afflicted with degenerative joint diseases.

ACKNOWLEDGEMENTS

This work was supported with funding from the National Institutes of Health (RO3 AR053668, RO1 AR52871), the University of Pennsylvania Institute on Aging, the National Science Foundation, and the Penn Center for Musculoskeletal Disorders.

REFERENCES

[1]   Macchiarini P, Jungebluth P, Go T, *et al.* Clinical transplantation of a tissue-engineered airway. Lancet 2008 Dec 13;372(9655):2023-2030.

[2]   Felson DT, Lawrence RC, Dieppe PA, *et al.* Osteoarthritis: new insights. Part 1: the disease and its risk factors. Ann Intern Med 2000 Oct 17;133(8):635-646.

[3]   Kurtz S, Ong K, Lau E, *et al.* Projections of primary and revision hip and knee arthroplasty in the United States from 2005 to 2030. J Bone Joint Surg Am 2007 Apr;89(4):780-785.

[4]   Friedenstein AJ. Precursor cells of mechanocytes. Int Rev Cytol 1976;47:327-359.

[5]   Bruder SP, Jaiswal N, Haynesworth SE. Growth kinetics, self-renewal, and the osteogenic potential of purified human mesenchymal stem cells during extensive sub-cultivation and following cryopreservation. J Cell Biochem 1997;64:278-294.

[6]   Clarke IC. Articular cartilage: a review and scanning electron microscope study. 1. The interterritorial fibrillar architecture. J Bone Joint Surg Br 1971 Nov;53(4):732-750.

[7]   Eyre DR. Collagen: molecular diversity in the body's protein scaffold. Science 1980 Mar 21;207(4437):1315-1322.

[8]   Muir H. The intracellular matrix in the environment of connective tissue cells. Clin Sci 1970 Feb;38(2):8P.

[9]   Lipshitz H, Etheredge R, 3rd, Glimcher MJ. Changes in the hexosamine content and swelling ratio of articular cartilage as functions of depth from the surface. J Bone Joint Surg Am 1976 Dec;58(8):1149-1153.

[10]   Maroudas A. Physicochemical properties of articular cartilage. In: Freeman MAR, Ed. Adult Articular Cartilage. 2nd ed. Kent: Pitman Medical 1979. p. 215-290.

[11]   Muir H. The chemistry of the ground substance of joint cartilage. In: Sokoloff L, Ed. The Joints and Synovial Fluid. New York: Academic Press 1980. p. 27-94.

[12]   Williamson AK, Chen AC, Sah RL. Compressive properties and function-composition relationships of developing bovine articular cartilage. J Orthop Res 2001 Nov;19(6):1113-1121.

[13]   Eyre DR. Collagens and cartilage matrix homeostasis. Clin Orthop and Relate Res 2004;427S:S118-S122.

[14]   Mankin HJ, Mow VC, Buckwalter JA, *et al.* Form and Function of Articular Cartilage. In: Simon SR, Ed. Orthopaedic Basic Science. Rosemont, IL: American Academy of Orthopaedic Surgeons 1994.

[15]   Eyre DR. Tye XI of 1alpha2alpha3alpha. In: Mayne R, Burgeson RE, Eds. Structure and Function of Collagen Types. New York: Academic Press 1987. p. 261-281.

[16]   Reginato AM, Olsen BR. The role of structural genes in the pathogenesis of osteoarthritic disorders. Arthritis Res 2002;4(6):337-345.

[17]   Hu K, Xu L, Cao L, *et al.* Pathogenesis of osteoarthritis-like changes in the joints of mice deficient in type IX collagen. Arthritis Rheum 2006 Sep;54(9):2891-2900.

[18]   Riesle J, Hollander AP, Langer R, *et al.* Collagen in tissue-engineered cartilage: types, structure, and crosslinks. J Cell Biochem 1998 Dec 1;71(3):313-327.

[19]   Stockwell RA. Biology of cartilage cells. Cambridge ; New York: Cambridge University Press 1979.

[20]   Malemud CJ, Goldberg VM. Future directions for research and treatment of osteoarthritis. Front Biosci 1999 Oct 15;4:D762-D771.

[21]   Stanton H, Rogerson FM, East CJ, *et al.* ADAMTS5 is the major aggrecanase in mouse cartilage in vivo and in vitro. Nature 2005 Mar 31;434(7033):648-652.

[22]   Karsenty G. An aggrecanase and osteoarthritis. N Engl J Med 2005 Aug 4;353(5):522-523.

[23]   Nagase H, Kashiwagi M. Aggrecanases and cartilage matrix degradation. Arthritis Res Ther 2003;5(2):94-103.

[24]   Weightman B. Tensile fatigue of human articular cartilage. J Biomech 1976;9:193-200.

[25]   Armstrong CG, Bahrani AS, Gardner DL. In vitro measurement of articular cartilage deformations in the intact human hip joint under load. J Bone Joint Surg Am 1979 Jul;61(5):744-755.

[26]   Paul JP. Forces transmitted by joints in the human body. Proc Instn Mech Engrs 1967;181 (3J):8.

[27]   Rydell N. Forces in the hip joint: Part (II) intravital measurements. In: Kenedi RM, Ed. Biomechanics and Related Bio-Engineering Topics. Oxford: Pergamon Press 1965. p. 351-357.

[28]   Dillman CJ. Kinematic analyses of running. Exerc Sport Sci Rev1975;3:193-218.

[29]   Ahmed AM, Burke DL, Yu A. In-vitro measurement of static pressure distribution in synovial joints--Part II: Retropatellar surface. J Biomech Eng 1983 Aug;105(3):226-236.

[30]   Brown TD, Shaw DT. In vitro contact stress distributions in the natural human hip. J Biomech 1983;16(6):373-384.

[31]   Brown TD, Shaw DT. In vitro contact stress distribution on the femoral condyles. J Orthop Res 1984;2(2):190-199.

[32]   Fukubayashi T, Kurosawa H. The contact area and pressure distribution pattern of the knee. A study of normal and osteoarthrotic knee joints. Acta Orthop Scand 1980 Dec;51(6):871-879.

[33] Huberti HH, Hayes WC. Patellofemoral contact pressures. The influence of q-angle and tendofemoral contact. J Bone Joint Surg Am 1984 Jun;66(5):715-724.

[34] Kurosawa H, Fukubayashi T, Nakajima H. Load-bearing mode of the knee joint: physical behavior of the knee joint with or without menisci. Clin Orthop 1980 Jun(149):283-290.

[35] Manouel M, Pearlman HS, Belakhlef A, *et al.* A miniature piezoelectric polymer transducer for in vitro measurement of the dynamic contact stress distribution. J Biomech 1992 Jun;25(6):627-635.

[36] Ateshian GA, Warden WH, Kim JJ, *et al.* Finite deformation biphasic material properties of bovine articular cartilage from confined compression experiments. J Biomech 1997 Nov-Dec;30(11-12):1157-1164.

[37] Athanasiou KA, Rosenwasser MP, Buckwalter JA, *et al.* Interspecies comparisons of in situ intrinsic mechanical properties of distal femoral cartilage. J Orthop Res 1991 May;9(3):330-340.

[38] Frank EH, Grodzinsky AJ. Cartilage electromechanics--I. Electrokinetic transduction and the effects of electrolyte pH and ionic strength. J Biomech 1987;20(6):615-627.

[39] Mow VC, Kuei SC, Lai WM, *et al.* Biphasic creep and stress relaxation of articular cartilage in compression? Theory and experiments. J Biomech Eng 1980 Feb;102(1):73-84.

[40] Chen SS, Falcovitz YH, Schneiderman R, *et al.* Depth-dependent compressive properties of normal aged human femoral head articular cartilage: relationship to fixed charge density. Osteoarthritis Cartilage 2001 Aug;9(6):561-569.

[41] Wang CC, Guo XE, Sun D, *et al.* The functional environment of chondrocytes within cartilage subjected to compressive loading: a theoretical and experimental approach. Biorheology 2002;39(1-2):11-25.

[42] Akizuki S, Mow VC, Muller F, *et al.* Tensile properties of human knee joint cartilage: I. Influence of ionic conditions, weight bearing, and fibrillation on the tensile modulus. J Orthop Res 1986;4(4):379-392.

[43] Grodzinsky AJ, Roth V, Myers E, *et al.* The significance of electromechanical and osmotic forces in the nonequilibrium swelling behavior of articular cartilage in tension. J Biomech Eng 1981 Nov;103(4):221-231.

[44] Roth V, Mow VC. The intrinsic tensile behavior of the matrix of bovine articular cartilage and its variation with age. J Bone Joint Surg Am 1980 Oct;62(7):1102-1117.

[45] Schmidt MB, Mow VC, Chun LE, *et al.* Effects of proteoglycan extraction on the tensile behavior of articular cartilage. J Orthop Res 1990 May;8(3):353-363.

[46] Woo SL, Akeson WH, Jemmott GF. Measurements of nonhomogeneous, directional mechanical properties of articular cartilage in tension. J Biomech 1976;9(12):785-791.

[47] Huang C-Y, Stankiewicz A, Ateshian GA, *et al.* Tensile and compressive stiffness of human glenohumeral cartilage under finite deformation. Proc Bioeng Conf, ASME BED 1999;42:469-470.

[48] Mow VC, Guo XE. Mechano-electrochemical properties of articular cartilage: their inhomogeneities and anisotropies. Annu Rev Biomed Eng 2002;4:175-209.

[49] Chahine NO, Wang CC, Hung CT, *et al.* Anisotropic strain-dependent material properties of bovine articular cartilage in the transitional range from tension to compression. J Biomech 2004 Aug;37(8):1251-1261.

[50] Broom ND. Further insights into the structural principles governing the function of articular cartilage. J Anat 1984 Sep;139 (Pt 2):275-294.

[51] Gomez S, Toffanin R, Bernstorff S, *et al.* Collagen fibrils are differently organized in weight-bearing and not-weight-bearing regions of pig articular cartilage. J Exp Zoo 2000;287:346-352.

[52] Below S, Arnoczky SP, Dodds J, *et al.* The split-line pattern of the distal femur: a consideration in the orientation of autologous cartilage grafts. J Arthros Rel Surg 2002;18(6):613-617.

[53] Lee RC, Frank EH, Grodzinsky AJ, *et al.* Oscillatory compressional behavior of articular cartilage and its associated electromechanical properties. J Biomech Eng 1981 Nov;103(4):280-292.

[54] Park SY, Hung CT, Ateshian GA. Mechanical response of bovine articular cartilage under dynamic unconfined compression loading at physiological stress levels. J Biomech 2003;12(1):391-400.

[55] Cohen B, Lai WM, Mow VC. A transversely isotropic biphasic model for unconfined compression of growth plate and chondroepiphysis. J Biomech Eng 1998 Aug;120(4):491-496.

[56] Soulhat J, Buschmann MD, Shirazi-Adl A. A fibril-network-reinforced biphasic model of cartilage in unconfined compression. J Biomech Eng 1999 Jun;121(3):340-347.

[57] Soltz MA, Ateshian GA. Interstitial fluid pressurization during confined compression cyclical loading of articular cartilage. Ann Biomed Eng 2000 Feb;28(2):150-159.

[58] Bursac P, McGrath CV, Eisenberg SR, *et al.* A microstructural model of elastostatic properties of articular cartilage in confined compression. J Biomech Eng 2000 Aug;122(4):347-353.

[59] Huang CY, Mow VC, Ateshian GA. The role of flow-independent viscoelasticity in the biphasic tensile and compressive responses of articular cartilage. J Biomech Eng 2001 Oct;123(5):410-417.

[60]   Li L, Shirazi-Adl A, Buschmann MD. Investigation of mechanical behavior of articular cartilage by fibril reinforced poroelastic models. Biorheology 2003;40(1,2,3):227-233.

[61]   Park S, Ateshian GA. Dynamic response of immature bovine articular cartilage in tension and compression, and nonlinear viscoelastic modeling of the tensile response. J Biomech Eng 2006 Aug;128(4):623-630.

[62]   Laasanen MS, Toyras J, Korhonen RK, *et al.* Biomechanical properties of knee articular cartilage. Biorheology 2003;40(1-3):133-140.

[63]   Toyras J, Rieppo J, Nieminen MT, *et al.* Characterization of enzymatically induced degradation of articular cartilage using high frequency ultrasound. Phys Med Biol 1999 Nov;44(11):2723-2733.

[64]   Park S, Nicoll SB, Mauck RL, *et al.* Cartilage mechanical response under dynamic compression at physiological stress levels following collagenase digestion. Ann Biomed Eng 2008 Mar;36(3):425-434.

[65]   Soltz MA, Ateshian GA. Experimental verification and theoretical prediction of cartilage interstitial fluid pressurization at an impermeable contact interface in confined compression. J Biomech 1998 Oct;31(10):927-934.

[66]   Wayne JS, Brodrick CW, Mukherjee N. Measurement of articular cartilage thickness in the articulated knee. Ann Biomed Eng 1998 Jan-Feb;26(1):96-102.

[67]   Macirowski T, Tepic S, Mann RW. Cartilage stresses in the human hip joint. J Biomech Eng 1994 Feb;116(1):10-18.

[68]   Eckstein F, Tieschky M, Faber SC, *et al.* Effect of physical exercise on cartilage volume and thickness in vivo: MR imaging study. Radiology 1998 Apr;207(1):243-248.

[69]   Mow VC, Hou JS, Owens JM, *et al.* Biphasic and quasilinear viscoelastic theories for hydrated soft tissues. In: Mow VC, Ratcliffe A, Woo SLY, Eds. Biomechanics of diarthrodial joints. New York: Springer-Verlag 1990. p. 215-260.

[70]   Soltz MA, Ateshian GA. A Conewise Linear Elasticity mixture model for the analysis of tension-compression nonlinearity in articular cartilage. J Biomech Eng 2000 Dec;122(6):576-586.

[71]   Gilbert SJ. Developmental Biology. 6th ed. New York: Sinauer Assoc.; 2000.

[72]   Zhou Z, Apte SS, Soininen R, *et al.* Impaired endochondral ossification and angiogenesis in mice deficient in membrane-type matrix metalloproteinase I. Proc Natl Acad Sci U S A 2000 Apr 11;97(8):4052-4057.

[73]   Jimenez MJ, Balbin M, Alvarez J, *et al.* A regulatory cascade involving retinoic acid, Cbfa1, and matrix metalloproteinases is coupled to the development of a process of perichondrial invasion and osteogenic differentiation during bone formation. J Cell Biol 2001 Dec 24;155(7):1333-1344.

[74]   Malemud CJ. Matrix metalloproteinases: role in skeletal development and growth plate disorders. Front Biosci 2006 May 1;11:1702-1715.

[75]   Iwamoto M, Tamamura Y, Koyama E, *et al.* Transcription factor ERG and joint and articular cartilage formation during mouse limb and spine skeletogenesis. Dev Biol 2007 May 1;305(1):40-51.

[76]   O'Keefe RJ, Loveys LS, Hicks DG, *et al.* Differential regulation of type-II and type-X collagen synthesis by parathyroid hormone-related protein in chick growth-plate chondrocytes. J Orthop Res 1997 Mar;15(2):162-174.

[77]   Koyama E, Shibukawa Y, Nagayama M, *et al.* A distinct cohort of progenitor cells participates in synovial joint and articular cartilage formation during mouse limb skeletogenesis. Dev Biol 2008 Apr 1;316(1):62-73.

[78]   Hyde G, Boot-Handford RP, Wallis GA. Col2a1 lineage tracing reveals that the meniscus of the knee joint has a complex cellular origin. J Anat 2008 Nov;213(5):531-538.

[79]   Mitrovic D. Development of the articular cavity in paralyzed chick embryos and in chick limb buds cultured on chorioallantoic membranes. Acta Anat 1982;112(4):313-324.

[80]   Persson M. The role of movement in the development of sutural and diarthrodial joints tested by long-term paralysis of chick embryos. J Anat 1983;213:391-399.

[81]   Mikic B, Isenstein AL, Chhabra AB. Mechanical modulation of cartilage structure and function during embryogenesis of the chick. Ann Biomed Eng 2004;32(1):18-25.

[82]   Mikic B, Johnson TL, Chhabra AB, *et al.* Differential effects of embryonic immobilization on the development of fibrocartilaginous skeletal elements. J Rehabil Res Dev 2000 Mar-Apr;37(2):127-133.

[83]   Pitsillides AA. Identifying and characterizing the joint cavity-forming cell. Cell Biochem Funct 2003;21:235-240.

[84]   Chen X, Macica CM, Nasiri A, *et al.* Regulation of articular chondrocyte proliferation and differentiation by indian hedgehog and parathyroid hormone-related protein in mice. Arthritis Rheum 2008 Dec;58(12):3788-3797.

[85]   Archer CW, Dowthwaite GP, Francis-West PH. Development of synovial joints. Birth Def Res (Part C) 2003;69:144-155.

[86]   Pacifici M, Koyama E, Iwamoto M. Mechanisms of synovial joint and articular cartilage formation: recent advances, but many lingering mysteries. Birth Def Res (Part C) 2005;75:237-248.

[87]   Athanasiou KA, Zhu CF, Wang X, *et al.* Effects of aging and dietary restriction on the structural integrity of rat articular cartilage. Ann Biomed Eng 2000 Feb;28(2):143-149.

[88]   Kempson GE. Age-related changes in the tensile properties of human articular cartilage: a comparative study between the femoral head of the hip joint and the talus of the ankle joint. Biochim Biophys Acta 1991 Oct 31;1075(3):223-230.

[89]   Kempson GE. Relationship between the tensile properties of articular cartilage from the human knee and age. Ann Rheum Dis 1982 Oct;41(5):508-511.

[90]   Gepstein A, Shapiro S, Arbel G, *et al.* Expression of matrix metalloproteinases in articular cartilage of temporomandibular and knee joints of mice during growth, maturation, and aging. Arthritis Rheum 2002;46(12):3240-3250.

[91]   Gepstein A, Arbel G, Blumenfeld I, *et al.* Association of metalloproteinases, tissue inhibitors of matrix metalloproteinases, and proteoglycans with development, aging, and osteoarthritis processes in mouse temporomandibular joint. Histochem Cell Biol 2003 Jul;120(1):23-32.

[92]   Williamson AK, Chen AC, Masuda K, *et al.* Tensile mechanical properties of bovine articular cartilage: variations with growth and relationships to collagen network components. J Orthop Res 2003;21(5):872-880.

[93]   Jadin KD, Wong BL, Bae WC, *et al.* Depth-varying density and organization of chondrocytes in immature and mature bovine articular cartilage assessed by 3d imaging and analysis. J Histochem Cytochem 2005 Sep;53(9):1109-1119.

[94]   Williamson AK, Masuda K, Thonar EJ, *et al.* Growth of immature articular cartilage in vitro: correlated variation of tensile biomechanical and collagen network properties. Tissue Eng 2003;9(4):625-634.

[95]   Schaefer D, Martin I, Jundt G, *et al.* Tissue-engineered composites for the repair of large osteochondral defects. Arthritis Rheum 2002 Sep;46(9):2524-2534.

[96]   Vunjak-Novakovic G, Martin I, Obradovic B, *et al.* Bioreactor cultivation conditions modulate the composition and mechanical properties of tissue-engineered cartilage. J Orthop Res 1999 Jan;17(1):130-138.

[97]   Davisson T, Kunig S, Chen A, *et al.* Static and dynamic compression modulate matrix metabolism in tissue engineered cartilage. J Orthop Res 2002 Jul;20(4):842-848.

[98]   Rotter N, Bonassar LJ, Tobias G, *et al.* Age dependence of biochemical and biomechanical properties of tissue-engineered human septal cartilage. Biomaterials 2002 Aug;23(15):3087-3094.

[99]   Puelacher WC, Kim SW, Vacanti JP, *et al.* Tissue-engineered growth of cartilage: the effect of varying the concentration of chondrocytes seeded onto synthetic polymer matrices. Int J Oral Maxillofac Surg 1994 Feb;23(1):49-53.

[100] Yates KE, Allemann F, Glowacki J. Phenotypic analysis of bovine chondrocytes cultured in 3D collagen sponges: effect of serum substitutes. Cell Tissue Bank 2005;6(1):45-54.

[101] Nehrer S, Breinan HA, Ramappa A, *et al.* Canine chondrocytes seeded in type I and type II collagen implants investigated in vitro. J Biomed Mater Res 1997 Summer;38(2):95-104.

[102] Hauselmann HJ, Fernandes RJ, Mok SS, *et al.* Phenotypic stability of bovine articular chondrocytes after long-term culture in alginate beads. J Cell Sci 1994 Jan;107 (Pt 1):17-27.

[103] Paige KT, Cima LG, Yaremchuk MJ, *et al.* Injectable cartilage. Plast Reconstr Surg 1995 Nov;96(6):1390-1400.

[104] Rowley JA, Madlambayan G, Mooney DJ. Alginate hydrogels as synthetic extracellular matrix materials. Biomaterials 1999 Jan;20(1):45-53.

[105] Mauck RL, Seyhan SL, Ateshian GA, *et al.* Influence of seeding density and dynamic deformational loading on the developing structure/function relationships of chondrocyte-seeded agarose hydrogels. Ann Biomed Eng 2002 Sep;30(8):1046-1056.

[106] Mauck RL, Wang CC, Oswald ES, *et al.* The role of cell seeding density and nutrient supply for articular cartilage tissue engineering with deformational loading. Osteoarthritis Cartilage 2003 Dec;11(12):879-890.

[107] Brittberg M, Sjogren-Jansson E, Lindahl A, *et al.* Influence of fibrin sealant (Tisseel) on osteochondral defect repair in the rabbit knee. Biomaterials 1997 Feb;18(3):235-242.

[108] Nixon AJ, Fortier LA, Williams J, *et al.* Enhanced repair of extensive articular defects by insulin-like growth factor-I-laden fibrin composites. J Orthop Res 1999 Jul;17(4):475-487.

[109] Hunter CJ, Imler SM, Malaviya P, *et al.* Mechanical compression alters gene expression and extracellular matrix synthesis by chondrocytes cultured in collagen I gels. Biomaterials 2002 Feb;23(4):1249-1259.

[110] Kawamura S, Wakitani S, Kimura T, *et al.* Articular cartilage repair. Rabbit experiments with a collagen gel-biomatrix and chondrocytes cultured in it. Acta Orthop Scand 1998 Feb;69(1):56-62.

[111] Kisiday J, Jin M, Kurz B, *et al.* Self-assembling peptide hydrogel fosters chondrocyte extracellular matrix production and cell division: implications for cartilage tissue repair. Proc Natl Acad Sci U S A 2002 Jul 23;99(15):9996-10001.

[112] Elisseeff JH, Lee A, Kleinman HK, *et al.* Biological response of chondrocytes to hydrogels. Ann N Y Acad Sci 2002 Jun;961:118-122.

[113] Bryant SJ, Anseth KS. The effects of scaffold thickness on tissue engineered cartilage in photocrosslinked poly(ethylene oxide) hydrogels. Biomaterials 2001 Mar;22(6):619-626.

[114] Burdick JA, Peterson AJ, Anseth KS. Conversion and temperature profiles during the photoinitiated polymerization of thick orthopaedic biomaterials. Biomaterials 2001 Jul;22(13):1779-1786.

[115] Benya PD, Shaffer JD. Dedifferentiated chondrocytes reexpress the differentiated collagen phenotype when cultured in agarose gels. Cell1 982 Aug;30(1):215-224.

[116] Buschmann MD, Gluzband YA, Grodzinsky AJ, *et al.* Chondrocytes in agarose culture synthesize a mechanically functional extracellular matrix. J Orthop Res 1992 Nov;10(6):745-758.

[117] Ragan PM, Staples AK, Hung HK, *et al.* Mechanical compression influences chondrocyte metabolism in a new alginate disk culture system. Trans Orthop Res Soc 1998;23:918.

[118] Moutos FT, Freed LE, Guilak F. A biomimetic three-dimensional woven composite scaffold for functional tissue engineering of cartilage. Nat Mater 2007 Feb;6(2):162-167.

[119] Elisseeff J, McIntosh W, Fu K, *et al.* Controlled-release of IGF-I and TGF-beta1 in a photopolymerizing hydrogel for cartilage tissue engineering. J Orthop Res 2001 Nov;19(6):1098-1104.

[120] Betre H, Setton LA, Meyer DE, *et al.* Characterization of a genetically engineered elastin-like polypeptide for cartilaginous tissue repair. Biomacromolecules 2002 Sep-Oct;3(5):910-916.

[121] Nettles DL, Vail TP, Morgan MT, *et al.* Photocrosslinkable hyaluronan as a scaffold for articular cartilage repair. Ann Biomed Eng 2004 Mar;32(3):391-397.

[122] Burdick JA, Chung C, Jia X, *et al.* Controlled degradation and mechanical behavior of photopolymerized hyaluronic acid networks. Biomacromolecules 2005 Jan-Feb;6(1):386-391.

[123] Chung C, Erickson IE, Mauck RL, *et al.* Differential Behavior of Auricular and Articular Chondrocytes in Hyaluronic Acid Hydrogels. Tissue Eng 2008 Jul;14(7):1121-1131.

[124] Bryant SJ, Anseth KS, Lee DA, *et al.* Crosslinking density influences the morphology of chondrocytes photoencapsulated in PEG hydrogels during the application of compressive strain. J Orthop Res 2004 Sep;22(5):1143-1149.

[125] Bryant SJ, Chowdhury TT, Lee DA, *et al.* Crosslinking density influences chondrocyte metabolism in dynamically loaded photocrosslinked poly(ethylene glycol) hydrogels. Ann Biomed Eng 2004 Mar;32(3):407-417.

[126] Bryant SJ, Nuttelman CR, Anseth KS. The effects of crosslinking density on cartilage formation in photocrosslinkable hydrogels. Biomed Sci Instrum 1999;35:309-314.

[127] Ng KW, Kugler LE, Doty SB, *et al.* Scaffold degradation elevates the collagen content and dynamic compressive modulus in engineered articular cartilage. Osteoarthritis Cartilage 2008 Sep 16.

[128] Bryant SJ, Anseth KS. Controlling the spatial distribution of ECM components in degradable PEG hydrogels for tissue engineering cartilage. J Biomed Mater Res A 2003 Jan 1;64(1):70-79.

[129] Lutolf MP, Hubbell JA. Synthetic biomaterials as instructive extracellular microenvironments for morphogenesis in tissue engineering. Nat Biotechnol 2005 Jan;23(1):47-55.

[130] Lutolf MP, Lauer-Fields JL, Schmoekel HG, *et al.* Synthetic matrix metalloproteinase-sensitive hydrogels for the conduction of tissue regeneration: engineering cell-invasion characteristics. Proc Natl Acad Sci U S A 2003 Apr 29;100(9):5413-5418.

[131] Park Y, Lutolf MP, Hubbell JA, *et al.* Bovine primary chondrocyte culture in synthetic matrix metalloproteinase-sensitive poly(ethylene glycol)-based hydrogels as a scaffold for cartilage repair. Tissue Eng 2004 Mar-Apr;10(3-4):515-522.

[132] Butler DL, Goldstein SA, Guilak F. Functional tissue engineering: the role of biomechanics. J Biomech Eng 2000 Dec;122(6):570-575.

[133] Guilak F, Sah RL, Setton LA. Physical regulation of cartilage metabolism. In: Mow VC, Hayes WC, Eds. Basic orthopaedic biomechanics. 2nd ed. Philadelphia: Lippincott-Raven 1997. p. 179-207.

[134] Smith RL, Rusk SF, Ellison BE, *et al.* In vitro stimulation of articular chondrocyte mRNA and extracellular matrix synthesis by hydrostatic pressure. J Orthop Res 1996 Jan;14(1):53-60.

[135] Gemmiti CV, Guldberg RE. Fluid flow increases type II collagen deposition and tensile mechanical properties in bioreactor-grown tissue-engineered cartilage. Tissue Eng 2006 Mar;12(3):469-479.

[136] Hung CT, Mauck RL, Wang CC, *et al.* A paradigm for functional tissue engineering of articular cartilage via applied physiologic deformational loading. Ann Biomed Eng 2004 Jan;32(1):35-49.

[137] Mauck RL, Soltz MA, Wang CC, *et al.* Functional tissue engineering of articular cartilage through dynamic loading of chondrocyte-seeded agarose gels. J Biomech Eng 2000 Jun;122(3):252-260.

[138] Buschmann MD, Gluzband YA, Grodzinsky AJ, *et al.* Mechanical compression modulates matrix biosynthesis in chondrocyte/agarose culture. J Cell Sci 1995 Apr;108 (Pt 4):1497-1508.

[139] Waldman SD, Spiteri CG, Grynpas MD, *et al.* Long-term intermittent shear deformation improves the quality of cartilaginous tissue formed in vitro. J Orthop Res 2003 Jul;21(4):590-596.

[140] Shieh AC, Athanasiou KA. Principles of cell mechanics for cartilage tissue engineering. Ann Biomed Eng 2003;31:1-11.

[141] Chang SC, Rowley JA, Tobias G, *et al.* Injection molding of chondrocyte/alginate constructs in the shape of facial implants. J Biomed Mater Res 2001 Jun 15;55(4):503-511.

[142] Vunjak-Novakovic G, Obradovic B, Martin I, *et al.* Dynamic cell seeding of polymer scaffolds for cartilage tissue engineering. Biotechnol Prog 1998 Mar-Apr;14(2):193-202.

[143] Blunk T, Sieminski AL, Gooch KJ, *et al.* Differential effects of growth factors on tissue-engineered cartilage. Tissue Eng 2002 Feb;8(1):73-84.

[144] Gooch KJ, Blunk T, Courter DL, *et al.* IGF-I and mechanical environment interact to modulate engineered cartilage development. Biochem Biophys Res Commun 2001 Sep 7;286(5):909-915.

[145] Gooch KJ, Blunk T, Courter DL, *et al.* Bone morphogenetic proteins-2, -12, and -13 modulate in vitro development of engineered cartilage. Tissue Eng 2002 Aug;8(4):591-601.

[146] Mauck RL, Nicoll SB, Seyhan SL, *et al.* Synergistic action of growth factors and dynamic loading for articular cartilage tissue engineering. Tissue Eng 2003 Aug;9(4):597-611.

[147] Pei M, Seidel J, Vunjak-Novakovic G, *et al.* Growth factors for sequential cellular de- and re-differentiation in tissue engineering. Biochem Biophys Res Commun 2002 May 31;294(1):149-154.

[148] Lima EG, Bian L, Ng KW, *et al.* The beneficial effect of delayed compressive loading on tissue-engineered cartilage constructs cultured with TGF-beta3. Osteoarthritis Cartilage 2007 Sep;15(9):1025-1033.

[149] Byers BA, Mauck RL, Chiang IE, *et al.* Transient exposure to transforming growth factor beta 3 under serum-free conditions enhances the biomechanical and biochemical maturation of tissue-engineered cartilage. Tissue Eng Part A 2008 Nov;14(11):1821-1834.

[150] Bos PK, Verhaar JA, van Osch GJ. Age-related differences in articular cartilage wound healing: a potential role for transforming growth factor beta1 in adult cartilage repair. Adv Exp Med Biol 2006;585:297-309.

[151] Plaas AH, Sandy JD, Kimura JH. Biosynthesis of cartilage proteoglycan and link protein by articular chondrocytes from immature and mature rabbits. J Biol Chem 1988 Jun 5;263(16):7560-7566.

[152] Bian L, Angione S, Lima EG, *et al.* Tissue-engineered cartilage constructs using mature bovine chondrocytes: effects of temporal exposure to growth factors and dynamic deformational loading. Trans Orthop Res Soc 2007;32:1480.

[153] Benya PD, Shaffer JD. Dedifferentiated chondrocytes reexpress the differentiated collagen phenotype when cultured in agarose gels. Cell 1982;30:215-224.

[154] Martin I, Vunjak-Novakovic G, Yang J, *et al.* Mammalian chondrocytes expanded in the presence of fibroblast growth factor 2 maintain the ability to differentiate and regenerate three-dimensional cartilaginous tissue. Exp Cell Res 1999 Dec 15;253(2):681-688.

[155] Ahmed N, Gan L, Nagy A, *et al.* Cartilage tissue formation using redifferentiated passaged chondrocytes in vitro. Tissue Eng Part A 2009 Mar;15(3):665-673.

[156] Francioli SE, Martin I, Sie CP, *et al.* Growth factors for clinical-scale expansion of human articular chondrocytes: relevance for automated bioreactor systems. Tissue Eng 2007 Jun;13(6):1227-1234.

[157] Ng KW, O'Conor CJ, Lima EG, *et al.* Primed mature chondrocytes can develop an engineered cartilage with physiologic properties. Trans Orthop Res Soc 2008;33:in press.

[158] Estes BT, Wu AW, Storms RW, *et al.* Extended passaging, but not aldehyde dehydrogenase activity, increases the chondrogenic potential of human adipose-derived adult stem cells. J Cell Physiol 2006;209(3):987-995.

[159] Pittenger MF, Mackay AM, Beck SC, *et al.* Multilineage potential of adult human mesenchymal stem cells. Science 1999 Apr 2;284(5411):143-147.

[160] Prockop DJ. Marrow stromal cells as stem cells for nonhematopoietic tissues. Science 1997 Apr 4;276(5309):71-74.

[161] Erickson GR, Gimble JM, Franklin DM, *et al.* Chondrogenic potential of adipose tissue-derived stromal cells in vitro and in vivo. Biochem Biophys Res Commun 2002 Jan 18;290(2):763-769.

[162] Choi YS, Noh SE, Lim SM, *et al.* Multipotency and growth characteristic of periosteum-derived progenitor cells for chondrogenic, osteogenic, and adipogenic differentiation. Biotechnol Lett 2008 Apr;30(4):593-601.

[163] Sakaguchi Y, Sekiya I, Yagishita K, *et al.* Comparison of human stem cells derived from various mesenchymal tissues: superiority of synovium as a cell source. Arthritis Rheum 2005 Aug;52(8):2521-2529.

[164] Noth U, Osyczka AM, Tuli R, *et al.* Multilineage mesenchymal differentiation potential of human trabecular bone-derived cells. J Orthop Res 2002 Sep;20(5):1060-1069.

[165] Caplan AI. Mesenchymal stem cells. J Orthop Res 1991 Sep;9(5):641-650.

[166] Barry FP, Murphy JM, English K, Mahon BP. Immunogenicity of adult mesenchymal stem cells: lessons from the fetal allograft. Stem Cells Dev 2005 Jun;14(3):252-265.

[167] Worster AA, Brower-Toland BD, Fortier LA, *et al*. Chondrocytic differentiation of mesenchymal stem cells sequentially exposed to transforming growth factor-beta1 in monolayer and insulin-like growth factor-I in a three-dimensional matrix. J Orthop Res 2001;19(4):738-749.

[168] Awad HA, Wickham MQ, Leddy HA, *et al*. Chondrogenic differentiation of adipose-derived adult stem cells in agarose, alginate, and gelatin scaffolds. Biomaterials 2004 Jul;25(16):3211-3222.

[169] Mauck RL, Tuan RS. Chondrogenic differentiation and development of functional mechanical properties in MSC-laden agarose hydrogels. NIAMS Annual Retreat 2004;in press.

[170] Angele P, Schumann D, Nerlich M, *et al*. Enhanced chondrogenesis of mesenchymal progenitor cells loaded in tissue engineering scaffolds by cyclic, mechanical compression. Trans Orthop Res Soc 2004;29:835.

[171] Majumdar MK, Wang E, Morris EA. BMP-2 and BMP-9 promotes chondrogenic differentiation of human multipotential mesenchymal cells and overcomes the inhibitory effect of IL-1. J Cell Physiol 2001 Dec;189(3):275-284.

[172] Majumdar MK, Banks V, Peluso DP, *et al*. Isolation, characterization, and chondrogenic potential of human bone marrow-derived multipotential stromal cells. J Cell Physiol 2000 Oct;185(1):98-106.

[173] Ma H-L, Hung S-C, Lin S-Y, *et al*. Chondrogenesis of human mesenchymal stem cells encapsulated in alginate beads. J Biomed Mat Res 2003;64A:273-281.

[174] Martin I, Padera RF, Vunjak-Novakovic G, *et al*. *In vitro* differentiation of chick embryo bone marrow stromal cells into cartilaginous and bone-like tissues. J Orthop Res 1998 Mar;16(2):181-189.

[175] Caterson EJ, Nesti LJ, Li WJ, *et al*. Three-dimensional cartilage formation by bone marrow-derived cells seeded in polylactide/alginate amalgam. J Biomed Mater Res 2001 Dec 5;57(3):394-403.

[176] Caterson EJ, Li WJ, Nesti LJ, *et al*. Polymer/alginate amalgam for cartilage-tissue engineering. Ann N Y Acad Sci 2002 Jun;961:134-138.

[177] Nuttelman CR, Tripodi MC, Anseth KS. Synthetic hydrogel niches that promote hMSC viability. Matrix Biol 2005 May;24(3):208-218.

[178] Salinas CN, Cole BB, Kasko AM, *et al*. Chondrogenic differentiation potential of human mesenchymal stem cells photoencapsulated within poly(ethylene glycol)-arginine-glycine-aspartic acid-serine thiol-methacrylate mixed-mode networks. Tissue Eng 2007 May;13(5):1025-1034.

[179] Connelly JT, Garcia AJ, Levenston ME. Inhibition of in vitro chondrogenesis in RGD-modified three-dimensional alginate gels. Biomaterials 2007 Feb;28(6):1071-1083.

[180] Lee HJ, Yu C, Chansakul T, *et al*. Enhanced chondrogenesis of mesenchymal stem cells in collagen mimetic peptide-mediated microenvironment. Tissue Eng Part A 2008 Nov;14(11):1843-1851.

[181] Erickson IE, Huang AH, Chung C, *et al*. Differential Maturation and Structure-Function Relationships in MSC- and Chondrocyte-Seeded Hydrogels. Tissue Eng Part A 2009 Jan 2.

[182] Mauck RL, Yuan X, Tuan RS. Chondrogenic differentiation and functional maturation of bovine mesenchymal stem cells in long-term agarose culture. Osteoarthritis Cartil 2006 Feb;14(2):179-189.

[183] Kisiday JD, Kurz B, DiMicco MA, *et al*. Evaluation of medium supplemented with insulin-transferrin-selenium for culture of primary bovine calf chondrocytes in three-dimensional hydrogel scaffolds. Tissue Eng 2005 Jan-Feb;11(1-2):141-151.

[184] Kisiday JD, Kopesky PW, Evans CH, *et al*. Evaluation of adult equine bone marrow- and adipose-derived progenitor cell chondrogenesis in hydrogel cultures. J Orthop Res 2007 Oct 24.

[185] Mauck RL, Helm JM, Tuan RS. Chondrogenesis of human MSCs in a 3D self-assembling peptide hydrogel: functional properties and divergent expression profiles compared to pellet cultures. Trans ORS 2006;31:775.

[186] Holmes TC, de Lacalle S, Su X, *et al*. Extensive neurite outgrowth and active synapse formation on self-assembling peptide scaffolds. Proc Natl Acad Sci U S A 2000;97(12):6728-6733.

[187] Chung C, Mesa J, Miller GJ, *et al*. Effects of auricular chondrocyte expansion on neocartilage formation in photocrosslinked hyaluronic acid networks. Tissue Eng 2006 Sep;12(9):2665-2673.

[188] Li Y, Toole BP, Dealy CN, *et al*. Hyaluronan in limb morphogenesis. Dev Biol 2007 May 15;305(2):411-420.

[189] Toole BP. Hyaluronan: from extracellular glue to pericellular cue. Nat Rev Cancer 2004 Jul;4(7):528-539.

[190] Knudson CB, Knudson W. Hyaluronan and CD44: modulators of chondrocyte metabolism. Clin Orthop Relat Res 2004 Oct(427 Suppl):S152-62.

[191] Knudson CB. Hyaluronan receptor-directed assembly of chondrocyte pericellular matrix. J Cell Biol 1993 Feb;120(3):825-834.

[192] Morales TI, Hascall VC. Correlated metabolism of proteoglycans and hyaluronic acid in bovine cartilage organ cultures. J Biol Chem 1988 Mar 15;263(8):3632-3638.

[193] Chung C, Burdick JA. Enhanced chondrogenic differentiation of mesenchymal stem cells in hyaluronan hydrogels. Tissue Eng 2008;in press.

[194] Erickson IE, Chung C, Huang AH, *et al.* Hydrogel effects on long-term maturation of chondrocyte- and MSC-laden hydrogels. Trans of the 54th Annual Meeting of the Orthopaedic Research Society 2008.

[195] Sahoo S, Chung C, Khetan S, *et al.* Hydrolytically degradable hyaluronic acid hydrogels with controlled temporal structures. Biomacromolecules 2008 Apr;9(4):1088-1092.

[196] Huang AH, Yeger-McKeever M, Stein A, *et al.* Identification of molecular antecedents limiting functional maturation of MSC-laden hydrogels. Trans of the 54th Annual Meeting of the Orthopaedic Research Society 2008 (in press).

[197] Huang AH, Yeger-McKeever M, Stein A, *et al.* Tensile properties of engineered cartilage formed from chondrocyte- and MSC-laden hydrogels. Osteoarthritis Cartilage 2008 Sep;16(9):1074-1082.

[198] Ponticiello MS, Schinagl RM, Kadiyala S, *et al.* Gelatin-based resorbable sponge as a carrier matrix for human mesenchymal stem cells in cartilage regeneration therapy. J Biomed Mater Res 2000 Nov;52(2):246-255.

[199] Huang AH, Yeger-McKeever M, Stein A, *et al.* Tensile properties of engineered cartilage formed from chondrocyte- and MSC-laden hydrogels. Osteoarthritis Cartil 2008 Sep;16(9):1074-1082.

[200] Huang CY, Reuben PM, D'Ippolito G, *et al.* Chondrogenesis of human bone marrow-derived mesenchymal stem cells in agarose culture. Anat Rec A Discov Mol Cell Evol Biol 2004 May;278(1):428-436.

[201] Park H, Temenoff JS, Tabata Y, *et al.* Injectable biodegradable hydrogel composites for rabbit marrow mesenchymal stem cell and growth factor delivery for cartilage tissue engineering. Biomaterials 2007 Jul;28(21):3217-3227.

[202] Hui TY, Cheung KM, Cheung WL, *et al.* In vitro chondrogenic differentiation of human mesenchymal stem cells in collagen microspheres: influence of cell seeding density and collagen concentration. Biomaterials 2008 Aug;29(22):3201-3212.

[203] Kavalkovich KW, Boynton RE, Murphy JM, *et al.* Chondrogenic differentiation of human mesenchymal stem cells within an alginate layer culture system. In Vitro Cell Dev Biol Anim 2002 Sep;38(8):457-466.

[204] Tuli R, Tuli S, Nandi S, *et al.* Transforming growth factor-beta-mediated chondrogenesis of human mesenchymal progenitor cells involves N-cadherin and mitogen-activated protein kinase and Wnt signaling cross-talk. J Biol Chem 2003 Oct 17;278(42):41227-41236.

[205] Huang AH, Stein A, Yeger-McKeever M, *et al.* Transient exposure to TGF-beta3 improves mechanical properties of MSC-laden constructs. Proc BIO2008 Summer Bioengineering Conference 2008.

[206] Mauck RL, Byers BA, Yuan X, *et al.* Cartilage tissue engineering with MSC-laden hydrogels: effect of seeding density, exposure to chondrogenic medium, and dynamic loading. Proceedings of the 52nd Annual Orthopaedic Research Society Meeting, Chicago, IL 2006.

[207] Mehlhorn AT, Schmal H, Kaiser S, *et al.* Mesenchymal stem cells maintain TGF-beta-mediated chondrogenic phenotype in alginate bead culture. Tissue Eng 2006 Jun;12(6):1393-1403.

[208] Awad H, Halvorsen Y-DC, Gimble JM, *et al.* Effects of transforming growth factor beta1 and dexamethasone on the growth and chondrogenic differentiation of adipose-derived stromal cells. Tissue Eng 2003;9(6):1301-1312.

[209] Estes BT, Wu AW, Guilak F. Potent induction of chondrocytic differentiation of human adipose-derived adult stem cells by bone morphogenetic protein 6. Arthritis Rheum 2006 Apr;54(4):1222-1232.

[210] Huang AH, Motlekar NA, Stein A, *et al.* High-throughput screening for modulators of mesenchymal stem cell chondrogenesis. Ann Biomed Eng 2008 Nov;36(11):1909-1921.

[211] Elder SH, Goldstein SA, Kimura JH, *et al.* Chondrocyte differentiation is modulated by frequency and duration of cyclic compressive loading. Ann Biomed Eng 2001 Jun;29(6):476-482.

[212] Elder SH, Kimura JH, Soslowsky LJ, *et al.* Effect of compressive loading on chondrocyte differentiation in agarose cultures of chick limb-bud cells. J Orthop Res 000 Jan;18(1):78-86.

[213] Simmons CA, Matlis S, Thornton DJ, *et al.* Cyclic strain enhances matrix mineralization by adult human mesenchymal stem cells via the extracellular signal-regulated kinase (ERK1/2) signaling pathway. J Biomech 2003;36(8):1087-1096.

[214] Miyanishi K, Trindade MC, Lindsey DP, *et al.* Effects of hydrostatic pressure and transforming growth factor-beta 3 on adult human mesenchymal stem cell chondrogenesis in vitro. Tissue Eng 2006 Jun;12(6):1419-1428.

[215] Wagner DR, Lindsey DP, Li KW, *et al.* Hydrostatic pressure enhances chondrogenic differentiation of human bone marrow stromal cells in osteochondrogenic medium. Ann Biomed Eng 2008 May;36(5):813-820.

[216] Angele P, Yoo JU, Smith C, *et al.* Cyclic hydrostatic pressure enhances the chondrogenic phenotype of human mesenchymal progenitor cells differentiated in vitro. J Orthop Res 2003 May;21(3):451-457.

[217] Huang CY, Reuben PM, Cheung HS. Temporal expression patterns and corresponding protein inductions of early responsive genes in rabbit bone marrow-derived mesenchymal stem cells under cyclic compressive loading. Stem Cells 2005 Sep;23(8):1113-1121.

[218] Angele P, Schumann D, Angele M, *et al.* Cyclic, mechanical compression enhances chondrogenesis of mesenchymal progenitor cells in tissue engineering scaffolds. Biorheology 2004;41(3-4):335-346.

[219] Mouw JK, Connelly JT, Wilson CG, *et al*. Dynamic compression regulates the expression and synthesis of chondrocyte-specific matrix molecules in bone marrow stromal cells. Stem Cells 2007 Mar;25(3):655-663.

[220] Mauck RL, Byers BA, Yuan X, *et al*. Regulation of cartilaginous ECM gene transcription by chondrocytes and MSCs in 3D culture in response to dynamic loading. Biomech Model Mechanobiol 2007 Jan;6(1-2):113-125.

[221] McMahon LA, Campbell VA, Prendergast PJ. Involvement of stretch-activated ion channels in strain-regulated glycosaminoglycan synthesis in mesenchymal stem cell-seeded 3D scaffolds. J Biomech 2008;41(9):2055-2059.

[222] McMahon LA, Reid AJ, Campbell VA, *et al*. Regulatory effects of mechanical strain on the chondrogenic differentiation of MSCs in a collagen-GAG scaffold: experimental and computational analysis. Ann Biomed Eng 2008 Feb;36(2):185-194.

[223] Kearney EM, Prendergast PJ, Campbell VA. Mechanisms of strain-mediated mesenchymal stem cell apoptosis. J Biomech Eng 2008 Dec;130(6):061004.

[224] Huang CY, Hagar KL, Frost LE, *et al*. Effects of cyclic compressive loading on chondrogenesis of rabbit bone-marrow derived mesenchymal stem cells. Stem Cells 2004;22(3):313-323.

[225] Terraciano V, Hwang N, Moroni L, *et al*. Differential response of adult and embryonic mesenchymal progenitor cells to mechanical compression in hydrogels. Stem Cells 2007 Aug 16.

[226] Campbell JJ, Lee DA, Bader DL. Dynamic compressive strain influences chondrogenic gene expression in human mesenchymal stem cells. Biorheology 2006;43(3-4):455-470.

[227] Thorpe SD, Buckley CT, Vinardell T, *et al*. Dynamic compression can inhibit chondrogenesis of mesenchymal stem cells. Biochem Biophys Res Commun 2008 Dec 12;377(2):458-462.

[228] Wang CC-B, Guo XE, Sun D, *et al*. The functional environment of chondrocytes within cartilage subjected to compressive loading: theoretical and experimental approach. Biorheology 2002;39(1-2):39-45.

[229] Tan SC, Pan WX, Ma G, Cai N, *et al*. Viscoelastic behaviour of human mesenchymal stem cells. BMC Cell Biol 2008;9:40.

[230] Darling EM, Topel M, Zauscher S, *et al*. Viscoelastic properties of human mesenchymally-derived stem cells and primary osteoblasts, chondrocytes, and adpocytes. J Biomech 2008;41(2):454-464.

[231] Darling EM, Guilak F. A neural network model for cell classification based on single-cell biomechanical properties. Tissue Eng Part A 2008 Sep;14(9):1507-1515.

[232] Parekkadan B, Sethu P, van Poll D, *et al*. Osmotic selection of human mesenchymal stem/progenitor cells from umbilical cord blood. Tissue Eng 2007 Oct;13(10):2465-2473.

[233] Oswald ES, Chao PH, Hung CT. Trans ASME Summer Bioeng Conf (Vail Colorado) 2005 June 22-26.

[234] Guilak F, Tedrow JR, Burgkart R. Viscoelastic properties of the cell nucleus. Biochem Biophys Res Commun 2000;269(3):781-786.

[235] Pajerowski JD, Dahl KN, Zhong FL, *et al*. Physical plasticity of the nucleus in stem cell differentiation. Proc Natl Acad Sci U S A 2007 Oct 2;104(40):15619-15624.

[236] Maniotis AJ, Chen CS, Ingber DE. Demonstration of mechanical connections between integrins, cytoskeletal filaments, and nucleoplasm that stabilize nuclear structure. Proc Natl Acad Sci U S A 1997 Feb 4;94(3):849-854.

[237] Engler AJ, Sen S, Sweeney HL, *et al*. Matrix elasticity directs stem cell lineage specification. Cell 2006 Aug 25;126(4):677-689.

[238] Song L, Tuan RS. Transdifferentiation potential of human mesenchymal stem cells derived from bone marrow. Faseb J 2004 Jun;18(9):980-982.

[239] Pelttari K, Winter A, Steck E, *et al*. Premature induction of hypertrophy during in vitro chondrogenesis of human mesenchymal stem cells correlates with calcification and vascular invasion after ectopic transplantation in SCID mice. Arthritis Rheum 2006 Oct;54(10):3254-3266.

[240] Jukes JM, Both SK, Leusink A, *et al*. Endochondral bone tissue engineering using embryonic stem cells. Proc Natl Acad Sci U S A 2008 May 13;105(19):6840-6845.

[241] Mueller MB, Tuan RS. Functional characterization of hypertrophy in chondrogenesis of human mesenchymal stem cells. Arthritis Rheum 2008 May;58(5):1377-1388.

[242] Lima EG, Tan AR, Tai T, *et al*. Differences in interleukin-1 response between engineered and native cartilage. Tissue Eng Part A 2008 Oct;14(10):1721-1730.

[243] Yeger-McKeever M, Huang AH, Stein A, *et al*. Engineeered MSC-Laden Cartilage Constructs are Sensitive to Inflammatory Cytokine-Mediated Degradation. Proc BIO 2008 Summer Bioengineering Conference 2007:176186.

[244] Hwang NS, Varghese S, Puleo C, *et al*. Morphogenetic signals from chondrocytes promote chondrogenic and osteogenic differentiation of mesenchymal stem cells. J Cell Physiol 2007 Aug;212(2):281-284.

[245] Hwang NS, Varghese S, Lee HJ, *et al*. In vivo commitment and functional tissue regeneration using human embryonic stem cell-derived mesenchymal cells. Proc Natl Acad Sci U S A 2008 Dec 30;105(52):20641-20646.

[246] Hung CT, Lima EG, Mauck RL, *et al.* Anatomically shaped osteochondral constructs for articular cartilage repair. J Biomech 2003 Dec;36(12):1853-1864.

[247] Bian L, Angione SL, Lima EG, *et al.* Tissue-engineered cartilage constructs using mature bovine chondrocytes: effects of temporal exposure to growth factors and dynamic deformational loading. Trans Orthop Res Soc 2007;32:1480.

[248] Ng KW, O'Conor CJ, Lima EG, *et al.* Primed mature chondrocytes can develop an engineered cartilage with physiologic properties. Trans Orthop Res Soc 2008;33.

CHAPTER 6

Therapeutic Angiogenesis for Coronary Artery Disease: Clinical Trials of Proteins, Plasmids, Adenovirus and Stem Cells

Keith A. Webster*

Department of Molecular and Cellular Pharmacology and The Vascular Biology Institute, University of Miami School of Medicine, Miami, FL 33136, USA

Abstract: Therapeutic angiogenesis represents a molecular and cellular approach to the treatment of CAD that may be an alternative or additive to traditional pharmacology and interventional cardiology. The goal of angiogenic therapy is to activate endogenous angiogenic and arteriogenic pathways and stimulate revascularization of ischemic myocardial tissue. The feasibility of such a strategy has now been established through the results of studies over the past two decades, and clinical trials involving more than 1000 patients have been implemented. In this review we will discuss the results from these trials, tracing the progression of the technology from the delivery of recombinant proteins through gene and stem cell therapies. Critical evaluations reveal that neither proteins nor genes delivered by transient expression vectors provide an optimal therapy. Similarly, stem cell therapy is not achieving the level of improvement that was expected or predicted from preclinical results. The future of therapeutic angiogenesis lies in the use of permanent gene delivery vehicles expressing regulated genes and/or stem cells appropriately engineered with regulated genes.

INTRODUCTION

Incidence

Coronary artery disease continues to be the leading cause of morbidity and mortality in North America and Europe. This is despite significant advances in interventional cardiology and pharmacological treatments. Currently more than 12 million people in the United States have coronary artery disease (CAD), and more than 7 million have had a myocardial infarction. Chronic stable angina is the initial manifestation of CAD in approximately half of all presenting patients, and it is estimated that 16.5 million Americans currently have stable angina. [1] Surgical interventions are increasing, there were 1.3 million inpatient cardiac catheterizations, and >1 million percutaneous transluminal coronary angioplasty (PTCA) and coronary artery bypass (CABG) procedures performed in 2000 in the United States. The economic cost of CAD in the United States is estimated to be greater than $120 billion per year.

Pharmacology

Four main pharmacological approaches are currently in use for treating ischemic heart disease [2], these include:

1) Angiotensin-converting enzyme (ACE) inhibitors that reduce peripheral vascular resistance.

2) Partial β-adrenergic agonists that can quench potentially lethal adrenergic surges while preserving β-adrenergic responses.

3) Calcium channel blockers that lower blood pressure, protect against adrenergic surges, and mediate vasodilation.

4) Lipid-lowering drugs, anti-platelet therapy (aspirin), and glucose-insulin-potassium infusion that prevent the progression of CAD, reduce thrombus formation, and positively modulate metabolism and blood flow during ischemia respectively. Newer procedures including anti-apoptosis reagents, antioxidants, preconditioning agents, and growth factors (IGF-1) have demonstrated strong cardioprotective actions in numerous preclinical studies and may be important next generation anti-ischemia therapies [3-6].

*Address correspondence to this author Keith A. Webster: Dept. of Molecular and Cellular Pharmacology and Vascular Biology Institute, University of Miami School of Medicine, 1600 NW 10th Ave, RMSB 6038, Miami, FL 33136, USA; Tel: 305.243.6779; Fax: 305.243.6082; Email: kwebster@med.miami.edu

Interventional Cardiology

Invasive procedures to treat severe CAD and angina including angioplasty with stent implantation, and CABG have been increasingly used for the past two decades [7]. These procedures are usually employed only when occluded arteries do not respond to thrombolytic therapy or when the ischemia is unstable and unresponsive to pharmacology. In CABG, sections of the patients' saphenous vein or internal thoracic artery are grafted around the occluded artery to bypass the occlusion and re-establish blood flow to the ischemic tissue. For single or double coronary arteries CABG has an operative success rate of more than 95% and the patency of thoracic artery grafts exceeds 90% at 10 years. Clearly other coronary arteries of patients receiving bypass grafts remain at risk, but morbidity and mortality are significantly improved following these procedures. PTCA has a similar 95% operative success rate, significantly improves morbidity and mortality, but suffers from a high rate of restenosis. This latter problem may be significantly alleviated through the catheter-mediated implanting of stents at the occlusion site [8]. Stent implantation reduces elastic recoil, plaque dissection, and the rate of restenosis. Conventional stents also suffer up to 20% restenosis and require repeat procedures but this is dramatically reduced by using drug-eluting stents [9]. Polymeric stents eluting sirolimus (rapamycin) or paclitaxel have been proven to reduce or eliminate intimal hyperplasia and in-stent restenosis in multiple clinical trials and are rapidly replacing conventional stents.

In combination with anticoagulant therapy and conventional drugs, invasive procedures are effective in reperfusing ischemic tissue and salvaging myocardium. They have contributed significantly to the vast improvement in the life expectancy of patients with heart disease that has occurred over the past two decades. On the negative side, these procedures are expensive and carry a risk of reperfusion damage [10-12]. In addition, a significant number of patients with ischemic heart disease are not candidates for revascularization and/or receive incomplete revascularization. CAD is a progressive disorder that is usually diffuse involving multiple regions of the vasculature and multiple stenoses. CAD is also usually associated with co-morbid conditions such as diabetes, obesity, hypertension and old age the effects of which are not restricted to specific regions of the vasculature. More than 10% of patients with symptomatic coronary artery disease are not suitable candidates for either PCTA or CABG [13, 14]. These patients are the primary candidates for the relatively new procedure called therapeutic angiogenesis. This procedure involves the delivery of pro-angiogenic growth factors to the myocardium of patients with CAD to stimulate collateral vessel production and hopefully resolve the ischemia.

THERAPEUTIC ANGIOGENESIS

Risk factors for both coronary and peripheral artery diseases include hereditary, age, diabetes, hypertension, lifestyle (smoking), and serum lipid composition [15-17]. Evidence from both animal and patient studies indicate that several of these risk categories, in particular age, diabetes, and hyperlipidemia are associated with depressed levels of angiogenic growth factors including vascular endothelial growth factor (VEGF) [18]. Growth factor deficiency and depressed angiogenic potential may therefore contribute to the establishment and progression of arterial disease. Preclinical studies initiated in the early 1990s provided conceptual proof for therapeutic angiogenesis, and supported the implementation of clinical trials of VEGF and fibroblast growth factor (FGF) [19-22]. Although these trials have generally been positive, the results are mixed in terms of the degree of therapeutic gain, and the dramatic responses seen in animal studies have so far not been reproduced clinically. There have been more than 1000 patient studies testing VEGF or FGF protein or genes and about 100 patient studies testing bone marrow derived stem cells. Here we will review the clinical trial results and discuss with hindsight what may realistically have been expected from the delivery methods used, and how these may be improved.

CLINICAL TRIALS

Fibroblast Growth Factor (FGF)

Protein Therapy

In the first therapeutic angiogenesis clinical study FGF-1 protein was injected directly into the left ventricles of 20 patients with three-vessel coronary artery disease that were undergoing venous bypass grafts [23]. For each patient, purified recombinant FGF-1, 10-μg/kg body weight, was injected at multiple sites close to the left anterior descending coronary artery (LAD) and distal to its anastomosis with the internal mammary artery (IMA).

Transfemoral intra-arterial digital subtraction angiography 12-weeks after surgery showed pronounced accumulation of contrast medium at the site of injection and extending peripherally around the LAD for 3-4 cm distal to the IMA/LAD anastomosis. At the site of injection a capillary network could be visualized sprouting out from the coronary artery into the myocardium. Stenoses distal to the anastomosis also appeared to be bridged by neovascularization. None of these effects were observed in patients receiving heat-denatured FGF. Follow up 3 years later confirmed the safety and apparent efficacy of FGF-1 therapy. The capillary network seen at 12-weeks persisted on angiography, and echocardiography suggested improved left ventricular ejection fraction (LVEF) [24].

Pilot phase I/II trials testing various dose and delivery methods have been reported for both FGF and VEGF. In a phase 1 randomized double-blind placebo controlled study, Laham et al implanted slow-release (3-4 weeks) heparin alginate microspheres containing 10 or 100 μg FGF in the epicardial fat overlying viable ischemic myocardium of 24 patients [25]. Nuclear and magnetic resonance imaging (MRI) perfusion scans were performed at onset and again at 90 days. All patients in the 100μg FGF treatment group reported improved symptoms at 90-days, whereas three of the seven control group patients experienced persistent symptoms and two required repeat revascularization. Nuclear perfusion imaging showed a significant reduction in the size of the ischemic target region in the 100μg FGF2 group, but not in the 10μg group. As in the first study, the benefits of FGF2 therapy were reported to be maintained at 3-year follow up [26]. Positive results from several pilot open-label dose-escalation studies of intracoronary single-bolus FGF2 delivery were reported that supported a larger phase II trial. In the preliminary studies a total of 91 patients received intracoronary infusions of FGF2 ranging from 0.33 to 100 g/kg [27-29]. Hypotension become dose limiting at 48 μg/kg and transient mild thrombocytopenia and proteinuria occurred in some subjects. One study reported improvements of LVEF, target wall thickening and myocardial perfusion as well as quality of life (angina frequency, treadmill exercise tolerance) at 3 and 6-month follow ups [27].

In the FGF Initiating RevaScularization Trial (FIRST) [30], 337 patients were enrolled in a multicenter, double-blind, phase II trial that examined three different concentrations (0.3, 3, and 30 g/kg) of single intracoronary infusions of FGF2 versus placebo controls. Efficacy was evaluated by exercise tolerance test, myocardial nuclear perfusion imaging, and quality of life questionnaires. Irrespective of dose, the mean change in exercise tolerance test time was not significantly different after 90 or 180 days between treatment and control groups. Angina frequency was significantly reduced at 90 days, but not 180 days and there was no significant difference in stress nuclear imaging. Follow up data at 32 months showed a trend for slightly sustained improvement in the treatment group [26].

Gene Therapy

Adenoviral delivery of the FGF-5 gene by intracoronary infusion in a porcine ameroid constriction model of myocardial ischemia was shown to alleviate ischemia and improve function [31]. This provided support for the Angiogenic Gene Therapy trial (AGENT), a dose escalating, double blinded, phase I/II trial of adenovirus (Ad5) encoding FGF-4 [32]. Seventy-nine patients were randomized to receive either placebo or one of 5 doses of Ad5-FGF-4 (3.3×10^9 to 3.3×10^{10} total viral particles) also delivered by intracoronary infusion. At 12-week follow-up, exercise tolerance was not significantly improved in the test groups compared with placebo, and there were no differences in stress-induced wall motion scores as measured by echocardiography. Although subgroup analyses suggested some improvement of the most severely effected patients, these effects were also very moderate.

VASCULAR ENDOTHELIAL GROWTH FACTOR (VEGF)

Protein Therapy

Several small pilot trials attested to the safety and tolerance of low dose recombinant VEGF administration by coronary infusion to patients with severe coronary artery disease [33-35]. These studies showed a trend for improved coronary flow and supported larger phase II trials. The VEGF in Ischemia for Vascular Angiogenesis (VIVA) trial [36] was a multicenter, randomized, double-blind, placebo-controlled study of intracoronary and intravenous rVEGF infusion. A total of 178 patients were randomized to low dose (17 ng/Kg), high dose (50 ng/Kg), or placebo. VEGF was delivered by an intracoronary infusion followed by intravenous infusions at three-day intervals. No significant improvements were reported in treadmill time or angina class in the treatment groups at 60 days or 1-year compared with placebo. Interestingly both treatment and placebos were significantly improved relative to controls indicating the powerful influence of placebo on CAD symptoms.

Gene Therapy

Positive results, although in some cases marginal, were obtained in multiple small trials of VEGF delivered as plasmid or adenovirus [37-39]. Several of these studies demonstrated slightly improved left ventricle ejection fractions and angiograms in treatment groups, and reduced anginal episodes at short-term follow up. Losordo et al [38] injected phVEGF$_{165}$ (plasmid) directly into the ischemic myocardium of 5 male patients with angina and documented CAD. A total of 125 μg of plasmid DNA was injected in 4 X 2-mL aliquots into the anterolateral left ventricular free wall via a mini left anterior thoracotomy. No apparent short or long-term side effects were associated with the procedures. The average postoperative hospital stay was 3.8 days. During 60 days of follow up, all patients reported significant reduction in angina; LVEF were unchanged or improved, and coronary angiography showed improved Rentrop scores in all treated patients. The low dose of DNA in these studies is noteworthy, only 125μg of VEGF plasmid was delivered to the ischemic myocardium whereas up to 4 mg was optimal for treating limb ischemia, and earlier studies indicated that doses of phVEGF$_{165}$ < 500μg were inactive in the limb muscles [40,41]. In a larger nonrandomized uncontrolled, dose escalating trial 25 patients received phVEGF$_{165}$ and were followed for 180 days. Safety and tolerance were confirmed, and improvements in collateral filling and SPECT-sestamibi perfusion were demonstrated at 60 days. In an attempt to target and contain transgene expression in the ischemic tissue, Vale et al used an electromechanical mapping (NOGA) catheter to identify viable tissue in ischemic hearts, and inject phVEGF$_{165}$ directly into the ischemic region. In the first, single blinded pilot study phVEGF$_{165}$, delivered by intramyocardial injections in 3 patients was compared to 3 patients that received placebo injections [37]. Significantly improved perfusion scores were reported in the treatment group at 90 days and a reduction in angina frequency and nitroglycerin use at one-year follow up. These results were supported in a larger phase II double-blind placebo controlled study in which 19 patients were assigned to phVEGF$_{165}$ or placebo both introduced using the NOGA technique [42]. Treatment groups showed improvements in exercise tolerance, anginal class, and a reduction in the area of ischemic myocardium at 12-week follow up. The recent Euroinject One study was a phase II randomized double-blind trial of percutaneous intramyocardial plasmid gene transfer of vascular endothelial growth factor (phVEGF-A(165) assessing myocardial perfusion, left ventricular function, and clinical symptoms.[43] In this study 80 "no-option" patients with severe stable ischemic heart disease, Canadian Cardiovascular Society functional class 3 to 4, were assigned randomly to receive system either 0.5 mg of phVEGF-A(165) (n = 40) or placebo plasmid (n = 40) in the myocardial region showing stress-induced myocardial perfusion defects. After three months, myocardial stress perfusion defects did not differ significantly between the VEGF gene transfer and placebo groups (38 +/- 3% and 44 +/- 2%, respectively). Similarly, semi quantitative analysis of the change in perfusion in the treated region of interest did not differ significantly between the two groups. Compared with placebo, VEGF gene transfer improved the local wall motion disturbances, assessed both by NOGA (p = 0.04) and contrast ventriculography (p = 0.03). Canadian Cardiovascular Society functional class classification of angina pectoris improved significantly in both groups but without difference between the groups. Five NOGA procedure-related adverse events were reported. The authors concluded that VEGF gene transfer did not significantly improve stress-induced myocardial perfusion compared with placebo but a significant improvement of regional wall motion may indicate a favorable anti-ischemic effect.

Therapeutic angiogenesis using adenoviral delivery of VEGF was tested in phase I and II trials. In the former 21 patients received Ad-VEGF$_{121}$ by direct intramyocardial injection; 15 patients received the therapy in conjunction with CABG and 6 received it as sole therapy [39]. Three patients in the former group each received $4x10^8$, $4x10^{8.5}$, $4x10^9$, $4x10^{9.5}$, and $4x10^{10}$ pu Ad-VEGF$_{121}$ and the latter patients each received $4x10^9$. Injections were directed to the regions of reversible ischemia, determined by ^{99m}Tc-sestambi perfusion scans. Trends toward improvement in angina classification and treadmill exercise testing were seen at six months in all groups and there was a suggestion of improved exercise tolerance in the gene therapy-only group. The study also reported improvements in wall motion at stress in the region of vector administration and increased collateral vessels in the majority of patients. There was no a significant adverse effect or increase of systemic VEGF associated with the treatments, but anti-adenoviral antibodies were detected in some subjects. The Kuopio Angiogenesis Trial (KAT) was a randomized, double-blinded trial of intracoronary infusion of the VEGF$_{165}$ cDNA at the time of PTCA and stenting [44]. A total of 109 patients were included in the study and 90% received stents. Thirty-seven patients received Ad-VEGF ($2x 10^{10}$ pfu), 28 patients received phVEGF (2 mg plasmid DNA in liposomes), and 38 control patients received Ringer's lactate. Follow-up time was 6 months. No adverse responses were reported and myocardial perfusion was significantly improved (only) in the Ad-VEGF treatments.

Conclusions from Protein and Gene-Therapy

The clinical responses to angiogenic growth factors delivered as protein, plasmid or adenoviral vector have been marginal. The best results appear to be in response to plasmid VEGF, possibly because plasmids promote longer duration of gene expression and there is more time for angiogenic response. There is scant evidence for arteriogenesis in any of the clinical trials to date. An optimist's view of the combined results from VEGF and FGF trials would support the therapeutic angiogenesis concept and conclude that the procedures used to implement the therapy are flawed. There are two broad possibilities that cannot yet be distinguished. One is that unlike healthy animal tissues the target tissues of patients are already defective in angiogenic responses and cannot respond to the exogenous growth factors because multiple components of vessel regeneration are missing. A second possibility is that cardiac muscle in the diseased tissue is responsive to pro-angiogenesis factors, but the delivery methods do not provide adequate temporal or directional cues for the establishment of new collateral networks with mature functional vessels. In either case some of these flaws may be overcome by introducing pluripotential stem cells into the diseased tissues with the capacity of differentiate into host tissues and simultaneously deliver pro-angiogenic cytokines.

CELL THERAPY

Preclinical Trials

Endothelial progenitor stem cells (EPCs) have been isolated from the peripheral blood and bone marrow of animals and humans and shown to incorporate into active sites of angiogenesis in models of ischemia [45]. EPCs promote angiogenesis in ischemic hearts of mice, rats, dogs, and pigs [46-48]. EPCs or bone marrow mononuclear cells (BM-MNCs) are usually delivered to the ischemic tissue as intramuscular grafts by direct injection. Numerous studies have demonstrated the potential of these cells to provide therapeutic benefit for myocardial ischemia. Intra-myocardial injection of BM-MNC following MI resulted in decreased infarct size and increased regional blood flow in a porcine model [49]. Similar results were reported in a rat model of MI where human BM-MNC- $CD34^+$ endothelial progenitors were injected into the tail vein [50]. The potential of bone marrow stromal cells (BMC) to develop into cardiomyocytes in vivo was also examined in rats [51]. Isolated bone marrow cells were expanded and labeled with the LacZ reporter gene ex vivo and infused into the aorta 2 weeks after coronary artery ligation. Histological analysis 4 weeks later indicated that the donor cells differentiated into cardiomyocyte-like cells, fibroblast, and endothelial cells in 8 out of 12 recipient rats. Further studies confirmed the potential of bone marrow -derived stem cells to produce functional cardiac cells as well as blood vessels [52]. Lineage negative (lin⁻), $c\text{-}kit^+$ bone marrow cells, a population of hematopoietic cells enriched for hematopoietic stem and progenitor cells, were isolated from male transgenic mice expressing enhanced green fluorescent protein (EGFP). MI was induced by coronary artery ligation and 3-5 hours later donor lin⁻; $c\text{-}kit^+$ hematopoietic cells were injected into the area adjacent to the infarct. Examination nine days later indicated that myocardial regeneration was obtained in 12 out of 30 recipient mice. In a second strategy, endogenous bone marrow cells were mobilized by infusion of granulocyte colony stimulating factor and stem cell factor. This treatment increased the in vivo population of stem cells able to contribute to myocardial repair [53]. Cytokine treatment significantly improved survival following MI and resulted in the formation of vascular structures and myocytes occupying an average of $76\pm11\%$ of the infarcted myocardium. Hemodynamics and left ventricle functions were significantly improved and scar formation was reduced. Two recent studies demonstrated the existence of cardiac stem cells in adult mouse hearts and their potential to regenerate and repair infarcted [54, 55] myocardium.

Clinical Trials

Several pilot phase 1 clinical trials reported positive results of autologous BM-MNC transplant into patients with ischemic heart disease. In the first study 10 patients undergoing PTCA were transplanted with autologous BM-MNC via a balloon catheter placed into the infarct-related artery during balloon inflation. At 3-months follow up the infarct region was significantly decreased compared with standard therapy and wall motion in the ischemic region, and hemodynamics were improved [56]. In a second study, bone marrow was aspirated from the iliac crest of six patients undergoing CABG, and MNC were isolated [57]. The day after isolation, immediately after CABG, 1×10^6 $AC133^+$ cells for each patient were injected by 10 injections of 0.2 mL each along the circumference of the infarct border. All patients survived the procedures and follow-up was implemented 9-16 months later. Transthoracic echocardiography revealed a gain in LVEF and improved diastolic ventricular dimensions in four patients, and SPECT-scans indicated markedly improved perfusion of the previously non-perfused or hypoperfused infarct zone in five patients. The authors acknowledge that they could not definitively attribute the positive effects to cell transplantation because all patients received simultaneous CABG. A third study included eight patients with stable angina that was refractory to maximum medical therapy. The ischemic regions were identified by electromechanical mapping, and a mixed population of autologous iliac crest bone marrow cells was injected into the ischemic region through the mapping (NOGA) catheter [58]. No adverse side effects of the procedures were reported. At 3 months follow up patients reported a reduction of anginal episodes and reduced use of nitroglycerine. MRI scans revealed no change of LVEF but significant improvement in radial wall motion and thickening during pharmacological stress, and slight improvement in perfusion parameters.

Assmus et al compared intracoronary infusion of bone marrow-MNC with peripheral blood derived progenitor cells in 20 patients with recent MI. They reported significant improvements of LVEF, wall motion in the infarct zone, and end-systolic LV volumes in both cell-therapy groups compared with a reference group [59]. Echocardiography and quantitative F-18-fluorodeoxyglucose-positron emission tomography revealed significantly improved contractile function, coronary blood flow reserve, and increased myocardial viability. In a similar study Perin et al enrolled 21 patients with end-stage ischemic heart disease in a prospective, nonrandomized, open-label study of bone marrow -MNC delivered by injection into ischemic myocardium by NOGA catheter [60]. Ischemic viable myocardium was identified by electromechanical mapping and patients underwent 2- and 4-month follow up. The study reported significant improvement of LVEF (20% to 29%; P= 0.003) and mechanical function of injected segments (P= 0.0005), as well as significant reduction of end-systolic volume (P=0.03). In the MAGIC cell randomized clinical trial, 27 patients with MI who underwent PTCA and stenting were randomized into 3 groups [61]. The first group received peripheral blood derived stem cells and daily subcutaneous injections of granulocyte-colony stimulating factor (G-CSF) to mobilize the stem cells. The second group received only G-CSF and the third group was control. Follow up was 6-months. The cell treatment group displayed significantly improved treadmill exercise capacity (450s to 578s; P=0.004), reduction of myocardial perfusion deficit (11.6% to 5.3%; P=0.02), and increased LVEF (48.7% to 55.1%; P=0.005) at 6-months compared with baseline. G-CSF was discontinued because it appeared to increase the incidence of in-stent restenosis.

In the REPAIR-MI [62] and REPAIR-CHF [63] studies, bone marrow or peripheral blood derived progenitor cells were administered via intracoronary infusion to patients who suffered recent or chronic (within 3 months) MI, respectively. In REPAIR-MI, 204 patients with acute myocardial infarction were randomly assigned to receive an intracoronary infusion of bone marrow derived progenitor cells or placebo medium into the infarct artery 3 to 7 days after successful reperfusion therapy. At 4 months the authors reported significant improvement of global left ventricular ejection fraction in the treatment group relative to placebo (mean [+/-SD] increase, 5.5+/-7.3% vs. 3.0+/-6.5%; P=0.01). Patients with a baseline LVEF at or below the median value of 48.9% derived the most benefit. At 1 year, the treatment group was associated with significant reductions in combined clinical end points including of death, recurrence of myocardial infarction, and any revascularization procedure. The authors concluded that intracoronary administration of bone marrow cells is associated with improved recovery of left ventricular contractile function in patients with acute myocardial infarction. Similar results were reported in a smaller study where 19 patients with AMI were infused with CD133+ BM cells [64]. The latter study concluded that patients with recent AMI, intracoronary administration of enriched CD133+ cells is associated with improved left ventricular performance and increased myocardial perfusion. They also reported increased incidence of coronary events associated with cell therapy. In REPAIR-CHF 75 patients with stable ischemic heart disease who had had a myocardial infarction within 3 months were randomly assigned to receive either no cell infusion (23 patients) or infusion of CPC (24 patients) or bone marrow cells (28 patients) into the patent coronary artery supplying the most dyskinetic left ventricular area. The patients in the control group were subsequently randomly assigned to receive CPC or bone marrow cells, and the patients who initially received bone marrow cells or CPC crossed over to receive CPC or bone marrow cells, respectively, at 3 months' follow-up. At 3 months follow up, LVEF was significantly greater among patients receiving bone marrow cells (+2.9 %) compared with CPC (-0.4 %, P=0.003) or no infusion (-1.2 %, P<0.001). In crossover patients, intracoronary infusion of bone marrow cells was associated with a significant increase in global and regional left ventricular function, regardless of whether patients crossed over from control to bone marrow cells or from CPC to bone marrow cells. The authors concluded that intracoronary infusion of progenitor cells is safe and feasible in patients with healed myocardial infarction and transplantation of bone marrow cells is associated with moderate but significant improvement in EF at 3 months.

CONCLUSIONS AND FUTURE PERSPECTIVES

Overall, the clinical trials of VEGF and FGF delivered as protein, or by plasmid or adenoviral vectors have fallen short of expectations. The success of neovascularization of diseased tissues is determined by numerous factors some of which are specific for the underlying pathology. Vessel development in the embryo involves three distinct steps referred to as vasculogenesis, angiogenesis, and Arteriogenesis [65]. These steps involve multiple sequentially activated factors and receptors as well as negative regulatory factors that are mutually dependent and coordinated. Vasculogenesis involves the assembly of endothelial cells into a primary vascular plexus followed by the incorporation of smooth muscle cells, monocytes and pericytes to form mature contractile vessels. Angiogenesis involves vascular sprouting from preexisting vessels, vascular fusion and intussusception to form a functional capillary network. Vasculogenesis and angiogenesis in both the embryo and adult tissues involve recruitment of endothelial and smooth muscle cells from pools of circulating progenitor cells that originate in the bone marrow. The homing signals that activate and promote the targeting of these cells involve concentration gradients of cytokines and angiogenic growth factors such as VEGF, HGF, SDF-1, and IGF-1. In arteriogenesis, the vascular network is further remodeled to form large collateral arteries. This process involves additional sprouting, longitudinal migration, proliferation, and recruitment of more endothelial and smooth muscle cells. The lamina elastic interna is degraded during the process of arteriogenesis; monocytes and macrophages are recruited to the vessel walls and the vessel diameter can increase by 2-20 folds. Each step in the generation of the mature vessel network is modulated by different sets of factors that are interrelated and precisely regulated both spatially and temporally.

The success of therapeutic angiogenesis in the treatment of CAD relies on the ability of the intervention to reactivate both angiogenesis and arteriogenesis, and to generate mature and stable conducting vessels. Most of the animal studies, and all of the patient studies to date have used single angiogenic factors; VEGF or FGF delivered as recombinant protein, or in plasmid or adenoviral vectors. In each case the duration of exposure of the ischemic tissue to growth factor is probably too short to allow arteriogenesis and may stimulate only a short burst of angiogenesis that cannot produce mature vessels. Studies from the author's laboratory argue in favor of this. Using a rabbit ischemic hindlimb model of PAD we found that Ad-VEGF stimulated a rapid proliferation of endothelium during the first week of treatment that coincided precisely with a transient rise of serum-VEGF. The new capillaries were not stable and rapidly disappeared, probably by apoptotic death 1-3 weeks after treatment [66, 67]. Other studies confirm that the exposure time to VEGF critically determines whether or not stable conducting vessels are produced [68], and a recent report showed that chronic VEGF expression in rat hindlimb delivered by AAV promoted arteriogenesis as well as angiogenesis [69]. We have confirmed this latter finding in the mouse and rabbit models (Webster, unpublished).

The use of permanent delivery vehicles such as AAV with tightly regulated expression and targeting of the angiogenic genes to the ischemic regions of tissue may alleviate the deficiencies of current therapeutic angiogenesis protocols. Such optimized delivery of appropriately regulated factors may stimulate arteriogenesis and provide chemoattractive signals for circulating PB-MNCs. Clinical trials of BM-MNCs or BM-mesenchymal stem cells (see accompanying chapter by Hare et al) currently look more promising than proteins or genes although this may change if the genes are delivered optimally. The relative efficacy of gene versus stem cell procedures cannot be determined because none of these procedures have been run in parallel. It seems likely that the optimal therapy will include both stem cells and genes delivered in a manner that will allow the genes to target and possibly regulate the activity of the cells. The future of this technology may indeed rest in stem cells appropriately engineered with disease-responsive and regulated genes [21,22,70].

REFERENCES

[1]   American College of Cardiology/American Heart Association Task Force on Practice Guidelines (Committee on the Management of Patients with Chronic Stable Angina). ACC/AHA 2002 guideline update for the management of patients with chronic stable angina. J Am Coll Cardiol 2003;41:159-168.

[2]   Ahmed A. American College of Cardiology/American Heart Association Chronic Heart Failure Evaluation and Management Guidelines: relevance to the Geriatric Practice. J Am Geriatr Soc 2003 Jan;51(1):123-126.

[3]   Laugwitz KL, Moretti A, Weig HJ, *et al.* M. Blocking caspase-activated apoptosis improves contractility in failing myocardium. Hum Gene Ther 2001 Nov 20;12,(17):2051-2063.

[4]   Rossig L, Hoffmann J, Hugel B, *et al.* Vitamin C inhibits endothelial cell apoptosis in congestive heart failure. Circulation 2001 Oct 30;104(18):2182-2187.

[5]   Frystyk J, Ledet T, Moller N, Flyvbjerg A, and Orskov H. Cardiovascular disease and insulin-like growth factor I. Circulation 2002 Aug20;106(8): 893-895.

[6]   Kukreja RC, Ockaili R, Salloum F, *et al.* Cardioprotection with phosphodiesterase-5 inhibition--a novel preconditioning strategy. J Mol Cell Cardiol 2004 Feb;36(2)36, 165-173.

[7]   Barakate MS, Hemli JM, Hughes CF, Bannon PG, Horton MD. Coronary artery bypass grafting (CABG) after initially successful percutaneous transluminal coronary angioplasty (PTCA): a review of 17 years experience. Eur J Cardiothorac Surg 2003 Feb(2):179-186.

[8]   Fattori R, Piva T. Drug-eluting stents in vascular intervention. Lancet 2003 Jan 18;361(9353):247-249.

[9]   Kleiman, NS, Patel, NC, Allen, KB, *et al.* Evolving revascularization approaches for myocardial ischemia. Am. J. Cardiol 2003 Nov 7;92(9B):9N-17N.

[10]   Gotto AM Jr. High-density lipoprotein cholesterol and triglycerides as therapeutic targets for preventing and treating coronary artery disease. Am Heart J 2002 Dec; 144(6 Suppl), S33-42.

[11]   Connolly DL, Lip GY, Chin BS. Antithrombotic strategies in acute coronary syndromes and percutaneous coronary interventions. BMJ 2002 Dec 144;325(7377): 1404-1407.

[12]   Mann MJ, Dzau VJ. Molecular approaches for the treatment of atherosclerosis. Cardiol Clin 2002 Nov;20(4):633-643.

[13]   Mukherjee D, Bhatt DL, Roe MT, Patel V, Ellis SG. Direct myocardial revascularization and angiogenesis - How many patients might be eligible? Am J Cardiol 1999 Sep 1d;84(5):598-600, A8.

[14]   Jones EL, Weintraub WS. The Importance of Revascularization during long-term follow-up after coronary artery operations. J Thoac Cardiovasc Surg 1996 Aug 112(2):227-237.

[15]   Schainfeld DO, Isner JM. Critical limb ischemia: nothing to give at the office? Ann Intern Med 1999 Mar 2; 130(5):442-444.

[16]   Isner JM. Manipulating angiogenesis against vascular disease. Hosp Pract (Minneap) 1999 Jun;34(6):69-74, 6, 9-80 passim.

[17]   Rivard A, Silver M, Chen D, *et al.* Rescue of diabetes-related impairment of angiogenesis by intramuscular gene transfer with Adeno-VEGF. Am.J.Pathol 1999 Feb;154(2):355-63.01.

[18]   Rivard A, Fabre JE, Silver M, *et al.* Age-dependent impairment of angiogenesis. Circulation 1999 Jan 5-12;99(1):111-120.

[19]   Melillo G, Scoccianti M, Kovesdi I, *et al.* Gene therapy for collateral vessel development. Cardiovasc Res 1997 Sep; 35(3):480-499.

[20]   Lewis BS, Flugelman MY, Weisz A, Keren-Tal I, Schaper W. Angiogenesis by gene therapy: a new horizon for myocardial revascularization. Cardiovasc Res 1997 Sep;35(3):490-497.

[21]   Webster KA. Therapeutic angiogenesis: a case for targeted, regulated gene delivery. Crit Rev Eukaryot Gene Expr 2000;10(2):13-25.

[22]   Webster KA. Therapeutic angiogenesis: a complex problem requiring a sophisticated approach. Cardiovasc Toxicol 2003;(3):283-298.

[23]   Schumacher B, Pecher P, von Specht BU, Stegmann T. Induction of neoangiogenesis in ischemic myocardium by human growth factors: first clinical results of a new treatment of coronary heart disease. Circulation 1998 Feb 24;97(7):645-50.

[24]   Pecher P Schumacher BA. Angiogenesis in ischemic human myocardium: clinical results after 3 years. Ann Thorac Surg 2000.May;69(5):1414-1419.

[25]   Laham RJ, Sellke FW, Edelman ER, *et al.* Local perivascular delivery of basic fibroblast growth factor in patients undergoing coronary bypass surgery: results of a phase I randomized, double-blind, placebo-controlled trial. Circulation 1999 Nov 2;100(18):1865-1871.

[26]   Ruel M, Laham RJ, Parker JA, *et al.* Long-term effects of surgical angiogenic therapy with fibroblast growth factor 2 protein. J Thorac Cardiovasc Surg 2002 Jul;124(1):28-34.

[27]   Laham RJ, Chronos NA, Pike M, *et al.* Intracoronary basic fibroblast growth factor (FGF-2) in patients with severe ischemic heart disease: results of a phase I open-label dose escalation study. J Am Coll Cardiol 2000 Dec;36(7):2132-2139.

[28]   Unger EF, Goncalves L, Epstein SE, *et al.* Effects of a single intracoronary injection of basic fibroblast growth factor in stable angina pectoris. Am J Cardiol 2000 Jun 15;85(12):1414-1419.

[29]   Udelson JE, Dilsizian V, Laham RJ, *et al.* Therapeutic angiogenesis with recombinant fibroblast growth factor-2 improves stress and rest myocardial perfusion abnormalities in patients with severe symptomatic chronic coronary artery disease. Circulation 2000 Oct 3;102(14):1605-1610.

[30]   Simons M, Annex BH, Laham RJ, *et al.* Pharmacological treatment of coronary artery disease with recombinant fibroblast growth factor-2: double-blind, randomized, controlled clinical trial. Circulation 2002 Feb 19;105(7):788-793.

[31]   Giordano, FJ, Ping, P, McKirnan, MD, *et al.* Intracoronary gene transfer of fibroblast growth factor-5 increases blood flow and contractile function in an ischemic region of the heart. Nat Med 1996 May 2(5):534-539.

[32]   Grines CL, Watkins MW, Helmer G, *et al.* Angiogenic gene therapy (AGENT) trial in patients with stable angina pectoris. Circulation 2002 Mar 19; 105(11):1291-1297.

[33]   Hendel RC, Henry TD, Rocha-Singh K, *et al.* Effect of intracoronary recombinant human vascular endothelial growth factor on myocardial perfusion: evidence for a dose-dependent effect. Circulation 2000 Jan 18;101(2):118-121.

[34]   Henry TD, Rocha-Singh K, Isner JM, *et al.* Intracoronary administration of recombinant human vascular endothelial growth factor to patients with coronary artery disease. Am Heart J 2001 Nov;142(5):872-880.

[35]   Henry TD, Rocha-Singh K, Isner JM, *et al.* Intracoronary administration of recombinant human vascular endothelial growth factor to patients with coronary artery disease. Am Heart J 2001 Nov;142(5):872-880.

[36]   HenryT, Annex B, Azrin M. Double blind placebo controlled trial of recombinant human vascular endothelial growth factor, the VIVA Trial. J Am Col. Cardiol 2001;33:384A.

[37]   Vale PR, Losordo DW, Milliken CE, *et al.* Randomized, single-blind, placebo-controlled pilot study of catheter-based myocardial gene transfer for therapeutic angiogenesis using left ventricular electromechanical mapping in patients with chronic myocardial ischemia. Circulation 2001 May 1;103(17): 2138-2143.

[38]   Losordo DW, Vale PR, Symes JF, D *et al.* Gene therapy for myocardial angiogenesis: initial clinical results with direct myocardial injection of phVEGF165 as sole therapy for myocardial ischemia. Circulation. 1998 Dec 22-29;98(25):2800-2804.

[39   Rosengart TK, Lee LY, Patel SR, *et al.* Six-month assessment of a phase I trial of angiogenic gene therapy for the treatment of coronary artery disease using direct intramyocardial administration of an adenovirus vector expressing the VEGF121 cDNA. Ann Surg 1999 Oct;230(4):466-470.

[40]   Baumgartner, I, Pieczek, A, Manor, O, *et al.* Constituive expression of phVEGF165 after intramusculer gene transfer promotes collateral vessel development in patients with critical limb ischemia. Circulation1998 Mar 31;97(12):1114-1123.

[41]   Tsurumi, Y, Takeshita, S, Chen, D, *et al.* Direct intramuscular gene transfer of naked DNA encoding vascular endothelial growth factor augments collateral development and tissue perfusion. Circulation 1996 Dec 15;94(12):281-290.

[42]   Losordo DW, Vale PR, Hendel RC, *et al.* Phase 1/2 placebo-controlled, double-blind, dose-escalating trial of myocardial vascular endothelial growth factor 2 gene transfer by catheter delivery in patients with chronic myocardial ischemia. Circulation 2002 Apr 30;105(17):2012-2018.

[43]   Kastrup, J; Jorgensen, E, *et al.* Direct intramyocardial plasmid vascular endothelial growth factor-A165 gene therapy in patients with stable severe angina pectoris A randomized double-blind placebo-controlled study: the Euroinject One trial. J Am Coll Cardiol 2005; Apr 5, 45(7):982-988.

[44]   Hedman M, Hartikainen J, Syvanne M. Safety and feasibility of catheter-based local intracoronary vascular endothelial growth factor gene transfer in the prevention of postangioplasty and in-stent restenosis and in the treatment of chronic myocardial ischemia: phase II results of the Kuopio Angiogenesis Trial (KAT). Circulation 2003 Jun 3, 107(21):2677-2683.

[45]   Asahara T, Murohara T, Sullivan A, *et al.* Silver M, van der Zee R, Li T, Witzenbichler B, Schatteman G, and Isner JM. Isolation of putative progenitor endothelial cells for angiogenesis. Scienc 1997 Feb 14;275(5302):964-967.

[46]   Hamano K, Li TS, Kobayashi T, *et al.* Therapeutic angiogenesis induced by local autologous bone marrow cell implantation. Ann Thorac Surg 2002 Apr;73(4):12103:1210-1215. 2002.

[47]   Clarke DL, Johansson CB, Wilbertz J, *et al.* Generalized potential of adult neural stem cells. Science 2000 Jun 2;288(5471):1660-1663.

[48]   Hamano K, Li TS, Kobayashi T, *et al.* The induction of angiogenesis by the implantation of autologous bone marrow cells: a novel and simple therapeutic method. Surgery 2001 Jul 130(1):4 44-54.

[49]   Kamihata H, Hiroaki M, Nishiue T, *et al.* Implantation of bone marrow mononuclear cells into ischemic myocardium enhances collateral perfusion and regional function via side supply of angioblasts, angiogenic ligands and cytokines. Circulation 2001 Aug 28;104(9):1046-1052.

[50]   Kocher AA, Schuster MD, Szabolcs MJ, *et al.* Neovascularization of ischemic myocardium by human bone-marrow-derived angioblasts prevents cardiomyocyte apoptosis, reduces remodeling and improves cardiac function. Nat Med 2001 Apr7 (4):430-436.

[51]   Wang JS, Shum-Tim D,Chedrawy E, Chiu RC. The coronary delivery of marrow stromal cells for myocardial regeneration: pathophysiologic and therapeutic implications. J Thorac Cardiovasc Surg 2001 Oct;122(4):6 699-705.

[52] Orlic D, Kajstura J, Chimenti S, *et al.* Bone marrow cells regenerate infarcted myocardium. Nature 2001 Apr 5;410(6829):701-705.

[53] Orlic D, Kajstura J, Chimenti S, *et al.* Mobilized bone marrow cells repair the infarcted heart, improving function and survival. Proc Natl Acad Sci U S A 2001 Aug 28;98(18):10344-10349.

[54] Beltrami AP, Barlucchi L, Torella D, *et al.* Adult cardiac stem cells are multipotent and support myocardial regeneration. Cell 2003 Sep 19;114(6):763-776.

[55] Oh H, Bradfute SB, Gallardo TD, *et al.* Cardiac progenitor cells from adult myocardium: homing, differentiation, and fusion after infarction. Proc Natl Acad Sci U S A 2003 Oct 14;100(21):12313-12318.

[56] Strauer, BE, Brehm, M, Zeus T, *et al.* Repair of infarcted myocardium by autologous intracoronary mononuclear bone marrow cell transplantation in humans. Circulation 2002 Oct 8;1006(15):1913-1918.

[57].Stamm C, Westphal B, Kleine HD, *et al.* Autologous bone-marrow stem-cell transplantation for myocardial regeneration. Lancet 2003 Jan 4;361(9351)45-46.

[58] Tse HF, Kwong YL, Chan JK, *et al.* Angiogenesis in ischaemic myocardium by intramyocardial autologous bone marrow mononuclear cell implantation. Lancet 2003 Jan 4;361 (9351):47-49.

[59] Assmus B, Schächinger, V, Teupe, C, *et al.* Transplantation of Progenitor Cells and Regeneration Enhancement in Acute Myocardial Infarction (TOPCARE-AMI). Circulation 2002 Dec 10;106(24):3009-3017.

[60] Perin EC, Dohmann HF, Borojevic R, *et al.* Transendocardial, autologous bone marrow cell transplantation for severe, chronic ischemic heart failure. Circulation. 2003 May 13;107(18):2294-2302

[61] Kang HJ, Kim HS, Zhang SY, *et al.* Effects of intracoronary infusion of peripheral blood stem-cells mobilised with granulocyte-colony stimulating factor on left ventricular systolic function and restenosis after coronary stenting in myocardial infarction: the MAGIC cell randomised clinical trial. Lancet 2004 Mar 6;363(9411):751-756.

[62] Schachinger V; Erbs S, Elsasser A, *et al.* Intracoronary bone marrow-derived progenitor cells in acute myocardial infarction. N Engl J Med 2006 Sep 21;355(12):1210-1221.

[63] Assmus B, Honold J, Schachinger V, *et al.* Transcoronary transplantation of progenitor cells after myocardial infarction. N Engl J Med 2006 Sep 21;355(12):1222-1232.

[64] Bartunek J, Vanderheyden M, Vandekerckhove B, *et al.* Intracoronary injection of CD133-positive enriched bone marrow progenitor cells promotes cardiac recovery after recent myocardial infarction: feasibility and safety. Circulation 2005 Aug 30;112(9 Suppl):I178-183.

[65] Carmeliet P. Angiogenesis in health and disease. Nat Med 2003 Jun;9(6):653-660.

[66] Gounis MJ, Spiga MG, Graham RM, *et al.* Angiogenesis is confined to the transient period of VEGF expression that follows adenoviral gene delivery to ischemic muscle. Gene Ther 2005 May; 12(9):762-771.

[67] Webster KA. Therapeutic angiogenesis: a complex problem requiring a sophisticated approach. Cardiovasc Toxicol 2003;3(3):283-298.

[68] Dor Y, Djonov V, Abramovitch R, *et al.* Conditional switching of VEGF provides new insights into adult neovascularization and pro-angiogenic therapy. EMBO J 2002 Apr 15;21(8):1939-1947.

[69] Chang DS, Su H, Tang GL, *et al.* Adeno-associated viral vector-mediated gene transfer of VEGF normalizes skeletal muscle oxygen tension and induces arteriogenesis in ischemic rat hindlimb.Mol Ther 2003 Jan;7(1):44-51.

[70] Yamashita K, Kajstura J, Discher DJ, *et al.* Reperfusion-activated Akt kinase prevents apoptosis in transgenic mouse hearts overexpressing insulin-like growth factor-1. Circ Res 2001 Mar 30;88(6):609-614.

Stem Cell and Regenerative Medicine, 2010, 75-99

CHAPTER 7

Use of Progenitor Cells in Pain Management

M.J. Eaton[1,*], Stacey Quintero Wolfe[2] and Eva Widerström-Noga[1,2,3]

[1]Department of Veterans Affairs Medical Center, Miami, Florida, 33136, USA; [2]Department of Neurological Surgery, University of Miami Leonard M. Miller School of Medicine, Miami, FL 33136, USA; [3]The Miami Project to Cure Paralysis, University of Miami Leonard M. Miller School of Medicine, Miami,FL 33136, USA

Abstract: The use of progenitor/stem cells to modulate the sensory systems in chronic pain is a new field in translational research. This follows 30 years of non-human cell therapy approaches to elucidate which tissue source, cell phenotype, neurotransmitter, or peptide might be antinociceptive in models of pain. Stem or progenitor approaches have been tested in cardiac myopathies, liver dysfunction, stroke, and genetic abnormalities, but almost none have applied progenitor cells to the relief of neuropathic, pain. Perhaps the best studied neural progenitor cell line NT2, has recently resulted in two NT2-derived cell lines: hNT2.17, secreting the inhibitory neurotransmitters GABA and glycine; and hNT2.19, secreting the neurotransmitter serotonin. Each of these NT2-lines has demonstrated antinociceptive potential in models of SCI-related neuropathic pain, in peripheral neuropathy, and diabetic neuropathic pain. These human progenitors may prove to be useful in the relief of chronic pain and open the way to other regenerative approaches to pain management.

INTRODUCTION

Treatment of sensory neuropathies that result in chronic pain, whether inherited (Keller BP 1999) [1], or caused by trauma (Schwartzman MCNA1999) [2], or the progress of diabetes (Benbow DM 1999) [3], or other disease states (Koltzenburg CON 1998) [4] is one of the most difficult problems in modern clinical practice. The prevalence of neuropathic pain has been conservatively estimated at 0.6% of the U.S. population (Bennett HP 1998) [5]. To the extent that low-back pain is sometimes neuropathic, the actual figure might be far higher. Neuropathic pain might realistically affect 1.5% of the total population nationwide and current pharmacologic treatments have often proven ineffective, or must be used at impractical dose levels, such as that seen with morphine or its analogues (Bowsher CONN 1993) [6]. Neuropathic pain is a common type of chronic pain with spinal cord injury (SCI), and results from the abnormal processing of sensory input due to damage to the nervous system (Dworkin CJP 2002) [7]. It is often difficult to identify a specific cause of neuropathic pain, which is frequently unresponsive to conventional methods of pain treatment (Yezierski JRRD 2009) [8]. SCI-related neuropathic pain (also called central, dysesthetic, or deafferentation pain) is primarily located at or below the level of injury and is often diffuse and poorly localized. Onset of SCI pain is usually weeks to months after injury (Siddall Pain 1999) [9] (Siddall Pain 2003) [10]. Few clinical pain trials have been conducted in persons with SCI pain although pain is perceived as one of the most difficult consequences of SCI to deal with (Widerstrom-Noga APMR 1999) [11]. So far no clinical trial has shown any drug to be effective for a significant number of people with SCI-related neuropathic pain. Even so, individuals with SCI have found pain relief, sometimes from a combination of drugs, sometimes from drugs in combination with physical therapy or other treatment modalities. The use of cell therapy, to release antinociceptive agents near the injured spinal cord and to provide ongoing pain relief, would be a logical next-step in the development of treatment modalities (Eaton EOBT 2004) [12] (Eaton JN 2006) [13] in order to limit the potential adverse effects often caused by systemic pharmacological administration. But there have been few clinical trials, especially for chronic pain, testing the transplant of cells or cell line to treat human disease (Sagen JRRD 2003) [14].

MECHANISMS OF NEUROPATHIC PAIN

Mechanisms associated with the onset and development of neuropathic pain (Melzack Science 1965) [15] (Basbaum

***Address correspondence to this author Mary J. Eaton:** Miami VAMC, D806C, 1201 NW 16th St, Miami, Fl 33125, USA; Tel: (305) 575-6995; Fax: (305) 575-3126; E-mail: meatonscience@gmail.com*

RAPM 1999) [16] (Campbell Neuron 2006) [17] (Garcia-Larrea PM 2008) [18] (Yezierski JRRD 2009) [19] can be described as the result of a restructuring and reset of normal responses to non-noxious or noxious sensory input, or even the generation of spontaneous stimulus-absent spontaneous pain, associated with maladaptive plasticity of the nervous system. A number of biochemical and cellular alterations have been described in animal models of neuropathic pain, but their relation with heterogeneous symptoms in humans is not well understood. These include central spinal sensitization, thought to be the cause of ongoing pain in humans (Siddall SC 1997) [20], even when the injury is peripheral in location (Yaksh PNAS USA 1999)[21]; ectopic discharges in damaged myelinated fibers (Abdulla JN 2001) [22]; abnormal activity in undamaged fibers (Suter Anesthesiology 2004) [23]; overexpression of calcium channels increasing the release of excitatory neurotransmitters (Li Pain 2006) [24] (Fuchs Anesthesiology 2007) [25]; and sympathetic sprouting towards the spinal ganglia (Woolf Science 2000) [26]. Blockade of N-type calcium channels is a current focus of many pharmaceutical agents (Yamamoto CTMC 2009) [27] (Schroeder MC 2006) [28], including the antiepileptic agents gabapentin and pregabulin, which preferentially bind $Ca2+$ channels (Bayer Neuropharmacology 2004) [29] (Gilron COA 2007) [30] (Bauer JN 2009) [31]. Also contributing to these modifications are attenuation of spinal inhibition by selective neuronal and neurotransmitter loss, seen in peripheral (Ibuki Neuroscience 1997) [32] (Satoh BR 1996) [33] (Eaton JCN 1998) [34] and central (Gwak JN 2006) [35] models of injury and pain. As well, the development of inflammatory phenomena, including cytokine secretion by macrophages and glial cells (Krenz JN 2000) [36] (Tsuda TN 2005) [37] contribute to the hypersensitivity that underlies the development of pain (Murphy EJN 1999) [38] (Sommer Anaesthesist 2001) [39]. Additionally, changes in the dorsal horn modify the activity of projections towards the brainstem and increase spinal hyperactivity still further by feedback loops(Yamashiro SFN 1997) [40], involving specific midbrain and cortical neuronal pathways (Zhang APS 1994) [41] (Helmchen NL 1995) [42] (Lenz Pain 1987) [43] (Morrow Pain 1998) [44] (Paulson Pain 2000) [45] These effects are delayed, suggesting that maintenance of spinal sensitization requires the involvement of mechanisms of descending facilitation involving the brainstem (Basbaum ARN 1984) [46] (Benarroch Neurology 2008) [47] (Behbehani PN 1995) [48] and anterior cingulate and insular cortical regions (Xie APS 2009) [49].

CLASSIFICATION OF NEUROPATHIC PAIN

Even though chronic neuropathic pain is often reported in SCI, traumatic brain injury (TBI), diabetic peripheral neuropathy (DPN), stroke, peripheral nerve injuries, cancer and a variety of other PNS and CNS disease states and injuries (Bennett Pain 2006) [50], and data is frequently collected on these presentations (Sawatzky SC 2008) [51], there is no agreed set of descriptors or standardized way to collect such data across diverse chronic pain populations. The use of standardized sets of outcome measures in clinical practice and in clinical trials would facilitate research collaboration between clinical centers and the translation, interpretation and application of results to improve the management of neuropathic pain. However, such standardized methods are only being recently developed to facilitate the quantification and description easier (Widerstrom-Noga SC 2008) [52] (Bouhassira Pain 2004) [53] (Treede Neurology 2008) [54]. Besides descriptors such as quality, temporal factors, location, intensity of pain, etc., one of the most important characteristics is the type of pain. Pain classification after SCI is partly based on the ASIA Impairment Scale (AIS) (Marino SCM 2003) [55]. For neuropathic pain to be classified as SCI-related a lesion or disease affecting the spinal cord or nerve roots must be present and the pain must fall within an expected anatomical location for that lesioned or diseased spinal cord or nerve roots. Neuropathic pain that cannot be attributed to a lesion or disease affecting the spinal cord or nerve roots is classified as "other" (neuropathic).

At-level (neuropathic) pain refers to neuropathic pain located in or near the neurological level of injury. It is perceived anywhere within the dermatome of the level of neurological injury and three dermatomes below this level. It may be perceived by the patient is often characterized as burning, electric or shooting. Sensory abnormalities, including allodynia (evoked pain in response to a stimulus that is not normally painful, such as touch) or hyperalgesia (exaggerated response to a stimulus that is normally painful) within the pain distribution are often found. The pain may be unilateral or bilateral in location.

Below-level (neuropathic) pain refers to neuropathic pain that is experienced more than three dermatomes below the neurological level of injury. Below level neuropathic pain is typically described by patients as burning, electric or shooting pain that may have a diffuse or regional distribution.

Other (neuropathic) pain includes neuropathic pains that are considered not to be caused by the spinal cord injury. Examples include both central and peripheral neuropathic pain associated with herpetic neuralgia, diabetic neuropathy, stroke and compressive mononeuropathies.

Other non-neuropathic pain types that occur after SCI include musculoskeletal pain in a region where there is at least some preserved sensation above, at or below the neurological level of injury and which is believed to be arising from musculoskeletal structures. This pain is commonly described as dull or aching and relieved by rest, muscle tenderness with pain relief in response to anti-inflammatory medications or evidence of skeletal pathology consistent with the pain presentation. Examples include spinal fractures, muscular injury, shoulder overuse syndromes and muscle spasms. Another example is visceral pain, located in the thorax or abdomen and believed to be generated in visceral structures. This type of pain may be perceived as dull, aching or cramping is associated with visceral pathology or dysfunction, for example, infection or obstruction. Examples include urinary tract infection, ureteric calculus and bowel impaction.

Unfortunately such pain after SCI is both disturbing and difficult (Felix JRRD 2007) [56], seriously interfering with most life activities, including quality and length of sleep (Widerstrom-Noga APMR 2001) [57], with symptoms persisting and even increasing over time (Cruz-Almeida J Rehabil Res Dev 2005) [58], conveying an overall perceived lack of ability to deal with such pain (Widerstrom-Noga APMR 1999) [59], and all endured with little effective treatment (Widerstrom-Noga Spinal Cord 2003) [60] available. Pharmacological interventions are rarely helpful for the long-term and are fraught with side-effects (Christo ACNA 2003) [61].

BEHAVIORAL OUTCOMES IN MODELS OF PAIN

The development of animal models of pain (Le Bars Pharamacol Rev 2001) [62] (Eaton JRRD 2003) [63] has allowed for the investigation of possible mechanisms, associated genetic basis (Delander APS 1997) [64] and the evaluation of potential therapeutics (Bennett BR 2000) [65] (Vierck Pain 2000) [66], including stem/progenitor cells (Klass AA 2007) [67] (Lin CT 2002) [68]. Each model mirrors the clinical appearance of many features of the particular syndrome, but few reproduce the myriad patient reports of either intensity or relevant contributing factors, especially in models of chronic neuropathic pain, including SCI. These models can be divided into acute, tissue injury, nerve injury, and central injury models. Most depend on and measure a behavioral hypersensitivity that develops over time to an injury (peripheral or central to the nervous system), or disease state that can be induced (diabetes, cancer, etc.). Almost all use noxious or non-noxious stimuli that are usually measured as a change in the threshold-of-response to the stimulus.

Acute tests, such as hot-plate, tail-flick, and paw pressure tests, require a high-intensity stimulus (such as thermal, mechanical, or chemical) but do not test a preinjured animal. The response measured (1) is immediate (or within seconds), (2) uses the Ad- and C-fiber input, and (3) is known to activate the spinal dorsal horn, the cells of which are nociceptive-specific and/or wide dynamic range neurons. In addition, the response is proportional to the frequency of stimulus and the fiber class of afferent input. Examples include those used for revealing the potency of opioid analgesics, useful for predicting analgesic effects in humans (Grumbach Pain 1966) [69].

Long-duration tests use an irritant, foreign chemical agent as the nociceptive stimulus. They differ from most other pain tests in that (1) they do not measure a threshold response; (2) they quantitatively measure the resulting behavior after the stimulus which varies in potency with time; and (3) they are not models of chronic pain, since the duration of the behaviors is short, usually minutes or tens of minutes. Hence, long-duration stimuli tests are considered models of tonic pain. They are usually based on intradermal or intraperitoneal injections of the agent. Examples include injection of formalin into a hindpaw, modeling arthritis or inflammatory processes (Otsuki BR 1986) [70] (Tonussi Pain 1992) [71] (Heapy BJ P1987) [72]. An important subtype of tonic pain is the writhing test, where the behaviors are used as evidence of peritoneovisceral or visceral pain associated with activation of visceral chemoreceptors after the intraperitoneal injection of agents that are irritating to serous membranes.

Pain caused by cardiac or vascular ischemia can also studied, and is a frequently occurring clinical problem which is suggested to be a possible target of stem/progenitor cell therapy (Marsala EJN 2004)[73](Saporta Neuroscience 1999)[74](Raval AJCD 2008)[75]. However ischemic pain is difficult to model and measure behaviorally in animals (Chen MP 2007) [76] (Qin CNR 2009) [77] (Li PR 2008) [78].

A variety of pain models have been developed that use an injury to a peripheral nerve, such as the sciatic nerve, to produce temporary or permanent behavioral hypersensitivity, such as tactile allodynia (non-noxious stimulus) or thermal hyperalgesia (a noxious stimulus). This hypersensitivity develops over several days after the injury and can lead to chronic pain (Zimmerman EJP 2001) [79]. Such behaviors are easily measured in a quantitative fashion with a Hargreaves device (Hargreaves Pain 1988) [80] for thermal hyperalgesia, or an automated von Frey device for tactile allodynia (Chaplan JNM 1994) [81]. When the injury is to the sciatic nerve, the animal=s hindpaw is used for these behavioral tests. Often contralateral paws are tested as the control for unilateral injury, but the inherent assumption for this approach is that spinal or supraspinal mechanisms are not globally affected by a unilateral injury, which is often not based experimentally. Complete transection of a peripheral nerve, such as the sciatic, invariably leads to tactile allodynia and thermal hyperalgesia, as well as autotomy, excessive self-grooming that leads to bite wounds and self-amputation of digits. Even with some controversy, which questions whether autotomy behavior is a sign of pain, excessive grooming and autotomy following a nerve lesion are now considered to reflect neuropathic pain following a nerve lesion. Both autotomy and vocalization behaviors are considered signs of severe pain following nerve deafferentation and were used commonly in the earliest studies of these injuries (Bennett Pain 1988) [82] (Wall Pain 1979) [83]. Partial nerve injuries, such as unilateral loose ligation, or chronic constriction injury (CCI) of the sciatic nerve results in the animal persistently holding the ipsilateral hindpaw in a guarded position. Depending on the tightness of ligation, the allodynia and hyperalgesia can resolve in about 8 weeks, or persist for many months. Bennett originally reported that this model likely involved the presence of spontaneous pain, since appetite was suppressed, along with the frequent occurrence of spontaneous nocifensive behaviors, but such non-evoked behaviors are neither common nor easily measurable. This model has been used in a great number (>400) and variety of studies since its first description: (1) to examine the development of spinal and supraspinal sensitization following CCI (Kontinen AA 2002) [84] (Aley Neuroscience 2002) [85] (Danziger Pain 2001) [86] (Novakovic JN 1998) [87]; (2) elucidate its genetic basis (Kim BRMBR 2002) [88] (Kim Neuroreport 2001) [89] (Dai Pain 2001) [90] (Draisci BR 1991) [91]; and (3) to examine a number of potential therapeutic interventions (Eaton JPNS 2000) [92] (Cejas Pain 2000) [93] (Eaton GT 2002) [94] for the partial nerve-injury related pain.

Three recent nerve injury models reproduce the development of certain types of neuropathic pain in humans: diabetic neuropathy (streptozotocin (STZ)-induced diabetes (Courteix Pain 1994) [95]), chemotherapy-induced neuropathy (Bhagra COR 2007) [96] and oncology-related immuno-therapy (anti-ganglioside (GD2) antibody (Slart Pain 1997) [97]). STZ is able to induce diabetes mellitus in experimental animals through its toxic effects on pancreatic beta cells, where a single dose (50 mg/kg, i.p) leads to the development of allodynia with 10 days (Field Pain 1999) [98]. Mechanical allodynia is the mostly commonly reported outcome to STZ injections, and this model for painful diabetic neuropathy has been used to examine effectiveness of analgesics, such as morphine (Courteix Pain 1994) [95], as well as for the elucidation of cellular mechanisms involved (Aley Neuroscience 2002) [85].

The clinical presentation of chronic central pain, especially after spinal cord injury (SCI), is common but under-reported, especially among SCI persons, and chronic central neuropathic pain has proven difficult to treat. In animal models of central pain that depend on evoked nociception after SCI, allodynia and hyperalgesia are dependent on direct observation and measurement of nocifensive behaviors such as withdrawal of a stimulated limb or tail. However, in humans, especially those with below-level pain after complete spinal transection, there can be a dissociation between reported chronic pain and elicited nociception (Bowsher JNNP 1996) [99], so animal models which use limb withdrawal to tactile or thermal stimuli must be interpreted with caution (Vierck Pain 2000) [100]. As reported in humans after SCI, abnormal sensations and dysthesias are common features (Putke SC 2002) [101] of pain, and in animal models of central pain overgrooming and/or autotomy reflects the presence of abnormal sensations, and is regarded as an indication of dysthesia/pain (Vierck Pain 2000)[100](Widerstrom-Noga CJP 2003) [102]. Recent and commonly evaluated regeneration models of SCI, namely weight-drop contusion and complete transection are relatively difficult to use for the study of behavioral hypersensitivity, such as allodynia and hyperalgesia, given the variability in outcomes, unless the lesion is extensive, in the case on contusive SCI. However, contusion injury and central cord lesions have been demonstrated to induce lowered thresholds for nocifensive behavior with stimulation of at-level dermatomes and tactile allodynia in skin responses (Hubscher JN 1999) [103] (Lindsey NNR 2000) [104], and in a few cases use of paw withdrawal responses or vocalization to paw pressure in a moderate contusion (Siddall NR 1995) [105]

(Hulsebosch JN 2000) [106]. A useful model of neuropathic pain following SCI is the recently described focal chemical lesion of the cord following injection of a glutamate receptor agonist (Yezierski JN 1993) [107] (Yezierski Pain 1998) [108]. This model not only allows for quantitative assessment of behavioral hypersensitivity after injury but, with focused spinal microinjections of the excitotoxic agent, also permits an investigation of the cellular mechanisms in the cord that might be associated with the onset of pain. As well, this excitotoxic SCI pain model has been used to evaluate the effects of cell transplantation of primary adrenal chromaffin tissue to reverse the chronic behavioral allodynia and hyperalgesia (Brewer BR 1998) [109] that chemical lesioning of the dorsal horn pain processing centers produces. The model makes use of intraspinal injection of the glutamate receptor agonist, quisqualic acid (QUIS) just above the lumbar segments which control sensory function in the hindlimbs, which leads to predictable and quantifiable temporal profile of pain behaviors, without the complications of a loss in motor systems, paralysis, or loss of bowel and bladder function. Typical with this model is tactile allodynia and thermal hyperalgesia, with the development of progressive, severe grooming behaviors in the dermatomes associated with the QUIS injection. Most animals require euthanasia within 30 days of the lesion. However, as with this model, the spread of secondary injury over time to spinal segments rostral and caudal to the injury site is critical to the nature and distribution of SCI pain (Yezierski PBR 2000) [110]. With the addition of kaolin to QUIS injections, this is also a reproducible model for progressive syringomyelia and pain after SCI (Yang Spine 2001) [111], where arachnoiditis is also a feature.

Lesions of the anterolateral column in monkeys and rats results in overgrooming and autotomy caudal to the lesion (Levitt Pain 1981) [112] (Ovelmen-Levitt SFN 1995) [113], with deafferentation of rostral targets and interruption of the spinolthalamic tract important to the development of below-level neuropathic pain in humans. Transection of a single antereolateral quadrant reliably results in contralateral hypoalgesia, but some patients develop contralateral and ipsilateral dysesthesias and pain or allodynia and hyperalgesia (Vierck AE 2000) [114]. A similar animal model, with T13 unilateral spinal hemisection, rats develop bilateral tactile allodynia in both forelimb and hindlimbs (Christensen JN 1997) [115], with evidence for bilateral spinal reorganization (Christensen EN 1997) [116] following injury. Dorsal column interruption may also contribute to below-level pain that develops after SCI in humans (Nathan Brain 1986) [117], with allodynia and hyperalgesia seen after stimulation caudal and ipsilateral to dorsolateral column lesions in monkeys (Vierck NYP 1986) [118]. Animal models have contributed much to the understanding of the mechanisms of pain in humans and current clinical treatments are based, in part, on those studies. But the future of effective strategies, such as stem/progenitor regenerative therapies, requires the use of these models to screen novel, safe and useful approaches in a pre-clinical setting.

STEM/PROGENITOR CELLS FOR THERAPEUTIC INTERVENTION

An increasing number of articles describing regenerative methods to improve function after injury and in certain disease states have appeared in the last few years. Most are related to transplants with stem cells, progenitors, and bone marrow and nontransplants. Stem cell transplants can be ranked in the following descending order of preference; bone marrow-derived cells, neural stem cells, human umbilical cord blood cells, embryonic stem cells, and myoblasts. Bone marrow derived cells and human umbilical cord blood cell have been used for various disease fields. The non-stem cell transplantation group is made up primarily of islet cells, followed by biomaterials, and other cells or tissues from a variety of source (Park MSM 2008) [119]. With their more limited multipotency, the use and potential of progenitor cells for improving function has still made significant progress recently (Kozlova MBM 2009) [120] (Goligorsky Nephrology 2009) [121], especially in the potential for renal and cardiac regeneration and reduction of ischemia (Stamm TACD 2009) [122] (Jevon CP 2008) [123]. But another critical potential to be fulfilled is in the area of the management of chronic, and especially neuropathic, pain.

STEM/PROGENITOR CELLS FOR PAIN

Regenerative approaches to treat pain is a very new field, but built on multiple decades of cell therapy studies (Hentall PBR 2000) [124] using primary tissues (Sagen JN 1993) [125], cells (Decosterd Pain 1998) [126], and more recently animal cell lines (Takahashi Peptides 1995) [127] as the sources for a graft source. Such earlier approaches have provided considerable information that can apply to development of stem/progenitor sources and their application in clinical studies. First is the understanding that current pharmacological therapies are often ineffective over time for a great number of patients. Although there are a variety of useful surgical and pharmacologic interventions (including electric stimulation, implantable mechanical pumps and a myriad of drugs for pain relief) cell and molecular technologies represent a new frontier in pain medicine and are worth pursuing, even with the considerable expense required to develop new strategies. Second, the cellular phenotype of grafts required to treat pain is apparently very specific, based on the current understanding of the antinociceptive agents that might work in the myriad models of pain, namely opioids (Takahashi Peptides 1995)[127](Breivik AAS 2001) [128], spinal inhibitory neurotransmitters such as γ-aminobutyric acid (GABA) or galanin (Eaton JPNS 1999) [129] (Eaton CT 1999) [130] (Stubley JN 2001) [131], the sensory-modulating neurotransmitter 5HT (Eaton Pain 1997) [132] (Hains EN 2001) [133] (Hains Neuroscience 2003) [134] (Hains BR 2001) [135], neurotrophins such as BDNF (Cejas Pain 2000) [93] (Eaton GT 2002) [94], or peptides that reduce central sensitization (Siegan Neuroreport 1997) [136] (Gajavelli CT 2008) [137] (Hama Neuropharmacology 2009) [138], or their combination (Hama BR 2006) [139] in the same treatment paradigm. Thirdly, some sort of naturally- or agent-disimmortalizable human cell line would eventually be necessary, given the heterogeneity or inherent dangers associated with primary tissue sources. The disimmortalization strategy, using molecular excision of the immortalizing sequence (Eaton EN 2002) [140], has been modeled in disimmortalizable chromaffin cell lines (Eaton JCB 2000) [141] (Eaton IRPCAARU 2007) [142] for pain, but such an approach has proven too cumbersome for clinical use. Whatever final, and practical, clinical strategy such cell therapy may manifest, it will likely involve these principles.

STEM/PROGENITOR CELLS FOR PAIN IN ANIMAL STUDIES

In a recent report (Lin CT 2002) [143] utilizing the partial nerve injury with CCI to induce neuropathic pain, rat spinal embryonic progenitor cells (SPC) that used basic fibroblast growth factor-2 (FGF-2) for proliferation of the SPC *in vitro* were able to reduce thermal hyperalgesia after intrathecal transplant. Presumably, grafted cells had been induced to a GABAergic phenotype by FGF-2 *in vitro* and survived in its absence after transplant, maintaining their phenotype to modulate the neuropathic pain. The authors suggest that the grafts also increased the glycine content in the CSF of grafted animals, suggesting that if precursors could be induced to a phenotype that provides nociceptive inhibition, they would function much like cell minipumps, surviving in the intrathecal space. Also in the CCI model of peripheral pain, freshly isolated syngeneic marrow mononuclear cells were injected i.v. following the unilateral nerve injury and tactile allodynia and thermal hyperalgesia evaluated weekly. Marrow transplantation did not prevent pain, and 5 days after CCI all animals were equivalently lesioned. However, 10 days after CCI, rats that received marrow transplants demonstrated paw withdrawal response and paw withdrawal latency patterns indicating recovery from pain, whereas untreated rats continued to have significant pain behavior patterns. The mechanisms underlying this improvement following bone marrow injection are unknown. The authors speculate that the marrow cells functioned as anti-inflammatory, neuroprotective, and proangiogenic, modulating ischemic, inflammatory, and cytotoxic events in the pain that follows nerve constriction in this model. However, marrow transplants are also known to exacerbate diabetic neuropathy in a different model of pain (Terashima PNASUSA. 2005) [144]. In this case, marrow cells fused with peripheral neurons, stimulating apoptosis.

One cause of severe neuropathic pain is traumatic injury that involves SCI is spinal root avulsion, and replacement of DRG neurons could reduce that pain. A recent study investigated whether human neural stem/progenitor cells (hNSPCs) transplanted to the DRG cavity can serve as a source for repairing lost peripheral sensory connections (Akesson CT 2008) [145]. The hNSPCs robustly differentiate to neurons, which survive long-term transplantation. The neuronal population in the transplants was tightly surrounded by astrocytes, suggesting their active role in neuron survival. Furthermore, 3 months after grafting hNSPCs were found in the dorsal root transitional zone (DRTZ) and within the spinal cord. The level of differentiation of transplanted cells was high in the core of the transplants whereas cells that migrated to the DRTZ and spinal cord were undifferentiated, nestin-expressing precursors. However, hNSPCs are not sufficient to restore normal sensory function; additional factors are required to guide their differentiation to the desired type of neurons.

Another approach to pain reduction with regenerative methods is in the low back pain model, or intervertebral disc replacement (Hiyama CMB 2008) [146]. Because disc disease progenitor cells exist in degenerate human discs is accompanied by a loss of cells, there is considerable interest in regeneration of cells of both the annulus fibrosus (AF) and nucleus pulposus (NP). Apparently, progenitor cells exist in degenerate human discs (Risbud Spine 2007) [147], a result confirmed in degenerate discs extracted from rats. Cells isolated from degenerate human tissues expressed CD105, CD166, CD63, CD49a, CD90, CD73, p75 low affinity nerve growth factor receptor, and CD133/1, proteins that are characteristic of marrow mesenchymal stem cells. This suggests that these endogenous progenitors might be used to repair the intervertebral disc and ultimately reduce low back pain. In another study, human bone-marrow derived CD34(+) (hematopoietic progenitor cells) and CD34(-) (nonhematopoietic progenitor cells, including mesenchymal stem cells) cells were isolated, fluorescent-labeled, and injected into rat coccygeal discs. Only the CD34(-) cells survived and differentiated within the relative immune privileged the relative immune privileged nucleus pulposus of intervertebral disc degeneration in this rat disc degeneration model (Wei JOR 2009) [148]. Olfactory cells, adult tissue-derived stem cell derived from the olfactory mucosa, may be another useful source for disc repair (Murrell SJ 2009) [149], if they can differentiate into a nucleus pulposus chondrocyte phenotype *in vivo* after transplantation into the injured intervertebral The donor-derived cells expressing CT2 and CSPG markers, specific for the nucleus pulposus chondrocyte phenotype, was achieved in after delivery to the nucleus pulposus region of rats whose discs had previously been lesioned before transplant, suggesting their potential for relief of human disc regeneration and back pain relief.

STEM/PROGENITOR CELLS FOR PAIN IN CLINICAL STUDIES

If ischemia can be considered to be significant cause of pain in humans, use of stem/progenitor cells to indirectly relieve pain is another area for consideration (Li NL 2009) [150], although the optimal cell type, dose, delivery mode, and target patient population has not been defined. Reduced migratory function of circulating angiogenic progenitor cells (CPCs) with impaired neovascularization in patients with cardiovascular disease has been associated with reduced homing of circulating CPCs and the involvement of the kinin B2 receptor (B(2)R) in the recruitment of CPCs to sites of ischemia and in their proangiogenic action. In mice, blood mononuclear cells (MNCs) from syngenic B(2)R-deficient mice resulted in reduced homing of sca-1(+) and cKit(+)flk1(+) progenitors to ischemic muscles, impaired reparative neovascularization, and delayed perfusion recovery as compared with wild-type MNCs. CPCs from cardiovascular disease patients showed low B(2)R levels and decreased migratory bradykinin-induced migration (Krankel CR 2008) [151]. Autologous transplantation of granulocyte colony-stimulating factor (G-CSF)-mobilized peripheral blood mononuclear cells (PBMNCs) in the treatment of critical limb ischemia (CLI) of diabetic patients had significantly improved angiographic scores in the transplant group and had significantly improved lower limb pain and ulcers (Huang DC 2005) [152]. But G-CSF administration to mobilize these precursors has its own significant side effects (Hilbe BMT 2000) [153] (Bensinger SC 1995) [154], including severe pyogenic infection in healthy donors diagnosed immediately following stem cell mobilization with G-CSF. When G-CSF was given to normal donors for the collection of allogeneic or syngeneic peripheral blood stem cells (PBSCs) side effects included mild-moderate bone pain, edema and mild thrombocytopenia. The incidence of chronic graft-versus-host-disease (GVHD) is approximately 50% in the patient hosts (Bensinger SC 1995) [154]. Bone marrow (BM) or peripheral blood progenitor cell collection (PBPCC) itself is moderately painful (Auquier BMT 1995) [155], further increasing pain and discomfort in the patient receiving chemotherapy. Therapeutic efficacy of stem cell peripheral blood and bone marrow therapy has been associated with restoration of endothelial function, augmentation of microcirculatory blood flow, pain reduction, and significant increase in circulating CD133(+)VEGFR2(+) progenitors, known as cell effectors of angiogenesis, in a small study in with non-healing ischemic ulcers in systemic sclerosis (Nevskaya Rheumatology 2009) [156]. In another small study, seven patients with critical peripheral arterial occlusive disease were treated with an intra-arterial infusion of autologous circulating blood-derived progenitor cells. Pain-free walking distance increased, accompanied by a significant increase in the ankle-brachial index. Transcutaneous O(2), flow-dependent vasodilation, flow reserve in response to adenosine, and endothelium-dependent vasodilation were also observed (Lenk EHJ 2005) [157]. External counter pulsation therapy (ECPT) offers symptomatic relief and improves ischemia in patients with refractory angina pectoris. ECPT is associated with increased number and colony-forming capacity of circulating endothelial progenitor cells, which may be a way of increasing the ischemic reduction potential of these progenitor cells (Barsheshet Cardiology 2008) [158]. Peripheral blood progenitors have also been reported to reduce pain and induce remission in a case of adult-onset Still's disease, which had frequent and recurrent systemic articular flares and loss of some functional abilities, including joint swelling, and morning stiffness (Lanza BMT 2000) [159]. These limited applications suggest pain relief needs a more well-defined approach, modeled in the development of neural progenitors that have been recently developed.

THE NEUROPROGENITOR NT2CELL LINE FOR PAIN

More than two decades ago it was discovered that when treated with retinoic acid (RA), a human embryonal carcinoma cell line, NTera2cl.D/l (NT2), differentiates irreversibly into several morphologically and phenotypically distinct cell types, which include terminally differentiated postmitotic CNS neurons (Andrews LI 1984) [160] (Pleasure JNR 1993) [161]. Successive re-plating of RA-treated NT2 cells, in the presence of growth inhibitors, results in the isolation of purified human neurons (Andrews DB 1984) [162] that have been extensively characterized and tested *in vivo* in a number of animal models of traumatic injury and neurodegenerative disease (Pleasure JNR 1993) [161] (Borlongan EN 1998) [163] (Cheung Neuroreport 1996) [164] (Ferrare FEBSL 2000) [165] (Guillemain JCN 2000) [166] (Satoh JNM 2000) [167]. This NT2 human neural cell line has been used for a variety of studies that reveal not only the regulation of an neuronal phenotype by agents such as retinoic acid (Andrews DB 1984) [162] (Guillemain JNR 2003) [168] (Dmitrovsky OR 1990) [169], but has been well characterized for the expression of a variety of neural phenotypic properties (Gortz BR 2004) [170] and proteins (Megiorni NL 2005) [171] (Lee JN 1986) [172] with differentiation of the cells *in vitro* and *in vivo* (Daadi BRB 2001) [173]. The potential application of NT2 neurons in cell transplantation therapy for CNS disorders, and their use as vehicles for delivering exogenous proteins into the human brain for gene therapy, has been envisioned (Trojanowski EN 1997) [174]. Such NT2 neurons have been used in Phase I clinical trials for the treatment of stroke (Kondziolka Neurology 2000) [175] (Nelson AJP 2002) [176] (Meltzer Neurosurgery 2001) [177], and this cell line or its derivatives can likely be utilized for further reparative transplant strategies. The rate-limiting enzyme GAD, for GABA synthesis is present in differentiating NT2 neurons *in vitro* (Yoshioka BR 1997) [178] (Podrygajlo CTR 2009) [179], and GABA is one the phenotypes for NT2 cells differentiated and transplanted *in vivo* (Saporta BRB 2000) [180]. But the NT2 cell line has a great variety of phenotypes expressed in differentiated cells (Guillemain JCN 2000) [166] (Podrygajlo CTR 2009) [179], making it a less-than-ideal cell line for the specific antinociceptive phenotype expression that might be required for application in pain management. While induction of a GABAergic phenotype in neural stem cells is possible with a somewhat complicated method of sequential exposure to epigenetic signals *in vitro* (Bosch EN 2004) [181], the host graft environment does not always allow for induction of desirable phenotypes *in vivo* (Cao EN 2002) [182]. A stable, naturally-occurring, antinociceptive phenotype, such as GABA or 5HT, in a clinically useful human progenitor cell line, such as that derived from the NT2 cell line, is more desirable.

NT2-DERIVED CELL LINES FOR PAIN

Since the NT2 cell line contains a mixed phenotype population of cells, many of which would likely be antinociceptive based on multiple studies with rat cell lines, by this author and others in both central and peripheral models of neuropathic pain (Cejas Pain 2000) [93] (Eaton JPNS 1999) [129] (Eaton CT 1999) [130] (Eaton Pain 1997) [132] (Hains EN 2001) [133] (Hains Neuroscience 2003) [134] (Hains BR 2001) [135] (Duplan NL 2004) [183] (Hains NL 2002) [184], it was considered likely that individual cell lines could be subcloned from the NT2 parental cell line. Using ordinary subcloning techniques involving isolation of individual cells plated sparsely, allowing them to grow into colonies, surrounding these with cloning rings, and removing these colonies, individual cell lines were established. This rather laborious process resulted in a number of morphologically and immunohistochemically-distinct NT2 subclonal cell lines, numbered consecutively as they were isolated. Two of the cell lines were chosen for their potential to function as sources of neurotransmitters which might prove useful in further testing in animal models of pain, the hNT2.17 and hNT2.19 cell lines. Since they are derived from the neuroprogenitor parent cell line NT2, these are considered to be human neuroprogenitor cell lines, as well, resulting in a neuronal-limited phenotype, and will be described below. These human progenitor cell lines are being developed for clinical use. Their characterization, and use in animal models reflect what will be required of any similar regenerative cell therapy for FDA approval to treat pain (Sagen JRRD 2003) [14].

THE HNT2.17 CELL LINE FOR PAIN

Characterization and use of differentiated hNT2.17 was first described (Eaton JP 2007) [185] in a SCI model of behavioral hypersensitivity with tactile allodynia and thermal hyperalgesia, behaviors that model the painful allodynia and hyperalgesia reported by SCI patients with neuropathic pain (Felix JRRD 2009) [186]. Quantitative sensory testing, modeled in rat studies of SCI pain, is a reliable and valid adjunct measurement strategy for quantifying the neurological dysfunction associated with neuropathic pain in persons with SCI (Felix JRRD 2009)

[186]. The animal model used to measure SCI pain associated with the first descriptions of lumbar subarachnoid grafts of hNT2.17 cells (Eaton JP 2007) [185] (Eaton THPI 2007) [187] (Wolfe NL 2007) [188] (Wolfe CN 2007) [189] (Eaton JRRD 2009) [190] is excitotoxic SCI after spinal injection of the glutamate agonist quisqualic acid (QUIS), and has many advantages over other commonly-used SCI models, such as weight-drop contusion, clip-compression, focal-laser, or dorsal hemisection. These advantages include: (1) there is no effect of the spinal injection on motor behaviors, which is especially important when sensory evoked-responses are used as an outcome; (2) the excitotoxic SCI pain model has been used to evaluate the effects of cell transplantation to reverse the chronic behavioral allodynia and hyperalgesia (Yezierski Pain 1998) [108] that chemical lesioning of the dorsal horn pain processing centers produces; (3) there are no apparent complications of paralysis, or loss of bowel and bladder function (Yezierski JN 1993) [107]; (4) this is also a reproducible model for progressive syringomyelia and pain after SCI (Yang Spine 2001) [111]; and (5) the spread of secondary injury over time to spinal segments rostral and caudal to the injury site is critical to the nature and distribution of SCI pain (Yezierski PBR 2000) [110]. In our hands, the tactile allodynia and thermal hyperalgesia that results from QUIS injection are not only reproducible but permanent for at least three months after SCI.

An important first step in developing this cell line for clinical use is immunohistochemical and biochemical characterization. The rapid aggregation method (Cheung BT 1999) [191] was used for the preparation of cultures of differentiated hNT2.17 cells *in vitro* for characterization and transplant. The hNT2.17 cells are initially proliferated in culture, then exposed to retinoic acid (RA) and mitotic inhibitors for three weeks, before replating for a further two weeks of differentiation, in a standard tissue culture media without RA or inhibitors (Eaton JP 2007) [185]. During these last two weeks, and any point beyond, they are exclusively neuronal (Fig. **1**) and stain brightly for GABA and glycine (Fig. **2**), the two major inhibitory neurotransmitters of the spinal cord.

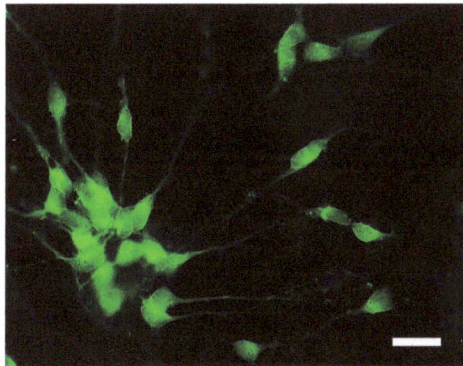

Figure 1: The neural marker neuron-specific enolase (NSE) in differentiated hNT2.17 cells.

The hNT2.17 cell line was treated for two weeks with retinoic acid and mitotic inhibitors and lifted to substrate-coated 8 well plastic TC slides for differentiation and immunohistochemistry for neuron-specific markers. As soon as 4 days *in vitro*, a variety of neural markers appeared, including human neuron-specific enolase (hNSE), this remained strong until at least 6 weeks of differentiation. Magnification bar= 20 μm.

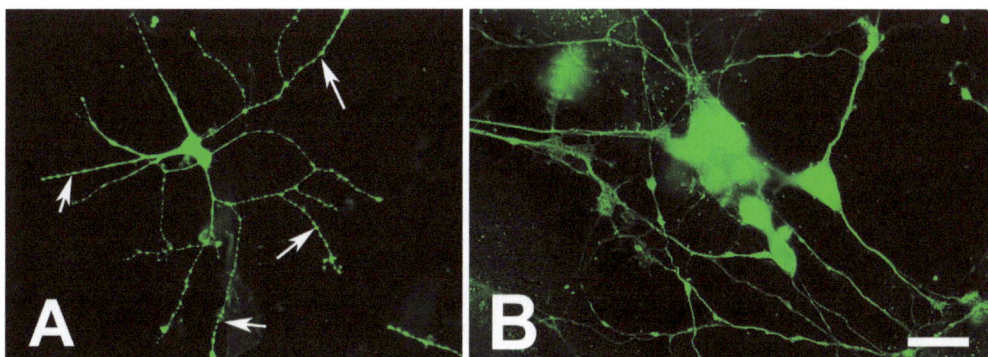

Figure 2: GABA and glycine in differentiated hNT2.17 cells.

The hNT2.17 cell line was treated for two weeks with retinoic acid and mitotic inhibitors and lifted to substrate-coated 8 well plastic TC slides for differentiation and immunohistochemistry for GABA and glycine. All the hNT2.17 cells stain very brightly for the inhibitory neurotransmitter GABA (A). Both the cell soma and extending fibers contain a strong GABA signal. As the fibers extend during differentiation, the fiber GABA signal becomes concentrated, punctate-like, in bouton-like structures, as early as 2 wks *in vitro* (A, arrows). Early in the differentiation period (B, 4 days of differentiation) and for at least 6 wks, all the hNT2.17 cells stain increasingly bright for the inhibitory neurotransmitter glycine. Both the cell soma and extending fibers contain a strong glycine signal. Like the GABA signal, as the fibers extend during differentiation, the glycine signal becomes concentrated, punctate-like, in bouton-like structures. Magnification bar= 20 μm.

When cells have been differentiated for two weeks in culture, they synthesize, secrete, and release measurable quantities of both GABA and glycine (Fig. **3**), examined with HPLC methods (Eaton JP 2007) [185].

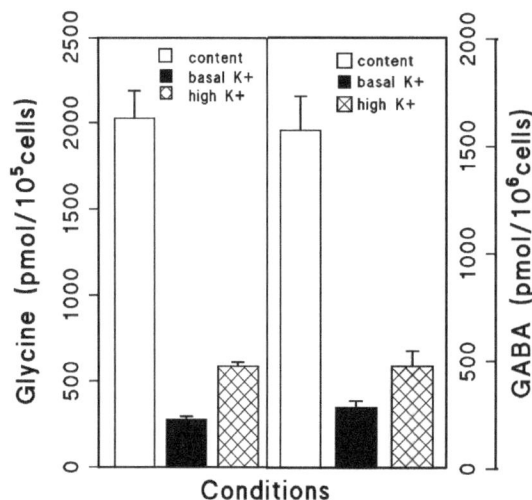

Figure 3: HPLC GABA and glycine content (synthesis), secretion and release in hNT2.17 cells *in vitro.*

The hNT2.17 cell line was differentiated, after RA and mitotic inhibitor treatment, for two weeks in 6-well substrate-coated plates before cell lysis and examination of cell content for glycine or GABA by HPLC methods. For glycine or GABA secretion (basal) and release (stimulated), sister cultures of the hNT2.17 cells were differentiated for two weeks before cells were exposed to basal (2.95 mM) or high (100mM) concentrations of KCl for potassium (K+)-stimulated release for glycine or GABA. Data represent the mean +/- SEM from 3-4 samples from 4 independent experiments for each neurotransmitter.

This inhibitory phenotype continues in 100% of grafted hNT2.17 cells, for at least two months after transplant in the QUIS model (Eaton JP 2007) [185]. It is likely that GABA and glycine are stored and released from the same vesicular compartment in the cells, since differentiated hNT2.17 cells co-localize GABA and glycine (Eaton JP 2007) [185] (Eaton JRRD 2009) [190] and express the vesicular inhibitory amino acid transporter VIATT. GABA, glycine, and VIATT are concentrated in bouton-like structures along the extended processes of the cells, suggesting mature synaptic elements in differentiated cells. In addition, the immunohistochemical signal for the neuronal glycine transporter, GlyT2 is present early after differentiation and the signal remains intense throughout differentiation. No other significant neurotransmitter markers have been found by immunohistochemical methods in the hNT2.17 cells during differentiation, such as catecholamine enzymes (tyrosine hyroxylase, dopamine beta-hyroxylase, phenylethanolamine N-methyltransferase); choline acetyltransferase; calcitonin gene-related peptide; substance P; galanin; or 5HT. Neither is there any signal for the NMDA receptor 1 or chromagranin (Eaton JP 2007) [185]. However, hNT2.17 contains low to moderate levels of a vasopressin and oxytocin signal. There also seems to be a low, but apparent signal for the inhibitory opioid peptide met-enkephalin and neuropeptide Y (NPY). These are present after at least 6 wks of differentiation. Met-enkephalin (Duplan NL 2004) [183] and NPY (Hua JPET 1991) [192] are important antinociceptive agents, and may contribute to the antinociceptive effects of grafted differentiated hNT2.17cells.

The question of possible tumorigenicity in the eventual clinical use of any differentiated NT2 cells is relevant to their characterization *in vitro* and *in vivo* (Newman SCD 2005) [193]. The parental NT2 cells are classified as embryonic carcinoma cells because they originate from testicular germ cells and express the same cell-surface antigens during proliferation. Exposure of NT2 (proliferating) cells to RA results in postmitotic hNT2 (or hNT2N) neural cells, which do not form tumors or revert to a neoplastic state with transplantation (Newman SCD 2005) [193] (Trojanowski EN 1993) [194]. When NT2-derived hNT2.17 cells are treated with RA and mitotic inhibitors and differentiated *in vitro*, they cease to express the tumor markers TGF-alpha (transforming growth factor) and FGF-4 (Eaton JP 2007) [185]. Also, bromodeoxyuridine (BrdU) immunostaining has been used as a marker for proliferating cells *in vitro* (Yong JNM 1987) [195] and *in vivo* (Brown JNT 1989) [196], since dividing cells incorporate BrdU-labeled uridine into newly made DNA. Differentiated hNT2.17 neurons cannot incorporate BrDU with differentiation, in contrast to the proliferating hNT2.17 cell line, suggesting that the differentiated hNT2.17 cells do not demonstrate any features of a tumor cell line, much like the NT2N (NT2 neuron) parent. Tumor proteins are abundant in the proliferating hNT2.17 cells, suggesting that only a differentiated hNT2.17 cell would be safe to transplant *in vivo*. The same observations were made with multiple graft studies with the NT2 cell line (Newman SCD 2005) [193], and grafts of non-RA treated NT2 cells can lead to tumors (Miyazono LI 1995) [197] (Hara PN 2008) [198]. Grafting well-differentiated hNT2.17 cells into the CNS does not form tumors; observations obtained from over 7 years of transplant studies with these cells in rats, and support the contention of safety for clinical use for these neuroprogenitors (Kondziolka Neurology 2000) [175]. Initial safety data as support for the eventual clinical graft of the differentiated hNT2.17 cells into the subarachnoid space needs to demonstrate that transplants do not lead to deleterious effects in the host.

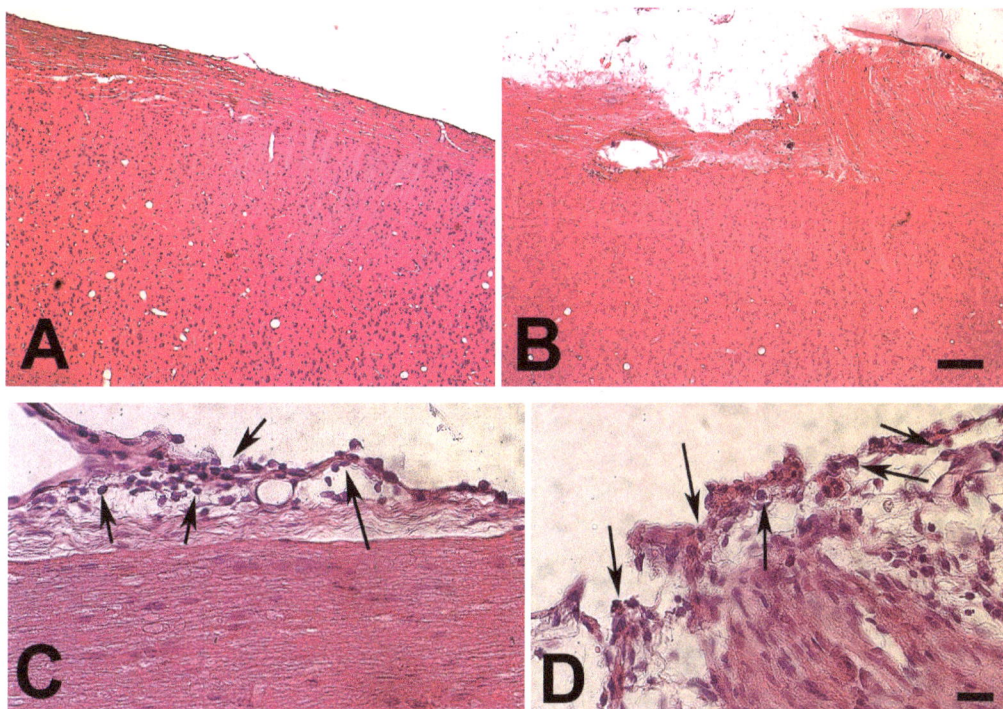

Figure 4: Spinal cord histopathology using hematoxyline/eosin (H&E) staining after transplants of hNT2.17 cells.

Rats were spinally injected with quisqualic acid (QUIS) and spinal cord sections were examined at 60 days after QUIS for evidence of dural tethering and arachnoidal proliferation and surviving hNT2.17 cell line grafts with H&E staining. The hNT2.17 (10^6 cells/injection), which had been differentiated for two weeks *in vitro*, were injected into the subarachnoid space two weeks after the QUIS lesion. All rats received 10 mg/Kg i.p.cyclospoorine A (CsA) at the time points corresponding to one day before and 14 days after cell transplant (daily injections). Spinal cords from naïve animals (A), QUIS-injected (B), naïve plus grafts (C), QUIS plus transplant (D) were visualized. Cell grafts were easily visible in naïve plus grafts (C, arrows) and QUIS plus transplant (D, arrows), but there was no additional cord damage associated with transplants. Magnification bar= 100 μm (A, B); magnification bar= 50 μm (C, D).

Pathologic comparison of the four groups revealed an obvious spinal lesion (Fig. **4**), dural tethering and arachnoidal proliferation in the QUIS injured animals (Fig. **4B**). No other groups (naïve or naïve plus transplant) showed gross dural tethering; however there was moderate microscopic arachnoid proliferation of QUIS plus hNT2.17 (Fig. **4D**) transplant group. There was minimal evidence of this proliferation in the naive plus transplant group at the laminectomy site, seen with H&E staining (Fig. **4C**), indicating safety of intrathecal hNT2.17 cell transplants. Initial safety data as support for the eventual clinical graft of the differentiated hNT2.17 cells into the subarachnoid space needs to demonstrate that transplants do not lead to deleterious effects in the host animal. The hNT2.17 cells were identified on H+E as small round basophilic cells without significant dendritic or axonal processes (Fig. **4C** and **D**). The H+E staining showed no difference between the cytoarchitecture of QUIS and QUIS plus transplant and showed no cord damage in the naive plus transplant cord group, compared to naive. Myelin staining showed significant demyelination in all animals undergoing a QUIS injury that did not improve with hNT2.17 transplants. No demyelination was seen in conjunction with cell grafts, again implying their safety as a graft source.

Aside from the issues of safety and phenotype of hNT2.17 cells, their value and feasibility for clinical use (Eaton JRRD 2009) [190] would be improved by their efficacy in various models of pain. Most reports with these GABA/glycine neuroprogenitors for pain attenuation use the excitotoxic QUIS SCI model of pain (Eaton JP 2007) [185] (Eaton THPI 2007) [187] (Wolfe NL 2007) [188] (Wolfe CN 2007) [189] (Eaton JRRD 2009) [190]. We have collected data in our laboratories, and with collaborators, that hNT2.17 grafts also attenuate pain in severe SCI contusion, unilateral chronic constriction injury (CCI) of the sciatic nerve and the STZ diabetic neuropathy model of pain. In the QUIS model, a complete examination of factors (Eaton JRRD 2009)[190] that influence attenuation of tactile allodynia and thermal hyperalgesia demonstrated that one week after lumbar transplant of these cells, behavioral hypersensitivity was permanently reversed. These antinociceptive hNT2.17 cell grafts demonstrated complete reversal of allodynia and hyperalgesia when transplanted acutely, but even showed significant improvement in pain-like behaviors when transplanted in a chronic injury. Maximal efficacy required a minimal course of cyclosporine A for immunosuppression two weeks after transplant for durable reversal of pain like behaviors. Grafts did not necessarily need to be placed near the SCI level to be effective; cervical graft location was as effective as lumbar placement. In addition, the transplantation of hNT2.17 cells demonstrated a dose-response effect, where a dose of 10^6 cells (or approximately 3 million/kg) potently and permanently reversed both tactile allodynia and thermal hyperalgesia within one week of transplant. Reduced graft doses did not permanently reverse behavioral hypersensitivity, suggesting that there is an optimal dose that can be used as clinically to treat SCI-associated neuropathic pain (Wolfe NL 2007)[188]. Significantly, hNT2.17 grafts also reduced spontaneous neuropathic pain, which manifests as excessive grooming or autophagia in this model (Eaton JRRD 2009) [190].

When used in the CCI model of peripheral nerve injury (Fig. **5**), hNT2.17 grafts reverse both tactile allodynia and thermal hyperalgesia, similar to the attenuation seen in the QUIS SCI model.

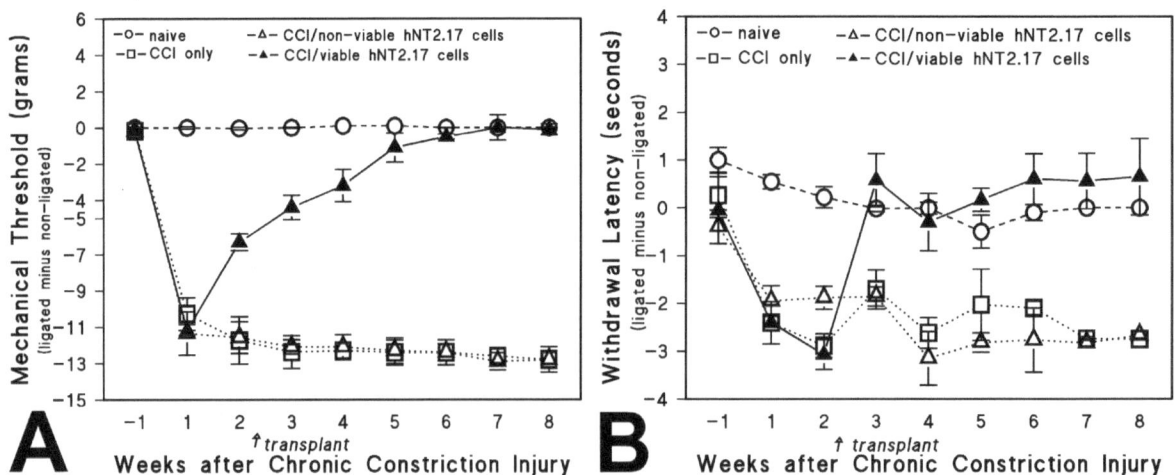

Figure 5: Attenuation of tactile allodynia and thermal hyperalgesia with transplant of hNT2.17 cells in the CCI model of pain.

Tactile allodynia (A) and thermal hyperalgesia (B) behaviors were examined for both a baseline period before unilateral chronic constriction injury (CCI) of the sciatic nerve and for 56 days following CCI. Animals were either left unoperated (naive), received the CCI, or transplanted with viable hNT2.17 or non-viable hNT2.17 cells two weeks following the CCI. Non-viable cells were prepared by suspension of the cells in water, centrifugation, and re-suspension in buffer before transplant. All rats received 10 mg/Kg i.p.CsA at the time points corresponding to one day before and 14 days after cell transplant (daily injections). Animals were tested for hindpaw withdrawal in to tactile (A) and thermal (B) stimuli for one week before and eight weeks following CCI and before and after transplants. The data reported are the mean +/- SEM of the difference values for ligated paw minus the sham-operated paw of 14 animals in each group. Only viable lumbar subarachnoid grafts ($1X10^6$ hNT2.17 cells) recovered normal behavioral responses following unilateral CCI of the sciatic nerve, compared to non-viable grafts or injury alone.

Similar results are seen when the hNT2.17 grafts are placed early after streptozotocin (STZ) -injection (Fig. **6**) in the diabetic neuropathy pain model.

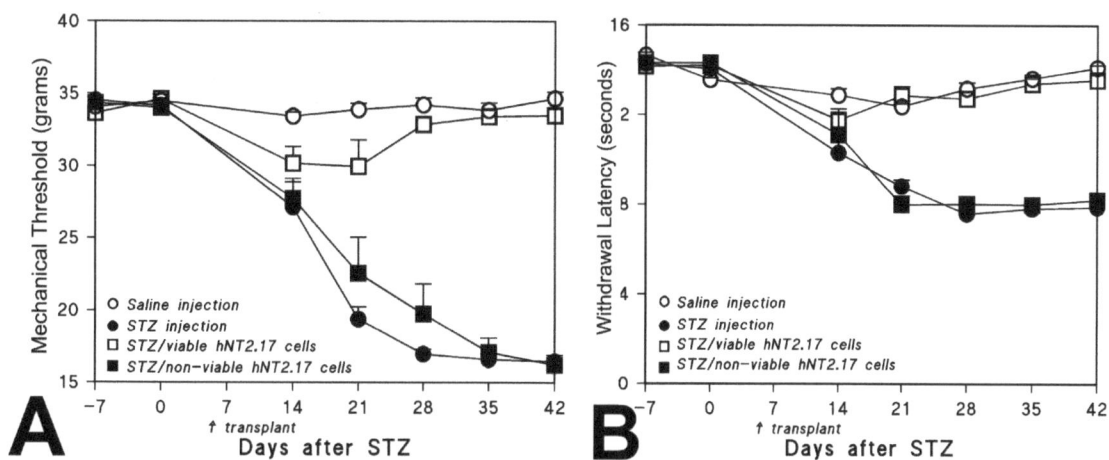

Figure 6: Attenuation of tactile allodynia and thermal hyperalgesia with transplant of hNT2.17 cells in the diabetic peripheral neuropathy (DPN) model of pain.

Tactile allodynia (A) and thermal hyperalgesia (B) behaviors were examined for both a baseline period before streptozotocin (STZ) injection and for 42 days following STZ. Two groups of STZ-injected rats were transplanted with either $1X10^6$ hNT2.17 viable or non-viable cells at 5 days following STZ, a time when the behavioral hypersensitivity to non-noxious tactile stimulation or noxious thermal stimulation was already apparent in the rats. Non-viable cells were prepared by suspension of the cells in water, centrifugation, and re-suspension in buffer before transplant. All rats received 10 mg/Kg i.p.CsA at the time points corresponding to one day before and 14 days after cell transplant (daily injections). In these three groups (non-transplanted and transplanted), both hindpaws develop (pooled data) increased hypersensitivity, but only the rats with viable hNT2.17 cell grafts recover permanent (near normal) tactile and thermal responses. Saline injected rats never develop tactile allodynia or thermal hyperalgesia and serve as positive controls. The data (mean +/- SEM) is from six rats in each group.

Interestingly, although the STZ-induced behavioral hypersensitivity is reversed by the grafts, hyperglycemia induced by STZ damage is not affected (Fig. **7**), while there is a reversal of the cachexia that is part of the diabetic syndrome (Fig. **8**).

Blood glucose levels were measured before and after a single i.v. injection of STZ (or saline) at 50 mg/Kg for 56 days after injection. As soon as 3 days after STZ, blood glucose increased to a permanent level of >250 mg/dL. Five days after STZ, some rats were transplanted with $1x10^6$ viable or non-viable hNT2.17 cells in the lumbar intrathecal space. Non-viable cells were prepared by suspension of the cells in water, centrifugation, and re-suspension in buffer before transplant. All rats received 10 mg/Kg i.p.CsA at the time points corresponding to one day before and 14 days after cell transplant (daily injections). Transplant of either viable or non-viable hNT2.17 cells had no effect on the increase in blood glucose levels that follows STZ injection. The data (mean +/- SEM) is from six rats in each group.

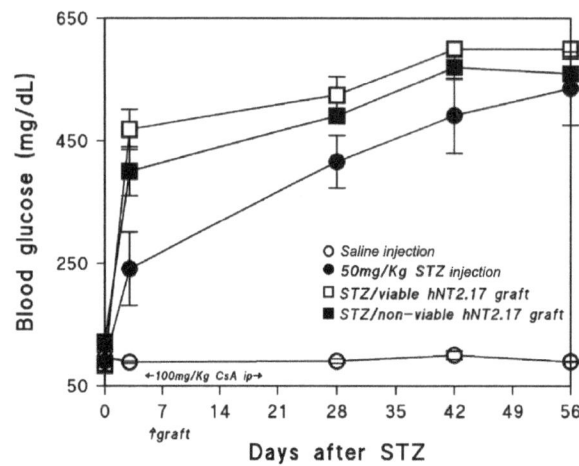

Figure 7: Hyperglycemia in diabetic peripheral neuropathy (DPN) not affected by hNT2.17 grafts.

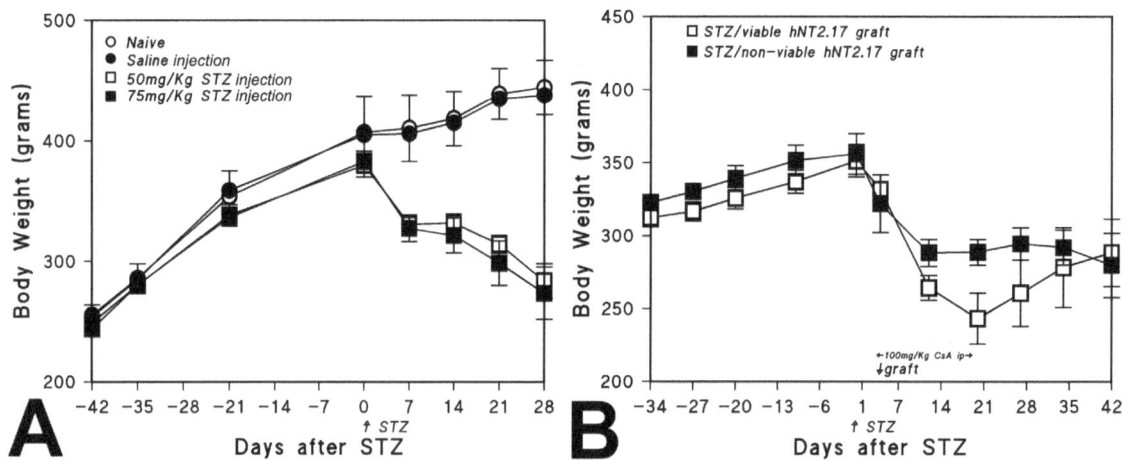

Figure 8: Cachexia in diabetic peripheral neuropathy (DPN) affected by hNT2.17 grafts.

Rats that received a single i.v. injection of STZ (50 or 75 mg/Kg) failed to gain body weight following injection (A), compared to naïve or saline injected rats. Rats that were grafted with 1×10^6 viable hNT2.17 cells in the lumbar intrathecal space 5 days after STZ began to gain body weight by the end of the 42 days period following STZ (B), compared to rats which received non-viable grafts of the same cells. Non-viable cells were prepared by suspension of the cells in water, centrifugation, and re-suspension in buffer before transplant. All rats (A, B) received 10 mg/Kg i.p.CsA at the time points corresponding to one day before and 14 days after cell transplant (daily injections). The data (mean +/- SEM) is from six rats in each group.

How such effects are initiated by hNT2.17 grafts in these models is not clear at this point, but other data suggest that these hNT2.17 grafts recover GABA expression in the spinal dorsal horn laminae I-III with lumbar subarachnoid transplant, much as that seen in the CCI model of pain, as well as reverse behavioral hypersensitivity (Ibuki Neuroscience 1997) [32] (Eaton JCN 1998) [34]. Reversal of the disinhibition that seems to accompany neuropathic pain with an outside source of antinociceptive inhibitory neurotransmitters is possible even with a single intrathecal injection of GABA (Eaton BR 1999) [200], or baclofen, in animal models (Bertman BR 1995) [201] and human pain studies (Herman CJP 1992) [202] (Taira SFN 1995) [203]. Baclofen is commonly used to treat spastcity, but is ineffective for pain at systemically tolerable doses. The use of GABA is impractical due to the short half-life and instability of a neurotransmitter. A cell-based source may prove more practical for pain relief, much as that seen in the clinical studies with chromaffin tissue or cells (Lazorthes ANS 1995) [204] (Lazorthes Pain 2000) [205] for the management of cancer pain. However, compared to primary tissue or cells, stable progenitor cell lines such as the NT2-derived cell lines, have many advantages.

THE HNT2.19 CELL LINE FOR PAIN

The hNT2.19 cell line was derived from the NT2 parent at the same time as the hNT2.17 cell line, but exhibits entirely unique and different characteristics from the inhibitory GABA and glycinergic hNT2.17 line. They are prepared for characterization and transplant by the same rapid aggregation method (Cheung BT 1999) [191], followed by RA and mitotic inhibitors for three weeks, before replating for a further two weeks of differentiation. Like the hNT2.17 they are exclusively neuronal, but express a serotonergic (5HT) phenotype *in vitro* (Fig. **9**).

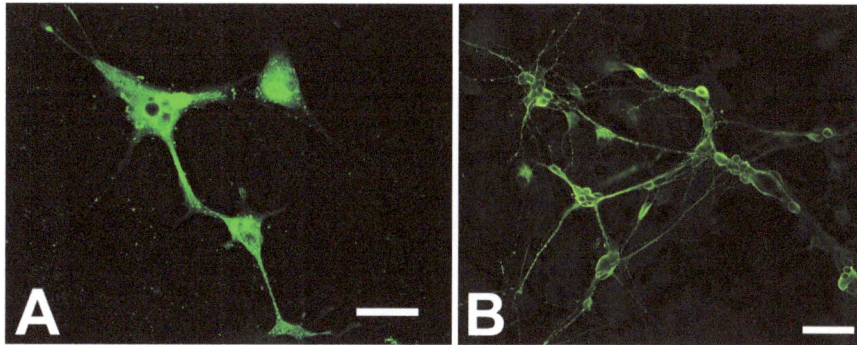

Figure 9: A neuronal serotonergic phenotype expressed by differentiated hNT2.19 cells.

The hNT2.19 cell line was treated for two weeks with retinoic acid and mitotic inhibitors. They were further differentiated for two weeks before an antibody stain for 5HT (A) and the human neuronal marker Tuj1 (B, human β-tubulin 3). The 5HT hNT2.19 cell line labeled for 5HT (A) has a very large nucleus, is generally multipolar, with short neurites and stains brightly for 5HT. The human neuronal marker Tuj1 is found early in all the cells (B, 4 days of differentiation), indicating all the cells human and exclusively neuronal in phenotype. Magnification bar= 10 μm (A); magnification bar= 20 μm (B).

Also, like the hNT2.17 cell line they are non-tumorogenic after differentiation. They are unable to take up BrDU during differentiation, suggesting they have lost the ability to proliferate after RA-induced differentiation (Fig. **10**).

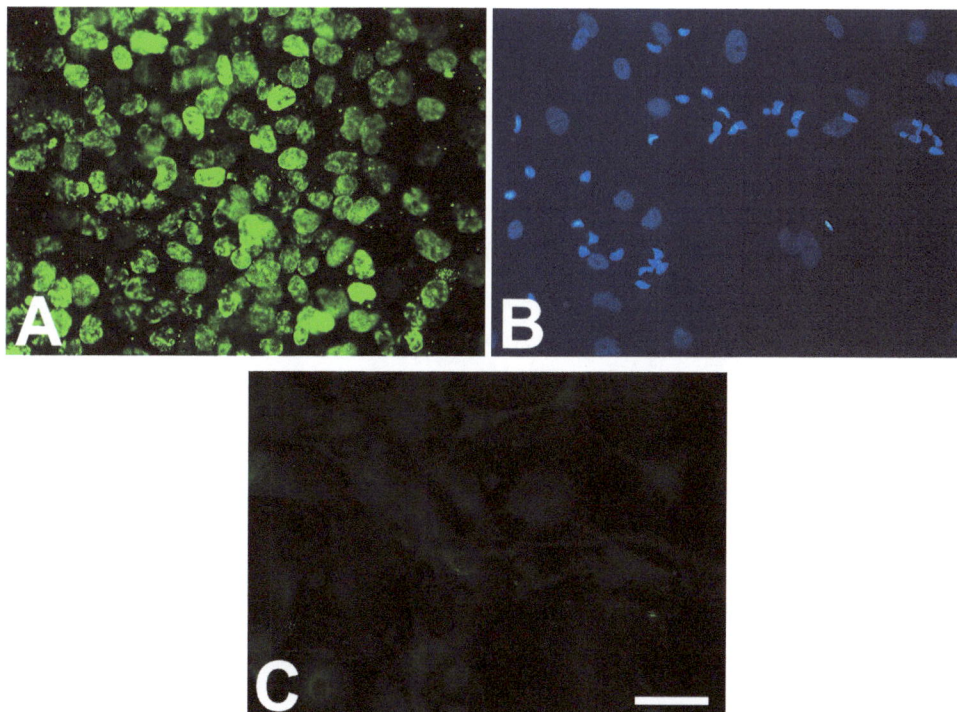

Figure 10: The BrdU, TGF-α, and FGF-4 signals in proliferating versus differentiating hNT2.19 cells invitro.

The hNT2.19 cells were either exposed to 1 uM bromodeoxyuridine (BrdU) during 3 days of proliferation (A) or for 1 week during differentiation (B, C) *in vitro*. With an antibody directed against BrdU to visualize BrdU staining, all proliferating cells incorporate abundant BrdU during proliferation (A). Viable differentiated cells were co-labeled with a DAPI stain (B), while the same field of differentiated cells did not incorporate any BrdU during differentiation (C). After two weeks of retinoic acid and mitotic inhibitors, the hNT2.19 cells cease dividing during differentiation. Magnification bar (D, G) =20 μm; Magnification bar (A) = 50 μm.

All current *in vitro* characterization data suggests they are a sister cell line to the GABAergic hNT2.17 cell line, but express a serotonergic phenotype *in vitro* and *in vivo*. HPLC methods to examine neurotransmitter synthesis, secretion, and release also reveal a serotonergic phenotype in differentiated hNT2.19 cells (Fig. **11**).

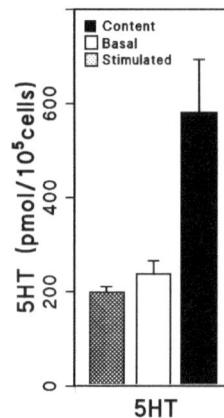

Figure 11: HPLC for serotonin in differentiated hNT2.19 cells.

The hNT2.19 serotonin cells were differentiated for two weeks in culture, following two weeks of exposure to RA and mitotic inhibitors. The cultures were either treated for 10 min with normal KCl buffer (basal), 100mM KCL/release buffer (stimulated), or sister cultures examined for GABA content by standard HPLC methods (content). Data are the mean +/- SEM of 4 replicates from 3 independent experiments. The hNT2.19 5HT cells synthesized, secreted and released measurable 5HT.

Our initial characterization and transplant use of hNT2.19 cells was to demonstrate their potential to improve motor behavioral recovery after severe contusive SCI (Eaton BBR 2008) [206], where the grafts were placed in an intraspinal location dorsal and caudal to the spinal lesion. Earlier studies have demonstrated that 5HT cell therapy requires a lumbar subarachnoid graft site to affect the behavioral hypersensitivity of neuropathic pain after SCI (Hains NL 2002)[184]. Our studies with lumbar subarachnoid grafts of hNT2.19 cells after severe contusion demonstrate potent antinociceptive effects (Fig. **12**).

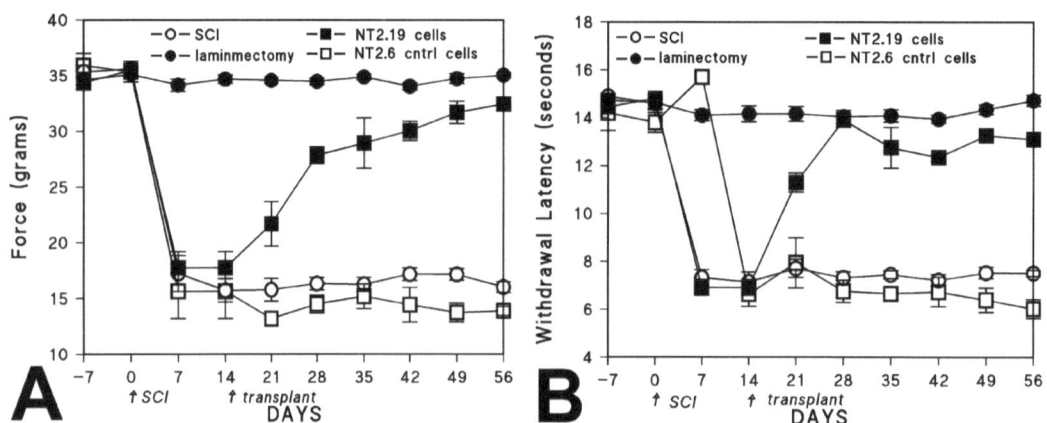

Figure 12: Sensory behaviors after severe contusive SCI and following transplant of hNT2.19 cells *in vivo*.

Rats were spinally impacted (NYU impactor, 25mm weight-drop) in a rat (severe contusion) model of SCI and chronic pain. All animals in the study received CsA (10mgKg) 1 day before and for 2 wks after the two week time-point when some animals were injected with hNT2.19 cells. Animals either left untreated, received the SCI alone or SCI plus laminectomy only or SCI plus viable or non-viable with hNT2.19 cells (10^6 cells/injection) into the subarchnoid space at two weeks after QUIS. Non-viable cells were prepared by suspension of the cells in water, centrifugation, and re-suspension in buffer before transplant. Animals were tested before the SCI (baseline) and once a week following SCI and treatments for hypersensitivity to tactile (A) or thermal (B) stimuli in hindpaws below the SCI. All animals were examined for chronic pain behaviors in the contralateral and ipsilateral hindpaws. Both ipsilateral and contralateral hindpaws recovered near-normal sensory responses to tactile and thermal stimuli after grafting the serotonergic hNT2.19 cells, compared to the SCI alone or transplant of non-viable hNT2.19 cells. SCI negatively affected hindpaw responses bilaterally, but the ipsilateral hindpaw is most affected by the severe contusion (shown here). Neither hindpaw recovers normal tactile or thermal responses after SCI alone or with transplant of non-viable hNT2.19 cells by 60 days after the injection. Data represent the mean value +/- SEM (n= 4-6 animals in each group) at each time point before and 63 days after QUIS. In a subarachnoid location, however, these grafts have no effect on motor dysfunction, suggesting optimal motor and sensory recovery after SCI would require a combination of subarachnoid, as well as intraspinal, grafts of these serotonergic hNT2.19 cells. Additionaly, a multi-modality treatment strategy of cell therapy and rehabilitation would likely improve graft effects (Berrocal JN 2007) [207].

CONCLUSIONS

Cell therapy for pain has a potential that will be fulfilled as other regenerative medicine approaches advance in tandem. The science of progenitor biology is developing rapidly (Wang Biofactors 2009)[208]. But, understanding how to determine and guide a specific progenitor phenotype for the development of useful antinociceptive cells is only a part of the problem. At least two other lines of research must be followed to achieve this goal. First, it needs to be determined exactly which cells or factors are needed to restore sensory function. One possibility is those cells that determine the recovery/regrowth of endogenous sensory fibers, as seen with the pioneering work with human neural stem/progenitor cells that can serve as a source for repairing lost peripheral sensory connections (Akesson CT 2008) [145]. Another possibility is a stem-cell based prosthetic device designed to integrate with nervous tissue (Purcell JNE 2009) [209]. Some of the most promising and effective candidates for inducing anti-nociception, especially neuropathic pain models, seem to be neurotransmitters, such as GABA and 5HT. Both these neurotransmitters which are intergral components of the normally functioning spinal cord sensory and motor systems, and can be administered to the specific and relevant injured areas via progenitor cellular minipumps such as the patented (Eaton USPO 2009)[210] hNT2.17 and hNT2.19 cell lines. Once it is further clarified which components or molecules are of primary importance for reducing nociceptive behaviors, other progenitor sources can be developed, including those from autologous non-embryonic parentage (Gregorian JN 2009)[211].

The second line of inquiry, and perhaps more difficult, is to understand what mechanisms are responsible for inducing pain after the various injuries and diseases involving the nervous system. If indeed most pain is more or less neuropathic in origin, there may be great similarities in the mechanisms of its establishment and perpetuation across diverse neurological injuries and disease states. It is common that some medications approved for one use are often prescribed off-label and provide a use for multiple types of pain. Because human pain, perhaps unlike that tested in animal studies, has a significant psychosocial component and can be significantly altered by social and psychological conditioning (Widerstrom-Noga JRRD 2009)[212](Molton JRRD 2009)[213], future clinical treatments should be interdisciplinary and target not only pathophysiological mechanisms but also psychosocial contributors of pain. Furthermore, no single restorative therapy is likely to work well for the all pain conditions; interventions must be tailored to individual patient requirements. Interestingly, genetic predictors of pain are beginning to be known (Edwards Curr Rheumatol Rep 2006) [214] (Kim JMG 2006) [215] and many answers may lie with genomic and proteonomic approaches, but cell therapy is a reasonable adjunct to other strategies, and will likely be useful components that persist for the foreseeable future as a means to treat pain.

ACKNOWLEDGEMENTS

This material was based on work supported by the Department of Veterans Affairs, Veterans Health Administration, Rehabilitation Research and Development Service (grants B4438I and B4862R); the American

Syringomyelia Alliance Project; the Column of Hope, Chiari and Syringomyelia Research Foundation; and the support of The Miami Project to Cure Paralysis and Department of Neurosurgery, Miller School of Medicine, Miami, Florida.

The authors have declared that no competing interests exist.

REFERENCES

[1] Keller MP, Chance PF. Inherited neuropathies: from gene to disease. Brain Pathol 1999;9:327-341.
[2] Schwartzman RJ, Maleki J. Postinjury neuropathic pain syndromes. Med Clin North Am 1999;83:597-626.
[3] Benbow SJ, Cossins L, MacFarlane IA. Painful diabetic neuropathy Diabet Med 1999;16:632-644.
[4] Koltzenburg M. Painful neuropathies. Curr Opin Neurol 1998;11:515-521.
[5] Bennett GJ. Neuropathic pain: new insights, new interventions. Hosp Prac 1998;33:95-114.
[6] Bowsher D. Pain syndromes and their treatment. Curr Opin Neurol Neurosurg 1993;6:257-263.
[7] Dworkin RH. An overview of neuropathic pain: syndromes, symptoms, signs, and several mechanisms. Clin J Pain 2002;18:343-349.
[8] Yezierski RP. Spinal and supraspinal mechanisms. J Rehabil Res Dev 2009;46(1):95-108.
[9] Siddall PJ, Taylor DA, McClellan JM, *et al.* Pain report and the relationship of pain to physical factors in the first 6 months following spinal cord injury. Pain 1999;81:187-197.
[10] Siddall PJ, McClelland JM, Rutkowski SB, *et al.* A longitudinal study of the prevalence and characteristics of pain in the first 5 years following spinal cord injury. Pain 2003;103:249-257.
[11] Widerstrom-Noga EG, Felipe-Cuervo E, Broton JG, *et al.* Perceived difficulty in dealing with consequences of spinal cord injury. Arch Phys Med Rehabil 1999;80:580-586.
[12] Eaton MJ. Cell therapy for neuropathic pain in spinal cord injuries. Expert Opin Biol Ther 2004;4(12):1861-1869.
[13] Eaton MJ. Cell and molecular approaches to the attenuation of pain after spinal cord injury. J Neurotrauma 2006;23:549-559.
[14] Sagen J. Cellular therapies for spinal cord injury: What will the FDA need to approve moving from the laboratory to the human? J Rehabil Res Dev 2003;40 (Suppl. 1):71-79.
[15] Melzack R, Wall PD. Pain mechanisms: A new theory. Science 1965;150:971-979.
[16] Basbaum AI. Spinal mechanisms of acute and persistent pain. Reg Anes Pain Med 1999;24:59-67.
[17] Campbell JN, Meyer RA. Mechanisms of neuropathic pain. Neuron 2006;52(1):77-92.
[18] Garcia-Larrea L, Magnin M. Pathophysiology of neuropathic pain: review of experimental models and proposed mechanisms. Presse Med 2008;37(2 Pt 2):315-340.
[19] Yezierski RP. Spinal and supraspinal mechanisms. J Rehabil Res Dev 2009;46(1):95-108.
[20] Siddall PJ, Taylor DA, Cousins MJ. Classification of pain following spinal cord injury. Spinal Cord 1997;35:69-75.
[21] Yaksh TL, Hua XY, Kalcheva I, *et al.* The spinal biology in humans and animals of pain states generated by persistent small afferent input. Proc Nat Acad Sci, USA 1999;96:7680-7686.
[22] Abdulla FA, Smith PA. Axotomy- and autotomy-induced changes in the excitability of rat dorsal root ganglion neurons. J Neurophysiol 2001;85(2):630-643.
[23] Suter MR, Papaloïzos M, Berde CB, *et al.* Development of neuropathic pain in the rat spared nerve injury model is not prevented by a peripheral nerve block. Anesthesiology 2004;101(3):806-807.
[24] Li CY, Zhang XL, Matthews EA, *et al.*Calcium channel alpha2delta1 subunit mediates spinal hyperexcitability in pain modulation. Pain 2006;125(1-2):20-34.
[25] Fuchs A, Rigaud M, Sarantopoulos CD, Filip P, Hogan QH. Contribution of calcium channel subtypes to the intracellular calcium signal in sensory neurons: the effect of injury. Anesthesiology 2007;107(1):117-127.
[26] Woolf CJ, Salter MW. Neuronal plasticity: increasing the gain in pain. Science 2000;288:1765-1768.
[27] Yamamoto T, Takahara A. Recent updates of N-type calcium channel blockers with therapeutic potential for neuropathic pain and stroke. Curr Top Med Chem 2009;9(4):377-395.
[28] Schroeder CI, Doering CJ, Zamponi GW, *et al.* N-type calcium channel blockers: novel therapeutics for the treatment of pain. Med Chem 2006;2(5):535-543.
[29] Bayer K , Ahmadi S, Zeilhofer HU. Gabapentin may inhibit synaptic transmission in the mouse spinal cord dorsal horn through a preferential block of P/Q-type Ca2+ channels. Neuropharm 2004;46(5):743-749.
[30] Gilron I. Gabapentin and pregabalin for chronic neuropathic and early postsurgical pain: current evidence and future directions. Curr Opin Anaesthesiol 2007;20(5):456-472.

[31]   Bauer CS, Nieto-Rostro M, Rahman W, *et al*. The increased trafficking of the calcium channel subunit alpha2delta-1 to presynaptic terminals in neuropathic pain is inhibited by the alpha2delta ligand pregabalin. J Neurosci 2009;29(13):4076-4088.

[32]   Ibuki T, Hama AT, Wang X-T, *et al*. Loss of GABA immunoreactivity in the spinal dorsal horn of rats with peripheral nerve injury and promotion of recovery by adrenal medullary grafts. Neuroscience 1997;76:845-858.

[33]   Satoh O, Omote K. Roles of monoaminergic, glycinergic and GABAergic inhibitory systems in the spinal cord in rats with peripheral mononeuropathy. Brain Res 1996;728:27-36.

[34]   Eaton MJ, Plunkett JA, Martinez MA, *et al*. Changes in GAD and GABA immunoreactivity in the spinal dorsal horn after peripheral nerve injury and promotion of recovery by lumbar transplant of immortalized serotonergic neurons. J Chem.Neuroanat 1998;16:57-72.

[35]   Gwak YS, Tan HY, Nam TS, *et al*. Activation of spinal GABA receptors attenuates chronic central neuropathic pain after spinal cord injury. J Neurotrauma 2006;23(7):1111-1124.

[36]   Krenz NR, Weaver LC. Nerve growth factor in glia and inflammatory cells of the injured rat spinal cord. J Neurochem 2000;74:730-739.

[37]   Tsuda M, Inoue K, Salter MW. Neuropathic pain and spinal microglia: a big problem from molecules in "small" glia. Trends Neurosci 2005;28 (2):101-107.

[38]   Murphy PG, Ramer MS, Borthwick L, *et al*. Endogenous interlukin-6 contributes to hypersensitivity to cutaneous stimuli and changes in neuropeptidesw associated with chronic nerve constriction in mice. Eur J Neurosci 1999;11:2243-2253.

[39]   Sommer C. Cytokines in neuropathic pain. Anaesthesist 2001;50:416-426.

[40]   Yamashiro K, Tomiyama N, Ishida A, *et al*. Characteristics of neurons with high-frequency discharge in the central nervous system and their relationship to chronic pain. Experimental and clinical investigations. Stereo Func Neurosurg 1997;68:149-154.

[41]   Zhang LX, Liu ZY. Effects of microiontophoretically applied GABA and 5HT on the electrical activities of neurons in nucleus parafascicularis of thalamus in rats. Acta Physiol Sin 1994;46:226-230.

[42]   Helmchen C, Fu QG, Sandkuhler J. Inhibition of spinal nociceptive neurons by microinjections of somatostatin into the nucleus raphe magnus and the midbrain periaqueductal gray of the anesthetized cat. Neurosci Lett 1995;187:137-141.

[43]   Lenz FA, Tasker RR, Dostrovsky JO, *et al*. Abnormal single-unit activity recorded in the somatosensory thalamus of a quadriplegic patient with central pain. Pain 1987;31:225-236.

[44]   Morrow TJ, Paulson PE, Danneman PJ, *et al*. Regional changes in forebrain activation during the early and late phase of formalin nociception: analysis using cerebral blood flow in the rat. Pain 1998;75:355-365.

[45]   Paulson PE, Morrow TJ, Casey KL. Bilateral behavioral and regional cerebral blood flow changes during painful peripheral mononeuropathy in the rat. Pain 2000;84:233-245.

[46]   Basbaum AI, Fields HL. Endogenous pain control systems: brainstem spinal pathways and endorphin circuitry. Ann Rev Neurosci 1984;7:309-338.

[47]   Benarroch EE. Descending monoaminergic pain modulation: bidirectional control and clinical relevance. Neurology 2008;71(3):217-221.

[48]   Behbehani MM. Functional characteristics of the midbrain periaqueductal gray. Prog Neurobiol 1995;46(6):575-605.

[49]   Xie YF, Huo FQ, Tang JS. Cerebral cortex modulation of pain. Acta Pharmacol Sin 2009;30(1):31-41.

[50]   Bennett MI, Smith BH, Torrance N, Lee AJ. Can pain can be more or less neuropathic? Comparison of symptom assessment tools with ratings of certainty by clinicians. Pain 2006;122(3):289-294.

[51]   Sawatzky B, Bishop CM, Miller WC. Classification and measurement of pain in the spinal cord-injured population. Spinal Cord 2008;46(1):2-10.

[52]   Widerstrom-Noga E, Biering-Sorensen F, Bryce T, *et al*. The International Spinal Cord Injury Pain Basic Data Set. Spinal Cord 2008;46:818-823.

[53]   Bouhassira D, Attal N, Fermanian J, *et al*. Development and validation of the Neuropathic Pain Symptom Inventory. Pain 2004;108(3):248-257.

[54]   Treede RD, Jensen TS, Campbell JN, *et al*. Neuropathic pain: redefinition and a grading system for clinical and research purposes. Neurology 2008;70(18):1630-1635.

[55]   Marino RJ, Barros T, Biering-Sorensen F, *et al*. International standards for neurological classification of spinal cord injury. J Spinal Cord Med 2003;26(suppl.1):S50-S56.

[56]   Felix ER, Cruz-Almeida Y, Widerstrom-Noga E. Chronic pain after spinal cord injury: what characteristics make some pains more disturbing than others? J Rehabil Res Dev 2007;44(5):703-715.

[57]   Widerstrom-Noga E, Felipe-Cuervo E, Yezierski RP. Chronic pain after spinal injury: interference with sleep and daily activities. Arch Phys Med Rehabil 2001;82:1571-1577.

[58]   Cruz-Almeida Y, Martinez-Arizala A, Widerstrom-Noga E. Chronicity of pain associated with spinal cord injury: A longitudinal Analysis. J Rehabil Res Dev 2005;42(5):585-594.

[59]   Widerstrom-Noga E, Felipe-Cuervo E, Broton JG, et al. Perceived difficulty in dealing with consequences of spinal cord injury. Arch Phys Med Rehabil 1999;80:580-586.

[60]   Widerstrom-Noga E, Turk DC. Types and effectiveness of treatments used by people with chronic pain associated with spinal cord injuries: influence of pain and psychosocial characteristics. Spinal Cord 2003;41:600-609.

[61]   Christo PJ. Opioid effectiveness and side effects in chronic pain. Anesthesiol Clin North Am 2003;21:699-713.

[62]   Le Bars D, Gozariu M, Cadden SW. Animal models of nociception. Pharamacol Rev 2001;53:597-652.

[63]   Eaton MJ. Common animal models of spasticity and pain. J Rehabil Res Dev 2003;40:41-54.

[64]   Delander GE, Schott E, Brodin E, Fredholm BB. Spinal expression of mRNA for immediate early genes in a model of chronic pain. Acta Physiol Scand 1997;161:517-525.

[65]   Bennett AD, Everhart AW, Hulsebosch CE. Intrathecal administration of an NMDA or a non-NMDA receptor antagonist reduces mechanical but not thermal allodynia in a rodent model of chronic central pain after spinal cord injury. Brain Res 2000;859:72-82-.

[66]   Vierck CJ, Siddall P, Yezierski RP. Pain following spinal cord injury: animal models and mechanistic studies. Pain 2000;89:1-5.

[67]   Klass M, Gavrikov V, Drury D, et al. Intravenous mononuclear marrow cells reverse neuropathic pain from experimental mononeuropathy. Anesth Analg 2007;104(4):944-948.

[68]   Lin CR, Wu PG, Shih HC, et al. Intrathecal spinal progenitor cell transplantation for the treatment of neuropathic pain. Cell Transplant 2002;11:17-24.

[69]   Grumbach L. The prediction of analgesic activity in man by animal testing. In: Knighton RS, Dumke PR, editors. Pain, 15th International Symposium, Detroit, 1964, Boston:Little Brown, 1966. pp. 163.

[70]   Otsuki T, Nakahama I, Niizuma H, et al. Evaluation of the analgesic effects of capsaicin using a new rat model for tonic pain. Brain Res 1986;365:235-240.

[71]   Tonussi CR, Ferreira SH. Rat knee-joint carrageenin incapacitation test: an objective screen for central and peripheral analgesics. Pain 1992;48:421-427.

[72]   Heapy CG, Jamieson A, Russell NJW. Afferent C-fibre and A-delta activity in models of inflammation. Br J Pharmacol 1987;90:164P.

[73]   Marsala M, Kakinohana O, Yaksh TL, et al. Spinal implantation of hNT neurons and neuronal precursors: graft survival and functional effects in rats with ischemic spastic paraplegia. Eur J Neurosci 2004;20:2401-2414.

[74]   Saporta S, Borlongan CV, Sanberg PR. Neural transplantation of human neuroteratocarcinoma (hNT) neurons into ischemic rats. A quantitative dose-response analysis of cell survival and behavioral recovery. Neuroscience 1999;91:519-525.

[75]   Raval AN. Therapeutic potential of adult progenitor cells in the management of chronic myocardial ischemia. Am J Cardiovasc Drugs 2008;8(5)315:326.

[76]   [76]Chen M, Tao Y-X, Gu JG. Inward currents induced by ischemia in rat spinal cord dorsal horn neurons Mol Pain 2007, 3:10.

[77]   Qin C, Du JQ, Tang JS, et al. Bradykinin is involved in the mediation of cardiac nociception during ischemia through upper thoracic spinal neurons. Curr Neurovasc Res 2009;6(2):89-94.

[78]   Li Y, Zhang J, Li L. Comparison of the therapeutic effects of different compositions of muskone in the treatment of experimental myocardial infarct in rats and analgesia in mice. Phytother Res 2008;22(9):1219-1223.

[79]   Zimmerman M. Pathobiology of neuropathic pain. Eur J Pharmacol 2001;429:23-37.

[80]   Hargreaves K, Dubner R, Brown F, et al. A new and sensitive method for measuring thermal nociception in cutaneous hyperalgesia. Pain 1988;32:77-88.

[81]   Chaplan SR, Bach FW, Pogrel JW, et al. Quantitative assessment of tactile allodynia in the rat paw. J Neurosci Meth 1994;53:55-63.

[82]   Bennett GJ, Xie Y-K. A peripheral mononeuropathy in rat that produces disorders of pain sensation like those seen in man. Pain 1988;33:87-107.

[83]   Wall PD, Devor M, Inbal R, et al. Autotomy following peripheral nerve lesions: experimental anesthesia dolorosa. Pain 1979;7:103-111.

[84]   Kontinen VK, Meert TF. Vocalization responses after intrathecal administration of ionotropic glutamate receptor agonists in rats. Anesth Analges 2002;95:997-1001.

[85]   Aley KO, Levine JD. Different peripheral mechanisms mediate enhanced nociception in metabolic/toxic and traumatic painful peripheral neuropathies in the rat. Neuroscience 2002;111:389-397.

[86]   Danziger N, Gautron M, Le Bars D, *et al*. Activation of diffuse noxious inhibitory controls (DNIC) in rats with an experimental peripheral mononeuropathy. Pain 2001;91:287-296.

[87]   Novakovic SD, Tzoumaka E, McGivern JG, *et al*. Distribution of the tetrodotoxin-resistant sodium channel PN3 in rat sensory neurons in normal and neuropathic conditions. J Neurosci 1998;18:2174-2187.

[88]   Kim DS, Choi Jo, Rim HD, *et al*. Downregulation of voltage-gated potassium channel alpha gene expression in dorsal root ganglia following chronic constriction injury of the rat sciatic nerve. Brain Res Mol Brain Res 2002;105:146-152.

[89]   Kim DS, Lee SJ, Park SY, *et al*. Differentially expressed genes in rat dorsal root ganglia following peripheral nerve injury. Neuroreport 2001;12:3401-3405.

[90]   Dai Y, Iwata K, Kondo E, *et al*. A selective increase in Fos expression in spinal dorsal horn neurons following graded thermal stimulation in rats with experimental mononeuropathy. Pain 2001;90:287-296.

[91]   Draisci G, Kajander KC, Dubner R, *et al*. Up-regulation of opioid gene expression in spinal cord evoked by experimental nerve injuries and inflammation. Brain Res 1991;560:186-192.

[92]   Eaton MJ. Emerging cell and molecular strategies for the study and treatment of painful peripheral neuropathies. J Peripher Nerv Sys 2000;5:59-74.

[93]   Cejas PJ, Martinez M, Karmally S, *et al*. Lumbar transplant of neurons genetically modified to secrete brain-derived neurotrophic factor attenuate allodynia and hyperalgesia after sciatic nerve constriction. Pain 2000;86:195-210.

[94]   [94]Eaton MJ, Blits B, Ruitenberg MJ, *et al*. Amelioration of chronic neuropathic pain by adeno-associated viral (AAV) vector-mediated overexpression of BDNF in the rat spinal cord. Gene Ther 2002;9:1387-1395.

[95]   Courteix C, Bardin M, Chantelauze C, *et al*. Study of the sensitivity of the diabetes-induced pain model in rats to a range of analgesics. Pain 1994;57:153-160.

[96]   Bhagra A, Rao RD. Chemotherapy-induced neuropathy. Curr Oncol Rep.2007;9(4):290-9.

[97]   Slart R, Yu AL, Yaksh TL, *et al*. An animal model of pain produced by systemic administration of an immunotherapeutic anti-ganglioside antibody. Pain 1997;69:119-125.

[98]   Field MJ, McCleary S, Hughes J, *et al*. Gabapentin and pregabalin, but not morphine and amitriptyline, block both static and dynamic components of mechanical allodynia induced by streptozocin in the rat. Pain 1999;80:391-398.

[99]   Bowsher D. Central pain: clinical and physiological characteristics. J Neurol Neurosurg Psychiatry 1996;61:62-69.

[100] Vierck CJ, Siddall P, Yezierski RP. Pain following spinal cord injury: animal models and mechanistic studies. Pain 2000;89:1-5.

[101] Putke JD, Richards JS, Hicken BL, *et al*. Pain classification following spinal cord injury: the utility of verbal descriptors. Spinal Cord 2002;40:118-127.

[102] Widerstrom-Noga E. Chronic pain and nonpainful sensations after spinal cord injury: is there a relation? Clin J Pain 2003;19:39-47.

[103] Hubscher CH, Johnson RD. Changes in neuronal receptive field characteristics in caudal brain stem following chronic spinal cord injury. J Neurotrauma 1999;16:533-541.

[104] Lindsey AE, LoVerso RL, Tovar CA, *et al*. An analysis of changes in sensory thresholds to mild tactile and cold stimuli after experimental spinal cord injury in the rat. Neurorehabil Neural Repair 2000;14:287-300.

[105] Siddall P, Xu CL, Cousins M. Allodynia following traumatic spinal cord injury in the rat. Neuro Report 1995;6:1241-1244.

[106] Hulsebosch CE, Xu GY, Perez-Polo JR, *et al*. Rodent model of chronic central pain after spinal cord contusion injury and effects of gabapentin. J Neurotrauma 2000;17:1205-1217.

[107] Yezierski RP, Santana M, Park SH, *et al*. Neuronal degeneration and spinal cavitation following intraspinal injections of quisqualic acid in the rat. J Neurotrauma 1993;10:445-456.

[108] Yezierski RP, Liu S, Ruenes GL, *et al*. Excitotoxic spinal cord injury: behavioral and morphological characteristics of a central pain model. Pain 1998;75:141-155.

[109] Brewer KL, Yezierski RP. Effects of adrenal medullary transplants on pain-related behaviors following excitotoxic spinal cord injury. Brain Res 1998;798:83-92.

[110] Yezierski RP. Pain following spinal cord injury: pathophysiology and central mechanisms. Prog Brain Res 2000;129:429-448.

[111] Yang L, Jones NR, Stoodley Ma, *et al*. Excitotoxic model of post-traumatic syringomyelia in the rat. Spine 2001;26:1842-1849.

[112] Levitt M, Levitt J. The deafferentation syndrome in monkeys: dysthesias of spinal origin. Pain 1981;10:129-147.

[113] Ovelmen-Levitt J, Gorecki J, Nguyen K, *et al*. Spontaneous and evoked dysesthesias observed in the rat after spinal cordotomies. Stereo Func Neurosurg 1995;65:157-160.

[114] Vierck CJ, Light AR. Allodynia and hyperalgesia within dermatomes caudal to a spinal cord injury in primates and rodents. In: Sandkuhler J, Bromm B, Gebhart GF, Eds. Nervous system plasticity and chronic pain., Amsterdam:Elsevier, 2000. pp. 411.

[115] Christensen MD, Hulsebosch CE. Chronic central pain after spinal cord injury. J Neurotrauma 1997;14:517-537.

[116] Christensen MD, Hulsebosch CE. Spinal cord injury and anti-NGF treatment results in changes in CGRP density and distribution in the dorsal horn in the rat. Exp Neurol 1997;147:463-475.

[117] Nathan PW, Smith MC, Cook AW. Sensory effects in man of lesions of the posterior columns and of some other afferent pathways. Brain 1986;109:1003-1041.

[118] Vierck CJ, Greenspan JD, Ritz LA, *et al.* The spinal pathways contributing to the ascending conduction and the descending modulations of pain sensations and reactions. In: Yaksh T, editor. Spinal systems of afferent processing, New York:Plenum, 1986. pp. 275.

[119] Park DH, Borlongan CV, Eve DJ, *et al.* The emerging field of cell and tissue engineering. Med Sci Monit 2008;14(11):RA206-220.

[120] Kozlova EN. Strategies to repair lost sensory connections to the spinal cord. Mol Biol (Mosk) 2008;42 (5)820:829.

[121] Goligorsky MS, Kuo MC, Patschan D, *et al.* Review article: endothelial progenitor cells in renal disease. Nephrology (Carlton) 2009;14(3):291-297.

[122] Stamm C, Choi YH, Nasseri B, *et al.* A heart full of stem cells: the spectrum of myocardial progenitor cells in the postnatal heart. Ther Adv Cardiovasc Dis 2009; May 14:3(3):215-29

[123] Jevon M, Dorling A, Hornick PI. Progenitor cells and vascular disease. Cell Prolif 2008;41(Suppl 1)-146.

[124] Hentall ID, Sagen J. The alleviation of pain by cell transplantation. Prog Brain Res 2000;127:535-550.

[125] Sagen J, Wang H, Tresco PA, *et al.* Transplants of immunologically isolated xenogeneic chromaffin cells provide a long-term source of pain-reducing neuroactive substances. J Neurosci 1993;13:2415-2423.

[126] Decosterd I, Buchser E, Gilliard N, *et al.* Intrathecal implants of bovine chromaffin cells alleviate mechanical allodynia in a rat model of neuropathic pain. Pain 1998;76:159-166.

[127] Takahashi K, Fujita T, Takeuchi T. Production of bioactive enkephalin from the nonendocrine cell lines COS-7, NIH3T3, Ltk-, C2C12. Peptides 1995;16:933-938.

[128] Breivik H. Opioids in cancer and chronic noncancer pain therapy: Indications and controversies. Acta Anesthesiol Scand 2001;45:1059-1066.

[129] Eaton MJ, Karmally S, Martinez MA, *et al.* Lumbar transplants of neurons genetically modified to secrete galanin reverse pain-like behaviors after partial sciatic nerve injury. J Peripher Nerv Syst 1999;4:245-257.

[130] Eaton MJ, Plunkett JA, Martinez MA, *et al.* Transplants of neuronal cells bio-engineered to synthesize GABA alleviate chronic neuropathic pain. Cell Transplant 1999;8:87-101.

[131] Stubley LA, Martinez M, Karmally S, *et al.* Only early GABA cell therapy is able to reverse neuropathic pain after partial nerve injury. J Neurotrauma 2001;18:471-477.

[132] Eaton MJ, Dancausse HR, Santiago DI, *et al.* Lumbar transplants of immortalized serotonergic neurons alleviates chronic neuropathic pain. Pain 1997;72:59-69.

[133] Hains BC, Johnson KM, McAdoo DJ, *et al.* Engraftment of immortalized serotonergic neurons enhances locomotor function and attenuates pain-like behavior following spinal hemisection injury in the rat. Exp Neurol 2001;171:361-378.

[134] Hains BC, Johnson KM, Eaton MJ, *et al.* Serotonergic neural precursor cell grafts attenuate bilateral hyperexcitability of dorsal horn neurons after spinal hemisection in rat. Neuroscience 2003;116:1097-1110.

[135] Hains BC, Fullwood SD, Eaton MJ, *et al.* Subdural engraftment of serotonergic neurons following spinal hemisection restores spinal serotonin, downregulates the serotonin transporter, and increases BDNF tissue content in the rat. Brain Res 2001;913:35-46.

[136] Siegan JB, Sagen J. A natural peptide with NMDA inhibitory activity reduces tonic pain in the formalin model. Neuroreport 1997;8:1379-1381.

[137] Gajavelli S, Castellanos DA, Furmanski O, *et al.* Sustained analgesic peptide secretion and cell labeling using a novel genetic modification. Cell Transplant 2008;17(4):445-455.

[138] Hama A, Sagen J. Antinociceptive effects of the marine snail peptides conantokin-G and conotoxin MVIIA alone and in combination in rat models of pain. Neuropharmacology 2009;56(2):556-563.

[139] Hama A, Basler A, Sagen J. Enhancement of morphine antinociception with the peptide N-methyl-D-aspartate receptor antagonist [Ser1]-histogranin in the rat formalin test. Brain Res 2006; 1095(1):59-64 2006.

[140] Eaton MJ, Herman JP, Jullien N, *et al.* Immortalized chromaffin cells disimmortalized with Cre/lox site-directed recombination for use in cell therapy for pain. Exp Neurol 2002;175:49-60.

[141] Eaton MJ, Frydel B, Lopez T, *et al.* Generation and initial characterization of conditionally immortalized chromaffin cells. J Cell Biochem 2000;79:38-57.

[142] Eaton MJ, Vaysse L, Herman JP, *et al.* Creation of immortalized chromaffin cell lines for clinical applications. IRPCA Adv Res Updates 2007;9 (1):13-26.

[143] Lin CR, Wu PG, Shih HC, Cheng *et al.* Intrathecal spinal progenitor cell transplantation for the treatment of neuropathic pain. Cell Transplant 2002;11:17-24.

[144] Terashima T, Kojima H, Fujimiya M, *et al.* The fusion of bone-marrow-derived proinsulin-expressing cells with nerve cells underlies diabetic neuropathy. Proc Natl Acad Sci U S A. 2005;102(35):12525-12530.

[145] Akesson E, Sandelin M, Kanaykina N, *et al.* Long-term survival, robust neuronal differentiation, and extensive migration of human forebrain stem/progenitor cells transplanted to the adult rat dorsal root ganglion cavity. Cell Transplant 2008;17 (10-11):1115-1123.

[146] Hiyama A, Mochida J, Sakai D. Stem cell applications in intervertebral disc repair. Cell Mol Biol (Noisy-le-grand). 2008;54(1):24-32.

[147] Risbud MV, Guttapalli A, Tsai TT, *et al.* Evidence for skeletal progenitor cells in the degenerate human intervertebral disc. Spine 2007;32(23):2537-2544.

[148] Wei A, Tao H, Chung SA, *et al.* The fate of transplanted xenogeneic bone marrow-derived stem cells in rat intervertebral discs. J Orthop Res.2009 Mar;27(3):374-379. 2009;27(3):374-379.

[149] Murrell W, Sanford E, Anderberg L, *et al.* Olfactory stem cells can be induced to express chondrogenic phenotype in a rat intervertebral disc injury model. Spine J 2009; [Epub ahead of print] doi:10.1016/j.spinee.2009.02.011

[150] Li Y, Chopp M. Marrow stromal cell transplantation in stroke and traumatic brain injury. Neurosci Lett 2009;456 (3):120-123.

[151] Krankel N, Katare RG, Siragusa M, *et al.* Role of kinin B2 receptor signaling in the recruitment of circulating progenitor cells with neovascularization potential. Circ Res 2008;103(11):1335-1343.

[152] Huang P, Li S, Han M, *et al.* Autologous transplantation of granulocyte colony-stimulating factor-mobilized peripheral blood mononuclear cells improves critical limb ischemia in diabetes. Diabetes Care 2005;28(9):2155-2160.

[153] Hilbe W, Nussbaumer W, Bonatti H, *et al.* Unusual adverse events following peripheral blood stem cell (PBSC) mobilisation using granulocyte colony stimulating factor (G-CSF) in healthy donors. Bone Marrow Transplant 2000;26(7):811-813.

[154] Bensinger WI, Appelbaum FA, Demirer T, *et al.* Transplantation of allogeneic peripheral blood stem cells. Stem Cells 1995;13(Suppl 3)63:70.

[155] Auquier P, Macquart-Moulin G, Moatti JP, *et al.* Comparison of anxiety, pain and discomfort in two procedures of hematopoietic stem cell collection: leukacytapheresis and bone marrow harvest. Bone Marrow Transplant 1995;16(4):541-547.

[156] Nevskaya T, Ananieva L, Bykovskaia S, *et al.* Autologous progenitor cell implantation as a novel therapeutic intervention for ischaemic digits in systemic sclerosis. Rheumatology (Oxford) 2009;48(1):61-64.

[157] Lenk K, Adams V, Lurz P, *et al.* Therapeutical potential of blood-derived progenitor cells in patients with peripheral arterial occlusive disease and critical limb ischaemia. Eur Heart J 2005;26(18):1903-1909.

[158] Barsheshet A, Hod H, Shechter M, *et al.* The effects of external counter pulsation therapy on circulating endothelial progenitor cells in patients with angina pectoris. Cardiology 2008;110(3):160-166.

[159] Lanza F, Dominici M, Govoni M, *et al.* Prolonged remission state of refractory adult onset Still's disease following CD34-selected autologous peripheral blood stem cell transplantation. Bone Marrow Transplant 2000;25(12):1307-1310.

[160] Andrews PW, Damjanov I, Simon D, *et al.* Pluripotent embryonal carcinoma clones derived from human teratocarcinoma cell line Tera-2. Lab Invest 1984;50:147-162.

[161] Pleasure SJ, Lee VM. NTera 2 cells: a human cell line which displays characteristics expected of a human committed neuronal progenitor cell. J Neurosci Res 1993;35:585-602.

[162] Andrews PW. Retinoic acid induces neuronal differentiation of a cloned human embryonal carcinoma cell line *in vitro*. Dev Biol 1984;103:285-293.

[163] Borlongan CV, Tajima Y, Trojanowski JQ, *et al.* Transplantation of cryopreserved human embryonal carcinoma-derived (NT2N cells) promotes functional recovery in ischemic rats. Exp Neurol 1998;149:310-321.

[164] Cheung WM, Chu AH, Leung MF, Ip NY. Induction of trk receptors by retinoic acid in a human embryonal carcinoma cell line. Neuroreport 1996;7:1204-1208.

[165] Ferrare A, Ehler E, Nitsch RM, *et al.* Immature human NT2 cells grafted into mouse brain differentiate into neuronal and glial cell types. FEBS Letts 2000;486:121-125.

[166] Guillemain I, Alonoso G, Patey G, *et al.* Human NT2 neurons express a large variety of neurotransmission phenotypes *in vitro*. J Comp Neurol 2000;422:380-395.

[167] Satoh J, Kuroda Y. Differential gene expression between human neurons and neuronal progenitor cells in culture: an analysis of arrayed cDNA clones in NTera2 human embryonal carcinoma cell line as a model system. J Neurosci Methods 2000;94:155-164.

[168] Guillemain I, Fontes G, Privat A, *et al.* Early programmed cell death in human NT2 cell cultures during differentiation induced by all-trans-retinoic acid. J Neurosci Res 2003;71:38-45.

[169] Dmitrovsky E, Moy D, Miller WH, *et al.* Retinoic acid causes a decline in TGF-alpha expression, cloning efficiency, and tumorigenicity in a human embryonal cancer cell line. Oncogene Res 1990;5:233-239.

[170] Gortz P, Fleischer W, Rosenbaum C, *et al.* Neuronal network properties of human teratocarcinoma cell line-derived neurons. Brain Res 2004;1018:18-25.

[171] Megiorni F, Mora B, Indovina P, *et al.* Expression of neuronal markers during NTera2/cloneD1 differentiation by cell aggregation method. Neurosci Lett 2005;373:105-109.

[172] Lee VM, Andrews PW. Differentiation of NTERA-2 clonal human embryonal carcinoma cells into neurons involves the induction of all three neurofilament proteins. J Neurosci 1986;6:514-521.

[173] Daadi MM, Saporta S, Willing AE, *et al. In vitro* induction and *in vivo* expression of bcl-2 in the hNT neurons. Brain Res Bull 2001;56:147-152.

[174] Trojanowski JQ, Kleppner SR, Hartley RS, *et al.* Transfectable and transplantable postmitotic human neurons: potential "platform" for gene therapy of nervous system diseases. Exp Neurol 1997;144:92-97.

[175] Kondziolka D, Wechsler L, Goldstein S, *et al.* Transplantation of cultured human neuronal cells for patients with stroke. Neurology 2000;55:565-569.

[176] Nelson PT, Kondziolka D, Wechsler L, *et al.* Clonal human (hNT) neuron grafts for stroke therapy: neuropathology in a patient 27 months after implantation. Am J Pathol 2002;160:1201-1206.

[177] Meltzer CC, Kondziolka D, Villermagne VL, *et al.* Serial [18F] fluorodeoxyyglucose positron emission tomography after human neuronal implantation for stroke. Neurosurgery 2001;49:586-592.

[178] Yoshioka A, Yudkoff M, Pleasure D. Expression of glutamic acid decarboxylase during human neuronal differentiation: studies using the NTera-2 culture system. Brain Res 1997;767:333-339.

[179] Podrygajlo G, Tegenge MA, Gierse A, *et al.* Cellular phenotypes of human model neurons (NT2) after differentiation in aggregate culture. Cell Tissue Res 2009;336(3):439-452.

[180] Saporta S, Willing AE, Colina LO, *et al. In vitro* and *in vivo* characterization of hNT neuron neurotransmitter phenotypes. Brain Res Bull 2000;53:263-268.

[181] Bosch M, Pineda JR, Sunol C, *et al.* Induction of a GABAergic phenotype in a neural stem cell line for transplantation in an excitotoxic model of Huntington's disease. Exp Neurol 2004;190:42-58.

[182] Cao QL, Howard RM, Dennison JB, *et al.* Differentiation of engrafted neuronal-restricted precursor cells is inhibited in the traumatically injured spinal cord. Exp Neurol 2002;177(2):349-359.

[183] Duplan H, Li RY, Vue C, *et al.* Grafts of immortalized chromaffin cells bio-engineered to improve Met-enkephalin release also reduce formalin-evoked c-fos expression in rat spinal cord. Neurosci Lett 2004;370:1-6.

[184] Hains BC, Yucra JA, Eaton MJ, Hulsebosch CE. Intralesion transplantation of serotonergic precursors enhances locomotor recovery but has no effect on development of chronic central pain following hemisection injury in rats. Neurosci Lett 2002;324:222-226.

[185] Eaton MJ, Wolfe SQ, Martinez MA, *et al.* Subarachnoid transplant of a human neuronal cell line attenuates chronic allodynia and hyperalgesia after excitotoxic SCI in the rat. J Pain 2007;8(1):33-50.

[186] Felix ER, Widerstrom-Noga E. Reliability and validity of quantitative sensory testing in persons with spinal cord injury and neuropathic pain. J Rehabil Res Dev 2009;46(1):69-84.

[187] Eaton MJ, Sagen J. Cell therapy for models of pain and traumatic brain injury. In: Sanberg PR, Davis CD, Eds. Cell Therapy for Brain Repair, Totowa, NJ:The Humana Press, Inc., 2007. pp. 199.

[188] Wolfe SQ, Salzberg M, Cumberbatch NMA, *et al.* Optimizing the transplant dose of a human neuronal cell line to treat SCI pain in the rat. Neurosci Lett 2007;414:121-125.

[189] Wolfe SQ, Cumberbatch NMA, Menendez I, Martinez M, Eaton MJ. Intrathecal transplantation of a human neuronal cell line for the treatment of neuropathic pain in a spinal cord injury model. Clinical Neurosurg 2007;54:220-225.

[190] Eaton MJ, Wolfe SQ. Clinical Feasibility for Cell Therapy Utilizing a Human Neuronal Cell Line to Treat Neuropathic Pain-like Behaviors following SCI in the rat. J Rehabil Res Dev 2009;46 (1):145-65

[191] Cheung WM, Fu WY, Hui WS, Ip NY. Production of human CNS neurons from embryonal carcinoma cells using a cell aggregation method. BioTechniques 1999;26:946-954.

[192] Hua XY, Boublik JH, Spicer MA, *et al.* The antinociceptive effects of spinally administered neuropeptide Y in the rat: Systemic studies on structure-activity relationship. J Pharm Exp Ther 1991;258:243-248.

[193] Newman MB, Misiuta I, Willing AE, *et al*. Tumorgenicity issues of embryonic carcinoma-derived stem cells: relevance to surgical trials using NT2 and hNT neural cells. Stem Cells Devel 2005;14:29-43.

[194] Trojanowski JQ, Mantione JR, Lee JH, *et al*. Neurons derived from a human tetratocarcinoma cell line establish molecular and structural polarity following transplantation into the rodent brain. Exp Neurol 1993;122:283-294.

[195] Yong VW, Kim SU. A new double labelling immunofluorescence technique for the determination of proliferation of human astrocytes in culture. J Neurosci Meth 1987;21:9-16.

[196] Brown DB, Stanfield BB. The use of bromodeoxyuridine-immunohistochemistry to identify transplanted fetal brain tissue. J Neural Transplant 1989;1(3-4):135-139.

[197] Miyazono M, Lee VM, Trojanowski JQ. Proliferation, cell death, and neuronal differentiation in transplanted human embryonal carcinoma (NTera2) cells depend on the graft site in nude and severe combined immunodeficient mice. Lab Invest 1995;73(2):273-283.

[198] Hara K, Yasuhara T, Maki M, *et al*. Neural progenitor NT2N cell lines from teratocarcinoma for transplantation therapy in stroke. Prog Neurobiol 2008;85(3):318-334.

[199] Eaton MJ, Martinez MA, Karmally S. A single dose of intrathecal GABA permanently reverses neuropathic pain after nerve injury. Brain Res 1999;835:334-339.

[200] Bertman LJ, Advokat C. Comparison of the antinociceptive and antispastic action of (-)-baclofen after systemic and intrathecal administration in intact, acute and chronic spinal rats. Brain Res 1995;684:8-18.

[201] Herman RM, D'Luzansky SC, Ippolito R. Intrathecal baclofen suppresses central pain in patients with spinal lesions. A pilot study. Clin J Pain 1992;8:338-345.

[202] Taira T, Kawamura H, Tanikawa T, *et al*. A new approach to control central deafferentation pain: spinal intrathecal baclofen. Stereo Funct Neurosurg1 1995;65:101-105.

[203] Lazorthes Y, Bes JC, Sagen J, *et al*. Transplantation of human chromaffin cells for control of intractable cancer pain. Acta Neurochir Suppl 1995;64:97-100.

[204] Lazorthes Y, Sagen J, Sallerin B, *et al*. Human chromaffin cell graft into the CSF for cancer pain management: a prospective phase II clinical study. Pain 2000;87:19-32.

[205] Eaton MJ, Pearse DD, McBroom JS, *et al*. The combination of human neuronal serotonergic cell implants and environmental enrichment after contusive SCI improves motor recovery over each individual strategy. Behav Brain Res 2008;194(2):236-241.

[206] Berrocal Y, Pearse DD, Singh A, *et al*. Social and environmental enrichment improves sensory and motor recovery after severe contusive spinal cord injury in the rat. J Neurotrauma 2007;24 (11):1761-1772.

[207] Wang K, Wong YH. G protein signaling controls the differentiation of multiple cell lineages. Biofactors 2009;35(3):232-238.

[208] Purcell EK, Seymour JP, Yandamuri S, Kipke DR. *In vivo* evaluation of a neural stem cell-seeded prosthesis. J Neural Eng 2009;6(2):026005.

[209] Eaton, MJ, inventor. Isolated/cloned NT2 cell lines expressing serotonin and GABA. United States patent US 7485457. February 3, 2009.

[210] Gregorian C, Nakashima J, Le Belle J, *et al*. Pten deletion in adult neural stem/progenitor cells enhances constitutive neurogenesis. J Neurosci 2009;29(6):1874-1886.

[211] Widerstrom-Noga E. Pain: A multidimensional problem of national priority. J Rehabil Res Dev 2009;46(1):vii-ix.

[212] Molton IR, Stoelb BL, Jensen MP, Ehde DM, Raichle KA, Cardenas DD. Psychosocial factors and adjustment to chronic pain in spinal cord injury: Replication and cross-validation. J Rehabil Res Dev 2009;46(1):31-42.

[213] Edwards RR. Genetic predictors of acute and chronic pain. Curr Rheumatol Rep 2006;8(6):411-417.

[214] Kim H, Mittal DP, Iadarol MJ, Dionne RA. Genetic predictors for acute experimental cold and heat pain sensitivity in humans. J Med Gen 2006;43(8):e40.

CHAPTER 8

Neural Stem Cells: New Hope for Successful Therapy

Denis English[1,*], Akshay Anand[2], Rama S.Verma[3] and Stefan Glück[4]

[1]Department of Neurosurgery, Foundation for Developmental Research, University of South Florida College of Medicine, Tampa, FL, USA; [2]Department of Neurology, Post Graduate Institute of Medical Education and Research, Chandigarh, India; [3]Stem Cell and Molecular Biology Laboratory, Department of Biotechnology, Institute of Technology-Madras, Chennai, India and [4]Sylvester Comprehensive Cancer Center, Division of Hematology/ Oncology, Department of Medicine, Miller School of Medicine, University of Miami, Miami, FL, USA

Abstract: The devastation caused by disruption of the central nervous system and the increased prevalence of chronic neural diseases in our aging population led to enthusiastic and rapid acceptance of neural stem cells as an effective tool to reverse central nervous system pathology over a decade ago. Shortly after human embryonic stem cells were identified, results which held that functional neurons generated from stem cells reversed severe damage to the central nervous system were widely disseminated and avidly endorsed. Subsequent reports claimed neural localization and proliferation of adult stem cells, trans-differentiation of mesenchymal stem cells into functional neurons, and stunning therapeutic effects of human neural stem cells in animal models.

Despite these claims, effective therapy with neural stem cells has not been realized. Early results have been attributed to factors released by infused cells and investigator bias but not to tissue regeneration. The identity of stem cell progeny identified as neurons by antigen expression and morphology has been questioned, leading to the re-interpretation of these results by many of the investigators who first reported them. Therapeutic expectations have subsided while reports of success in animal models continue to appear. The thought that neural stem cells, as currently defined, will reverse brain injury or pathology has been largely dismissed.

Despite these diminished expectations, herein we note that regenerative cells, or structures that mimic the function regenerative cells possess, are present in germinal areas of the adult human brain, albeit in limited numbers. Evidence does suggest that damaged brain tissue does, in some patients, regenerate with recovery of lost function. These cellular entities have not been widely studied, characterized or cultured, but they may be similar to structures generated in neural tissue of primitive vertebrates which have a remarkable capability to regenerate intact, functional brain. These structures can potentially be expanded using methods that differ vastly from stem cell culture methods employed to date. Successfully expanded and stored, these structures may provide an effective means to regenerate brain tissue after stroke and traumatic brain injury in humans.

INTRODUCTION

During fetal development, embryonic stem cells give rise to neural progenitors which provide the basis of the central nervous system or CNS, a network of highly specialized and heterogeneous neurons that extend axons into tunnels forged by macrophage – like "Schwann" cells as well as dendrites in opposing directions. Emanating from a central cell body, interconnected axons and dendrites effectively connect virtually all tissues of the body to a single focus of the central nervous system—the brain. When we study functions of the brain, our brains are doing the study. We may thereby appropriately question the investigators' objectivity. Neural activity seems to exert a defining role not only in our actions but also in events that occur during embryonic development of blood vessels and many –perhaps all-- other tissues.

The brain is truly a remarkable organ. Protected by a fortified skeletal shield, it is highly resistant to injury. Separated from the circulation by an ill-defined barrier, the brain is remarkably resistant to infection or autoimmune disease. However, these protections allowed evolution not endow central nervous system cells the healing mechanisms available to cells of all other organs. Brain damage results in irreversible dysfunction in humans, and neural diseases are not readily amendable to therapy.

*Address correspondence to this author Denis English: Florida Foundation for Developmental Research PO Box 1561, Palmetto, FL 34420, 813-355-1994, USA: E-mail: dkenglish@msn.com

However, in primitive vertebrates, complete restoration of neural activity is often observed after prolonged periods of hypoxia or hypothermia. Since the CNS of these animals is also protected by well developed skeletal and circulatory barriers, we wondered what was gained when this capacity was lost. What forces impinged during evolution to limit neural regenerative potential as vertebrates advanced?

Perhaps none. The human brain is unique in its compulsion to explore the existence of its host; to reach out to areas not previously encountered; to scrutinize its composition and function. Evolution is not merely reflected by enhanced adaptation. As we learn ways to prolong our life-span, evolution takes a new turn. Not only do the most fit survive. Progeny most able to adapt, as well those best able to protect their parents, achieve an advantage that within a single generation ensures the preservation of this genetic trait as it promotes the unique characteristics humans hold; a compulsion to advance society as a unit, to explore our very existence, to "go where none has gone before", and recently to identify and utilize "stem cells" that reg.enerate tissues, lost to the ravages of aging or disease. Evolution has a curious manner of anticipating its own result, a trait that accelerates fundamental evolutionary processes. Evolutionary forces may probably left regenerative neural cells or neural structures in the human brain for our own survival advantage. In fact, it is difficult to envision how evolution would not reach this endpoint, given the importance of the brain in survival.

NEURAL STEM CELLS

By definition, neural stem cells [NSCs] consist of a self renewing population of cells that give rise to neurons, astrocytes and glia while they maintain themselves during life [1-3]. These cells have been widely postulated to proliferate, differentiate, and regenerate damaged neural tissue [eg. see refs 4-9], even though regeneration of damaged cells of the CNS has rarely been demonstrated in preclinical models [10]. Neural stem cells have been reported to reside both in hematopoietic tissues and in the CNS of animals and man. Defined by their ability to give rise to neurons and neurospheres in culture, neural stem cells have been postulated to exist in preparations of mesenchymal stem cells [MSCs, 10- 21], a unique population of cells derived from highly adherent yet poorly characterized cells of the bone marrow stroma [22]. MSC's can be recovered from marrow stroma, adipose tissue, synovial membranes, cord blood, amniotic fluid and blood [reference 23 and references therein].

Although MSCs are thought arise from the mesoderm, they have been postulated to generate cells of the endoderm and ectoderm by the process of transdifferentiation [24-26]. Default differentiation of MSCs leads to osteoblasts, condrocytes and adipocytes in vitro [22, 23]. Progeny of human MSCs have been identified in brains of mice and other animals after IV infusion. Identification of these cells as neural cells initially relied on immune localization of antigens previously considered specific for neural tissue, such as nestin [27-31]. Differentiation of neurons from stem cells was further "verified" by morphology, wherein cultured MSC derivatives were observed to emit projections that resembled those of neurons.

However, it is now clear that many antigens once considered specific for neural tissue are expressed by non-neuronal cells, including endothelial cells and monocytes [10, 32-34]. Morphologic changes resulting in the projection of structures that resemble those of neurons are observed when cells of many types die in culture. The generation of ectodermal cells by cells derived in and from the mesoderm is highly questionable. In vivo, such morphologic changes are not observed and the accumulation of MSC-derived progeny in brains, while widely held as proof of stem cell migration into brain tissue, has been dismissed as an experimental artifact. In contrast to morphology in culture, after transplantation, "neural stem cell progeny" which localize in the brain do not appear to bear any resemblance to neurons. In all reported studies, these cells are so few in number that their role in direct regeneration of lost tissues has been widely dismissed [10, 18].

The earliest evidence of post - natal neurogenesis was reported in 1938, based on cytological evidence of mitotic cells in the sub-ventricular zone of rodent brain. In 1983, Goldman and Nottebohm demonstrated the apparent genesis of neurons in the telencephalon of adult male songbirds [35]. These neurons were thought to be required for the production of new components the neural network were thought to generate in order to acquire the ability to compose the new songs the birds must sing each season in order to attract mates. This highly touted but rather short - sighted conclusion was quite liberally interpreted and led to the postulate that post - natal neurogenesis in fact occurs in avians and leads to advanced neural development. Similar reasoning would imply that stem cell-dependent neurogenesis occurs as we write this paper. Perhaps it does; but likely this provocative essay is fueled by good wine, and not by stem cell-dependent neurogenesis. The conclusion was premature, as it did not link with any degree of certainty neurogenesis to the new compositions. Simple learning could explain these results, as could many other factors.

NEURAL MATURATION VS NEURAL REGENERATION

The source of new neurons observed by many must also be re-examined in light of stunning recent studies showing that under adverse conditions, neuronal projections of certain primitive vertebrates avidly and quickly condense into the central cell body within the neural cavity. These cell bodies then condense individually and do not appear to constitute a functional brain; rather the neural cavity appears to become almost devoid of cells during sustained hypothermia or hypoxia. This result was vividly demonstrated in a recent study by Kersaraju and Milton [36]. The investigators wondered how certain turtles survived submerged for weeks and even months in the absence of oxygen. After this prolonged anoxia, when the submerged turtle emerges they almost immediately re-acquire full functionality. A simple experiment cast a new light on the consequences of the protective processes involved. Previous studies had implicated altered glucose metabolism and ATP utilization in adaptation to hypoxia, but these studies did not identify how the anoxic brain cells survived nor define if the changes observed led to or resulted from anoxia. Kersaraju and Milton described results of a simple experiment which demonstrated that practically all of the brain tissue appeared to be totally lost soon after turtles were submersed [36]. Neural projections collapsed upon their cell bodies which condensed to small rounded structures not resembling neural cells. The animals' brain cavity appeared to be devoid of all structures but small granules. These structures developed to afford sustained protection to the animals' brain during prolonged hypoxia and hypothermia. The condensed cell bodies retained full viability and their morphology, projections and function rapidly returned upon exposure to air. Examination of regenerative structures isolated from brains of submerged turtles or other anoxia – resistant vertebrates holds promise for defining a novel population of cells that may be useful therapeutically, even if the cells are not true stem cells.

Why did human brain lose this protective process during evolution? Perhaps it did not. Several studies have demonstrated enhanced generation of neural stem cells in response to low oxygen tension in culture [37-39]. The response seems to be confined to a rare population of cells in the subventricular zone, a purported focus of neurogenesis in the adult brain. The new cells may reflect properties held by primitive animal brain regenerative cells as a remnant of evolution. If this is the case, isolation and expansion of these structures from human brains may afford a new therapeutic approach. How can such cells be isolated and expanded? A logical approach would involve determination of the human equivalent of these structures by examination of brains of humans or other animals deprived of oxygen. Such deprivation may serve to amplify the structures endogenously with retention of regenerative capabilities. It may be possible to restore full functionality using such cells expanded under hypoxic conditions when a permissive environment is restored.

Similarly, regeneration of nerves in the peripheral nervous system of humans results from elongation of axons from a viable cell body and does not reflect regeneration of intact new tissue, as commonly assumed. The axons forge new connections with their target tissues, but fail to generate new transmitter-dependent neural connections. Thus, regeneration claimed to result from "stem cell" proliferation must be shown to not result from differentiation of precursors, restoration of function of protected cells or axonal elongation. While this may not be possible, other structures may provide protection and regeneration by differentiation, and may thereby achieve therapeutic goals desired.

Studies such as those which indicate that adult neural stem cells indeed form functional neurons must therefore be carefully re-evaluated to determine if the regenerative cells were actual "stem cells" or altered neural cells which had "de-differentiated" to survive. These may be present in enhanced levels in the subventricular zone, cerebral cortex and hippocampus of the adult brain, which have been identified to possess neural stem cells [40-44]. When the brain is exposed to an adverse environment, such as it is when these cells are harvested for use in the very experiments designed to characterize their presence, numbers, functions and characteristics, stem cells-if present-may change dramatically. This fact is never considered by stem cell researchers; no study has addressed the possibility that the invasive procedures used to isolate cells that are later characterized as "stem cells" may well impact the cell they seek to define. Indeed, stem cells are thought to avidly migrate to sites of trauma and wounding; trauma and wounding result from virtually all procedures used to isolate stem cells from humans as well as experimental animals.

PROBLEMS WITH PRESENT APPROACHES

While stem cell therapy is said to be based on results with hematopoietic cells, we [45] and others have found that culture of hematopoietic cells even for brief periods rapidly results in the cells' failure to engraft. Thus, experiments to expand human hematopoietic progenitors in culture have not been successful even though cells with a phenotype identical to that of what we consider the hematopoietic stem cell possesses are amplified. Similarly, a single clone of cells of a component of the hematopoietic system is not able to restore loss of that individual component. When progeny of MSCs are used for therapeutic trials, typically these are infused as a single unit derived from a clone generated in culture that reflects the cells the investigator wishes to restore. This approach would not restore specific defects in hematopoiesis. For example, neutropenia cannot be reversed by infusion of expanded myeloid precursors [46]. Anemia is not treatable with erythrocyte progenitors. The entire system must be replaced to reverse specific defects within it and it must be replaced with cells that have not been cultured, for reasons that remain to be defined. Yet approaches to stem cell therapy rely on the method of infusion of a derivative of a single colony of cells generated from a mesenchymal stem cell, or other stem cell in culture.

This approach does not reflect the successful approach developed for restoration of the entire hematopoietic system or specific components of it. Fresh cells – perhaps stored after cryopreservation — are the only clinically acceptable cells for use in hematopoietic restoration. The dramatically different approach most often used for evaluation of tissue regeneration using progeny of MSCs or other cultured cells in no way reflects the successful methodology used for hematopoietic reconstitution. In addition, in the few reports that indicate stem cell - dependent tissue regeneration other than that of the hematopoietic system, freshly harvested cells were used; these cells lost their ability to regenerate tissue when cultured. Comparison of fresh and cultured cells showed little changes; among these was enhanced expression of CD-105 by cultured cells, a transforming growth factor receptor. Further, it is noteworthy that adherent hematopoietic stem cells that resemble fibroblasts were identified by their ability to generate all components of the hematopoietic system in culture and to restore hematopoiesis in ablated animals. These cells, initially identified by Huss and associates, resemble MSC's and may in fact be a subpopulation of MSCs. They are effective in restoration of all components of the hematopoietic system but only in chimeric models; i.e., injected alone, they fail to restore hematopoiesis to an ablated animal. If mixed with fresh, viable hematopoietic stem cells after genetic marking, they apear to contribute to all components of the hematopoietic system restored after transplantation, leading to their acceptance as adherent and expandable hematopoietic stem cells. They are anything but.

As convincing as these results seem to be, no report shows restoration of hematopoiesis with similar cultured cells injected alone, and no clinical trials have indicated any therapeutic potential of these cells alone. The CD-34 negative adherent "hematopoietic stem cell" has led to much speculation and increased enthusiasm for restorative therapy with MSCs in other systems, but their limitations are consistently overlooked. If such cells were able to restore hematopoiesis directly, therapeutic avenues involving genetic engineering before culture or selection of mutant-reversed cells would provide material for autologous hematopoietic transplants as a curative process for any and all hematopoietic defects resulting from nucleotide mutations, such as adenosine deaminase deficiency or sickle cell anemia. These expectations, considered to be near at hand a few years ago, remain elusive. We suggest that they will, since fundamental concepts are flawed.

WHERE NEURAL STEM CELLS RESIDE

Studies of antigen expression and other characteristics have led to the identification of the subventricular zone as well as the ventricular zone and cerebral cortex as foci of neural stem cells, as discussed above. A leading expert in the field has estimates that approximately 10,000 neural stem cells reside in the ciliary epithelium of human retina and another 100,000 in human central nervous system [Mahendra Rao, personal communication]. This is certainly not a large number of cells. However, if these rare cells are true regenerative neural stem cells, they should be studied for their ability to be expanded in culture for therapy. Neural stem cells have been said to produce "neuroblasts" or neurospheres derived from the neural crest [46, 47]. These cells are thought to migrate along discrete pathways, such as the rostral migratory stream into the olfactory bulb where they form mature neurons which mediate the sense of smell [48, 49]. However, the assumption that neuroblasts arise from neural stem cells is based only on inference, since no test is available to define a neural stem cell.

DETECTION, MANIPULATION AND EARLY EXPECTATIONS OF NEURAL STEM CELLS

For many years, accepted dogma held that neurons do not regenerate in the injured or diseased human brain. However, early reports of effective therapy resulting from local implantation of human stem cells led to rapidly embraced concept that neural stem cells not only existed but rapidly regenerated functional neurons that established new functional connections.

The earliest of these reports led to a plethora of expectations. Investigators reported that spinal cord - injured rats were rescued from paralysis by local instillation of fetal stem cells. While this study was not published in any scientific journal, it quickly swept the lay media and captured the imagination of scientists as well. In a stunning video presented on popular evening news shows in the United States against a backdrop of a radiograph of the severed spine of the late actor, Christopher Reeves, rats treated with human fetal stem cells after a paralytic spinal injury played joyfully in their cage, eating aggressively and frantically exercising on that little wheel that revolves endlessly as rats seeks whatever it is that healthy rats seek while turning that wheel. In contrast, animals not treated with stem cells after injury remained paralyzed, with hardly the movement of an extended limb. Mr. Reeves watched the video presentation in awe, concluding that he would again walk. One highly visible, popular and questioning newscaster, Dan Rather, asked his science advisor, John Stossel, a highly respected and credible journalist with very close ties to the scientific community, for his opinion. Mr. Stossel allowed little doubt; the technique held vast and incredible promise; it would only be a matter of time before these new magic bullets cured chronic diseases of aging as well as injuries to tissues as complex as the spinal cord.

Unfortunately, the heroic actor would never again walk. Unlike the injury he sustained in an equine accident, the stem cell - treated rats did not recover from a severed spinal injury, as clearly indicated by this widely disseminated video. The rats that remained paralyzed would soon recover as well as they were subjected to a mild, paralytic compression injury. Stem cells administered perhaps facilitated recovery by releasing growth factors or suppressing immune responses. No mention of this defining difference was given as the video was presented at scientific gatherings and seminars and to the lay public over a period of years. That being said, the composure of Mr. Reeves and his strength, endurance and will to survive after his spinal injury greatly helped many patients facing devastating diseases to better deal with the consequences; Christopher Reeves set the standard, and he remains a hero in the development of stem cell research.

This result of this carefully orchestrated presentation led most observers to believe that embryonic stem cells certainly held the ability to generate neural regenerative stem cells. Ironically, this thought, based on misleading data, gained wider acceptance when President Bush –after consulting scientists, religious leaders, political rivals and friends as well as the public and his own conscious--- responsibly decided to limit embryonic stem cell research to cell lines that were available, but would not permit the establishment of any new lines at the expense of a viable embryo. This proclamation limited the ability of scientists to show the true potential of embryonic or fetal stem cells. No scientist of note questioned the validity of early results for years, overlooking the nearly impossible series of events that would have to occur in order to effect precise reconnection of all nerves of a severed spine and restore function. Scientists as well as the lay public leapt to the conclusion that diseases of the brain would quickly be cured were it not for prohibitive regulations. Nancy Reagan supported the Democratic candidate for president who opposed President Bush in the 2004 presidential election only because the Democratic candidate supported embryonic stem cell research, thoroughly convinced that embryonic stem cells would have saved her husband, President Ronald Reagan, from the ravages of Alzheimer's disease [personal communication]. Individuals who supported embryonic stem cell research neglected to note and consider the very deep religious, personal and even scientific arguments against this research others just as validly held. Simply because they were absolutely certain that the technique held amazing potential, they supporters were blind to views of opponents. Many if not most individuals were led to believe that cures for neural, pulmonary, kidney, liver, eye, and virtually all other organs had in fact been developed; only governmental restrictions hampered their availability and use.

Profit-motivated biotechnology firms rationalized their failure to meet expectations they expressed when gaining funds from investors by suggesting that failure resulted from research restrictions. Individuals spent thousands of dollars to obtain stem cell transplants in a limited number of foreign countries, with no bona fide reports of success. When asked, the wife of President Bush, Laura Bush, inquired why the topic had become a political issue, as it was inarguable that the President's decision followed weeks of consultation and thought. Immediately prior to announcement of the ban, a select group of noted stem cell researchers met at the NIH headquarters in Bethesda Maryland, and avidly endorsed the compromise the President developed; not one expressed deep reservations, and the decision was widely endorsed by the stem cell community. Only one peer reviewed scientific journal, Stem Cells and Development (then known as the Journal of Hematotherapy and Stem Cell Research), expressed reservations editorially, noting that the existing cell lines were not "immortal", as advertised, and all would mutate and lose functional characteristics to mutations during the next 3 years. The editorial predicted with accuracy that of the 70 established embryonic stem cell lines the NIH had identified, less than 15 would retain viability before the next presidential election. Supposedly, 11 did; of these, none generated progeny that resembled that of freshly harvested embryonic stem cells.

In fact, the feelings of both First Ladies held immense yet opposing credibility. The scientific community stands to be faulted for not questioning the incredible results presented on news shows, and for basing developing dogma on these observations. Faced with lack of fresh material for embryonic stem cell studies, scientists turned their attention to "adult" stem cells, focusing on the mesenchymal stem cells (MSC) identified years earlier by Caplan [22]. These cells were virtually ignored as the hematopoietic stem cell (HSC) was the target of most investigations of adult stem cells. Based on years of prior work stimulated largely by the development of nuclear weapons, the HSC was defined as a cell that could restore the hematopoietic system of animals exposed to radiation or other hemato-toxic materials. The HSC was found to exist as a non-adherent, radiosensitive cell that resided in the bone marrow of humans and experimental animals. The cell was characterized and used to cure both leukemia and immune defects in terminally ill patients in 1962 by groups led by Dr. Robert A Good and Nobel Laureate E. Donnal Thomas. Highly profiled studies provided evidence that indicated the entire hematopoietic/immune system could be regenerated by a single cell, a cell termed "pluripotential", and which was thought to generate copies of itself as well as a more differentiated cell from one division. As the hematopoietic system in fact is an organ system, this work engendered expectations that similar cells which held the ability to regenerate intact somatic organs in their entirety existed, and could be used for a similar successful therapeutic effect. Initial studies indicated that such cells existed in bone marrow and to a lesser extent blood of healthy individuals. As the fury to find this cell grew unrestrained, one report claimed to "turn blood into brain"; surprisingly, this report was published in a very well regarded journal, and the public awaited this emerging therapy with restrained enthusiasm.

Soon after the ban on embryonic stem cell research went into effect, a rare subset of cells termed MAPCs or multi-potential adult progenitor cells was identified within populations of MSCs. These were portrayed to hold many of the characteristics of embryonic stem cells. Based on studies from a prominent lab at the University of Minnesota, these cells were also said to possess incredible regenerative capabilities of tissues from all germ lines. Mesodermal regeneration remained to target of most studies; endothelial progenitor cells were identified that were thought to be capable of facilitating the repair of torn vessels; cardiac muscle progenitors were claimed to be abundant in MSC preparations and were said to be strikingly effective in restoration of ischemic heart tissue after myocardial infarction. Virtually every field of clinical medicine held to the hope of regenerative stem cell therapy; yet no therapeutically effective approach had been provided. Dogma touting the wonders of stem cells developed despite the publication of alternative explanations for the apparent regeneration reported by the controversial process of post-natal transdifferentiation, a process wherein cells of one germ line transforms to generate cells of another. Few scientists of note questioned these remarkable developments, which continued to be reported, unhindered by lack of confirmation. The field was exploding and unrestrained. Science and businesses merged, providing a new motive to industrious researchers. Inevitably, however, doubters coalesced their efforts leading to the foundation of Stem Cells and Development, a journal that questioned the basic tenants of stem cell research [50]. At its onset, the Journal surveyed leading investigators in the field, initially asking two simple questions; what is a stem cell [51,52] and why hasn't stem cell transplantation worked to date [53]? No consistent answer was obtained.

Presently, regeneration of any tissue, let alone organ, with stem cells remains an elusive goal. Techniques used to reach this goal may be flawed, as all are based on the concept that a single cell can yield progeny to generate an entire organ, a conclusion based on results of hematopoietic stem cell transplantation. This conclusion can be held to question, as the result was obtained in a limited number of experiments which relied on an indirect approach to assess hematopoietic system regeneration. In no reproduced experiment did injection of a single cell rescue an animal from the lethal effects of total marrow ablation. Models wherein a single cell is expanded by colony growth in vitro and the cells of that colony are mixed with freshly harvested marrow cells of a genetically similar animal result in expression of genes of the colony forming cell by some cells of all components of the hematopoietic system are consistent with the underlying hypothesis, but may arise from factors that lead to an inaccurate conclusion. All organ systems are comprised of cells that vary widely in their composition, and the thought that even a simple organ, for example skin, can be regenerated by a single cell, expanded or not, seems untenable. The question of why apparently incredible results of early studies of stem cell researchers were avidly published and stood unchallenged by the scientific community is not perplexing; it is informative as it reveals major flaws in presently accepted modes of scientific communication. These flaws must be addressed, as valuable resources are diverted to studies based on erroneous results. Communication of results is an essential component of the research process, not merely its endpoint. Rather, effective, reliable and clear presentation of key results stands as the starting point of investigations which result in therapeutic advance. It is evident that fundamental tenants of scientific communication must change to increase the credibility of reported results; the accuracy of interpretations and predictions these results engender. Absent that, science shall become a business, and one which creates more problems than it solves. Why incredible results of early experiments in stem cell research were allowed to stand unchallenged poses perplexing and important questions. Yet, nothing has changed, as the number of publications and Journals that they appear in continues to increase almost exponentially and the problem becomes a medical issue. A medical issue that is undefined, not a focus of structured research and which holds ramifications that influence almost all aspects of scientific study.

TECHNIQUES USED IN NEURAL STEM CELL RESEARCH

Advances in high-resolution cellular imaging, combined with genetic manipulations in mice, novel fluorescent recombinant probes, and large-scale screening of gene expression have revealed multiple molecular mechanisms that may underlie structural and functional plasticity in the brain and retina. Understanding the biology of stem cells has been facilitated by the development of sophisticated tools, including new imaging techniques [54], advanced culture methods and fluorescent activated cell sorting, which characterize and isolate specific stem cell populations based on surface protein expression [55]. The complexity of NSCs, neural patterning and the formation of multiple populations of neurons, astrocytes, and oligodendrocytes rationalizes the need to intensify studies to characterize these cells and to define the microenvironment required to support them in the CNS.

In vitro differentiation assays are important in cell characterization, in detecting novel instructive molecules, and in generating specific cell types. Functional MRI (fMRI) is gaining recognition as a method to locate sites of brain repair and enhanced or diminished function [56]. Together, these techniques indicate that brain repair does occur, consistent with a physiological role of tissue - specific neural stem cells. However, it is important to note that repair as assessed by functional improvement does not evidence the involvement of any specific stem cell. It is perhaps just as likely that the determined patient trains undamaged areas of the brain to perform functions lost to injury and disease.

Separation of cells has been a key aspect of stem cell research. Milteny Biotech Inc. has recently developed a magnetic bead based assay that allows sorting of putative neural stem cells using a cocktail of antibodies specific for markers expected to be selectively expressed by these cells. Similarly, specific cells can be depleted before transplant to lessen undesirable effects [57-59]. Imaginative but simple methods have, in contrast, been developed to enhance recovery of stem cells from sources wherein the numbers of such cells are limited. Such an approach provided, for example, sufficient numbers of stem cells from the blood of a single umbilical cord to allow successful allogeneic transplantation, and remains the only approved method for this purpose today [60,61]. The method simply avoids any loss of cells from the fluid to be processed by entirely avoiding cell separation; all of the cells recovered in the initial extract are recovered, stored and infused into the recipient. Initially met with skepticism, the paucity of stem cells in a single umbilical extract rendered this approach necessary; no stem cell could be lost, and any cell enrichment or depletion technique inevitably results in some cell loss. Fortunately, contaminating erythrocytes, lymphocytes, neutrophils, platelets and other cells did not have any adverse effect on the transplant, which resulted in curative therapy for a child with Fanconi's anemia. The pioneering studies, led by Dr. Hal E Broxmeyer, initiated a new approach to hematopoietic stem cell transplants as well as to stem cell biology.

Automated closed systems are now widely employed to isolate stem cells from mobilized peripheral blood as well as marrow aspirates by a method that reduces the risk of contamination and enhances recovery. Most of these are based on the initial description of such an approach soon after the same investigators developed the processing methods for HSCs from cord blood for transplantation described above [62]. Closed systems are now commercially available and many employ technology developed with skill and precision by Baxter Inc., as well as specialized equipment from this corporation. Study of migration of stem cells requires accurate mapping of the traffic of the cells after infusion. Various methods of labeling have been used in animal models ranging from simple non-toxic dyes to sophisticated genetic tags. Positron emission tomography [PET] has acquired the unique distinction of defining the precise location of cells at sites of injury and disease. This endpoint has also been accomplished using MRI to trace pre-labeled cells in studies which have successfully located as few as 2 stem cells after transplantation [56].

FATE DECISIONS AND RHO FAMILY GTPASES AND DIVERSE STEM CELL FUNCTIONS

Stem cells that reside in the marrow must detach, mobilize, migrate to the circulation, adhere to the vascular bed at areas near the injured tissue, migrate into the affected zone, stop migrating and then proliferate and differentiate to generate new cells for structural regeneration. Some have termed the changing responses as "fate decisions" cells make. We emphasize however that the individual cell does not possess the capacity to make any decision; their function is dependent on exogenous factors and environmental components.

Yang and coworkers developed a focused microarray to compare protein expression of putative stem cell populations and defined by a 'molecular signature' common to all putative stem cell populations [63]. The group found certain ectodermal - associated genes to be down-regulated while genes needed for adherence and matrix signaling were expressed when embryonic stem cells were induced to form embryoid bodies. Other studies indicated opposite expression patterns when stem cells were cultured under different conditions, consistent with the theory that the stem cell is anything but a primitive cell. The cell holds the ability to express any gene; its differentiation depends on which focused set of genes is expressed. Default generation to cells of a neural phenotype has been observed from both embryonic and adult stem cells [64, 65] deprived of inducing growth factors, such as VEGF or EGF. As the neural ectoderm is perhaps the most complex system of the adult vertebrate, it is not surprising that its foundation would be formed early in development. Cells from the neural crest, a fascinating structure that develops when ecodermal folds coalesce, have been postulated to provide essential stem cells for many tissues [48, 49]. Indeed, the neural crest plays a key role in development but exactly how it exerts its effects remains mysterious. Surrounded by mesoderm, the neural crest is in a pivotal position to utilize divergent germ layer components as cells fuse to generate advanced progenitors.

In a little noticed but potentially defining study, Kratchmarova and coworkers showed differential induction of MSC differentiation was due to a tyrosine kinase-dependent process [66]. Knowing that EGF induces MSCs to differentiate into osteoblasts but the related growth factor, PDGF, does not, the authors compared tyrosine phosphorylated proteins expressed by the stem cells upon exposure to PDGF and EGF. PDGF induced the tyrosine phosphorylation of several proteins by a mechanism dependent of the unique enzyme, PI3' kinase, but EGF did not. When the authors treated MSCs with a specific PI3' kinase inhibitor, PDGF was capable of inducing osteogenic differentiation in a manner similar to that observed with EG.F. These results led the authors to conclude that PI3' kinase activation of tyrosine phosphorylation dampened the stem cell activity of proliferation.

We note that proliferation is the final function of a stem cell. Proliferation proceeds at the expense of functions necessary to make stem cells available, and as such, amplification of proliferation may not optimize stem cell therapy. In order for stem cells to proliferate in a setting that provides beneficial function, they must first mobilize, adhere and migrate to the site of action, all the while retaining their ability to differentiate. The former functions are dependent on processes promoted by the small GTPase, Rac, a member of the Rho family of small GTPase's. Cell functions dependent on Rac signaling include adherence, migration, margination and activation of certain enzyme systems, such as the NADPH oxidase. On the other hand, Rho effectors mediate differentiation and proliferation of stem cells after they reach their target. Rho signaling is dampened by PI3' kinase and enhanced by PKA, which acts as a point of switching of cell function from those that depend on Rac to those dependent on Rho signaling. These functions are tightly regulated by matrix interactions as a result of physical alterations secondary to adherence (or detachment) as well as by induction of matrix signaling pathways which often impinge upon the activity of PKA, PI3' kinase, integ.rin dependent kinase, focal adhesion kinase and as well as to alterations in src positioning and activity and the deployment of key intermediates such as CAS, Crk, Rho kinases, and Pak-1. These signaling intermediates exert their effects after cells encounter primary signaling initiators, specifically growth factors (such as the EG.F family, the FGF family and the TGF family), bone morphogenic protein family members, tissue specific growth factors (BNDF, NGF), as well as matrix components which dramatically alter the cells' function in response to any factor or co-factor.

Although a detailed biochemical discussion of cell function dictated by external clues transcends the scope of this essay, the results abstracted above provide a glimpse of the interconnected mechanisms that orchestrate optimal responses. As research progresses, we enter an era where cellular therapy may result in a means to reverse disorders of brain. However, it is naïve to think that this result will be achieved without clarification of the underlying biochemical events that dictate cell function. In this respect, while much remains to be known, many processes are well described. Reports of years past shed new light on functions we only now appreciate.

NEURAL STEM CELLS AND ANIMAL MODELS

Most of our preclinical knowledge of stem cell biology derives from disease models. Here we discuss some of the studies that shape future trends for clinical applications. Parkinson's disease is characterized by a selective loss of dopaminergic neurons and hence presents an attractive target for stem cell therapy. While there are reports that indicate functional recovery of animals models when similar neurons derived from ES cells were implanted into diseased brains, detailed analyses leads to the conclusion that these effects were not due to regeneration of tissue. Others have reported that human NSCs improve cognitive function of rats with traumatic brain injury. The grafted cells survived, differentiated into neurons and expressed and released GNDF.

Tang *et al.* [7] injected murine embryonic stem cell - derived neural precursors into the hippocampus of amyloid β-depleted rats and found marked decrease in escape latency and exploratory time, 2 well accepted measures of rat memory, 16 weeks after transplantation. Yamasaki *et al.* [67] used transgenic mice carrying cells with an inducible system to initiate the expression of the A chain of diphtheria toxin, leading to progressive loss of neurons within the hippocampus and resulting in specific memory impairment to demonstrate similar memory enhancement when endogenous NSCs were recruited to the hippocampus. These reports are but 2 examples of a multitude of reports that should be held to strict questions in interpretation. First, it is no easy task to assess the memory capability of any animal. Second, investigator bias certainly influences interpretation of results of single studies, especially in an era where profit motivates much of the research undertaken and careers depend on information disseminated to investors. This is a scientific fact, and one that needs to be evaluated in assessments of reports of neural stem cell therapeutic successes. Third, non-specific factors, such as cytokines and growth factors delivered by the infused cells influence the results in a manner that can be mimicked by immunosupressants, such as corticosteroids. Of the trials being conducted with adult of MSCs, one that has yielded the most promising results is the study of the utility of MSCs for prevention of graft vs. host disease following allogeneic bone marrow transplantation in cyclosporine - resistant individuals. Clearly, MSCs possess immunosuppressive activity. It has been long appreciated that immunosuppressants can lessen some effects of traumatic brain injury if delivered at the appropriate time and in amounts sufficient to suppress the immune system. While it may be premature to conclude that traumatic brain injury is enhanced by autoimmune responses, this is certainly a possibility after disruption of the "blood brain barrier".

Many other processes may contribute to the results reported to date, but no reproducible results indicate neural tissue regeneration and establishment of precise new neural connections in the benefits of stem cell therapy reported in pre-clinical models and inferred for therapeutic use. These considerations lead to an irrefutable conclusion that both the scientific community and lay public must now come to appreciate. That conclusion is that ***no stem cell-based therapy for neural disease has proven clinically effective to date.*** The lure of stem cells as a magic bullet for neural problems resulted from early claims of their ability to reverse brain and spinal cord injuries. Despite years of intense investigations by a number of highly motivated groups who have employed embryonic, fetal and adult stem cells, stem cells do not reverse neural injury or regenerate functional neural tissue when used in any manner yet reported.

THE ORGANIC BRAIN SYNDROMES

After traumatic brain injury or stroke, some patients show remarkable functional improvement over a prolonged period of time. It is convenient to attribute this result to stem cell mediated restoration of tissues and tissue function. However, while this is certainly possible, it is not the only explanation for recovery. For the purposes of this essay, organic brain syndromes are considered to be brain dysfunction resulting from a readily identifiable cause. Not included in this discussion are Alzheimer's, Parkinson's or genetic diseases. Mental illnesses including situational or biochemical depression, schizophrenia, bi-polar disorders are also not considered here. This discussion is limited to neural dysfunction resulting from traumatic brain injury and stroke, where the cause is apparent, physical and defined. We note that animal models used to assess stem cell repair of brain injury rely on traumatic brain injury in large part, and that traumatic brain injury is a leading cause of neural pathology that leads to devastating effects with few therapeutic options. The availability of neural stem cells seems to provide a high degree of promise for patients after neural assault, based on pre-clinical results. We here assess these results and the hope of stem cells for therapy of patients with "organic brain disease".

In the usual clinical scenario, a patient who sustained a severe but non-fatal head injury or stroke presents with confusion and retrograde amnesia often following a period of loss of consciousness. These patients may be relieved to be alive and cognizant, and often do not think they sustained any neural injury. The symptomatic effects of a non-fatal injury are, in the usual clinical setting, secondary to blood infiltration, edema, hypoxia or direct damage to neural tissue. In latter 3 instances, the symptoms may be delayed but soon become readily apparent and lead quite often to death. Most often, imaging and other immediately available, noninvasive tests confirm the pathology leading to the symptoms. Cerebral swelling may initially cause few noticeable effects, but leads to pronounced and fatal effects within days after traumatic brain injury. The damage caused by cerebral swelling can be alleviated if the cerebrum is opened to relieve pressure soon [within 20 minutes] after the injury. Fatal responses are not uncommon and are not delayed past a period of a few days. Second, frank blood infiltration through a broken skull or from a ruptured vessel (stroke, aneurism) causes immediate damage leading to altered motor abilities, acute and intense pain, confusion, remorse and finally death. Surgical intervention may help, but often the results are unfavorable.

Damage resulting from hypoxia is similarly immediately readily evident, as is damage from direct tissue injury, which often affects the frontal lobe resulting in memory loss as well as loss of judgment and the reversion of the patient to a childlike – if not vegetative state. Tissue destruction due to stroke (ischemia) and assault can influence neural function in many ways.

Organic brain syndrome secondary to a closed head injury results from sustained and slow infiltration of blood, usually across a small disruption of the forehead caused by the helmet worn by individuals involved in motorcycle accidents. Since the injury is not evident by blood loss or apparent by X-Ray or MRI imaging, and since the symptoms are invariably delayed, these patients face incredible problems as symptoms appear. These problems are enhanced by the mere fact that the patient doesn't have any idea of what is going on. Lack of blood from the damaged site and intact function of the patient in prior days, weeks or months lead observers to minimize the involvement of the injury when symptoms progress. Many patients are diagnosed as having sustained a "concussion", and are diagnosed as suffering "post-concussional syndrome". Organic brain injury results from much more that a concussion, the effects of the latter being totally reversible. Symptoms that develop after traumatic brain injury sufficient to cause organic brain disease are not reversible. Organic brain diseases result from irreversible damage to neural tissues, but manifest slowly and lead the patient's colleagues, friends, family and care-givers providers to of confusion, doubt and consequent disdain. As this happens, the patient invariably falls into a crevice of hopeless despair.

Early researchers concluded that patients could not recover fully from even mild to moderate neural injury that resulted in delayed symptoms [68]. However, the finding that some patients with severe traumatic brain injury as well as stroke - induced injury recovered led Raisman to postulate in 1978 that actual regeneration within the central nervous system does occur [69]. The Raisman postulate, which remains controversial, set the stage for the hope that regeneration could be accelerated by stem cell therapy, based on the assumption that the regeneration Raisman noted was due to the activity of stem cells. These stem cells were thought to reside in the brain itself, or alternatively postulated to be a component of the MSCs which reside within hematopoietic tissues. Recent evidence indicates that tissue - specific stem cells reside in the brain and that after assault, regenerate neural tissue. If this is the case, stem cell therapy may hold substantial potential for treatment of neural disorders caused by trauma, infection or disease. Indeed the spontaneous recovery of patients who sustained stroke or severe neural trauma is consistent with this view. However, recovery is rare, and several questions persist.

Thus, it is evident that patients who suffer the effects of severe brain injury never recover completely. These patients may show decreased aphasia and improved gait and dexterity as well as better judgment and decreased emotional distress, but not recover their ability to remember the previous day's events; to recall the details of their childhood; to be free of over-reaction to stimuli leading to inappropriate expressions of certain emotions or to regain their trust in others. While marked clinical improvement appears evident, patients retain many deficiencies and exhibit inappropriate fears. "Executive functioning" remains impaired as many patients simply assert what is on their minds, unhindered by prefrontal connections to the hippocampus that develop during maturation, networks successful individuals adeptly use to reach goals. The previously successful patient is often discharged when confidence that he will "say the right thing" is lost. They patient may easily become lost, fail to recall the names or phone numbers of all friends, and — even if they do not show it — exist in a state of confused desperation best characterized as "fearful dependence" on others. Dependence on others is an unavoidable consequence and the patient realizes it; however, patients with progressive organic brain disease often find themselves in a unique and inescapable paradox; either depend on others or die. Exploitation is not a consequence of organic brain disease; it is a symptom. By the time the once independent patient finds it impossible to "fend for himself", he has learned to not place his trust in anyone. Unlike other disabled individuals, victims of severe organic brain disease are met with distrust, disbelief and the neither inconsequential nor legal consequences of malicious rumor-mongering and mis-characterization.

Realizing the profound impact these factors have on recovery, Strub and Black [70] summarized a classification system based on physical factors that are usually available even months or years after the injury. Retrograde amnesia of over 30 seconds prior to the injury, loss of consciousness for over 7 hours and anteriograde amnesia of more than one week results from "severe" closed head trauma. Symptoms may be similar to that of post-concessional syndromes or mild head injury but which progress are often irreversible. The most obvious symptoms are aphasia and hemiparesis, irritability, loss of interest, lack of attention, amnesia, hostility, problems with pattern recognition, withdrawal, inappropriate fear and anxiety, inappropriate behavior, personality alterations, motor retardation, affective disturbances, involuntary emotional outbursts, confusion, sleep disturbances, hormone changes, dysarthria imbalance, ataxia, tremor and depression. Initial neuropsychological testing reveals significant deficits in WAIS Full Scale IQ to ranges between 65-75, often a lower Memory Quotient. Initial language and constructional ability may be normal but Trail Making Test performance often shows marked impairment. Of the WAIS parameters, verbal levels often exceed performance levels.

Treatment is complicated by several factors. First, patients are often referred for testing because of suspected mental illness. This may manifest as immature behavior, irritability, lack of recall, and disinterest. Often these and other mental responses are aggravated by the almost inadvertent and hostile relation many uneducated therapists develop toward the patient, which results when the therapist concludes the patient's hostility or other symptoms are elaborated in a deliberate attempt to resist help or to seek some financial gain. This is often enhanced by input from the patient's family and employer, who "in the interest of society", are appraised by the therapist of his suspicions and who then readily agree, and in doing so, add weight to the misdiagnosis. The curious fact that "higher" cognitive capacities of such patients are usually well preserved or even enhanced as the brain stem sustains the brunt of the damage sparing cortical functions further fuels the misdiagnosis. A typical question is "'how could the individual be suffering from effects of a severe brain injury when he can write top selling novels?". Such thoughts enhance suspicion. Sooner or later the patient becomes well aware of this, but is neither able nor does he particularly want to address this paradox.

Employers often have much to lose if a diagnosis of organic illness is made, and family members often refrain from any input due to doubt, frustration and the fear of impending financial and chronic emotional encumbrance.

Typically, they essentially abandon the patient, rationalizing this action by the thought that the patient is well equipped to survive on his own. Family members who are not in a position to abandon the patient, specifically spouses and offspring, often enjoin the therapist in promoting the false diagnosis of mental rather than organic disease in order to alleviate their own responsibilities, avoid financial encumbrance and to justify prior and planned actions taken at the expense of the compromised patient.

Damage to the midbrain during closed head injury is common, as the head moves violently causing the brain to rotate about its cranial vault distorting midbrain structures. Damage to the brain stem stroma results in loss of consciousness with concomitant damage to other structures in the area. Dementia is often diagnosed as a result of dysarthria, ataxia, tremor, occulomotor nerve damage and inability to sense changes in patterning, but this is usually not the case. Dysarthria makes these individuals appear demented, but cognitive function remains remarkably intact, and can usually be detected by appropriate methods. Patients typically remain aware of their environment, and many seem able to function normally in all situations. But they are not. Since these patients sustained significant trauma, memory defects and behavioral changes are unavoidable but manageable in a supportive environment. Straub and Black emphasize the irreversible aggravation of damage an unsupportive or doubting environment inevitably creates, as they emphasize the inability of psychiatrists to recognize the distinction between organic and mental illness of the central nervous system, as well as the financial advantage of a diagnosis of mental illness in the usual clinical setting (70).

Personality changes resulting in what family members and therapist consider to be inappropriate behavior characterized by apathy, irritability, euphoria and memory lapse are often misinterpreted as being intentional. Often this misinterpretation is bolstered by external factors and represents a callous and perhaps malicious mis-interpretation by a therapist who only needs to examine WAIS scores to dismiss this possibility, which can otherwise lead to drastic negative consequences, including institutionalization and treatment denied. Institutionalization should be avoided whenever possible for individuals who sustain traumatic brain damage; these patients should be released from the hospital as soon as possible after trauma. Identification of the source of behavioral changes as organic renders both the staff and patient more relaxed and results in a favorable environment for recovery to whatever extent is possible. Unfortunately, the prognosis is less favorable. In general, the overall outcome of severe closed head injury is as follows: half the patients die before leaving the hospital. Forty percent of the survivors die within 6 years of the accident. Of the remainder, 42% remain severely disabled and the rest moderately disabled for life. However of these, 17% experience what is considered to be a "good" recovery. Patients with anteriograde amnesia of over 3 weeks shall have continuing memory defects often aggravating mental problems. Amnesia of over 40 days results in the failure of most patients to return to work.

When a full rehabilitation effort is put forth, these statistics change. Fully half of the patients return to work albeit with a less responsible assignment due to disability. On the other hand, certain symptoms seem to be refractory to any therapeutic intervention in progressive disease, including gait difficulty and falling due to hydrocephalus, incontinence, and a progressive decrease in the level of consciousness.

According to Straub and Black, the most common and costly mistake made in the management of patients with even minor head trauma is the quick "brush off" many patients experience. Due to negative radiological findings and other factors, the patient is thought to hold no squeal from brain trauma and is told to return to work, where he cannot perform. The patient then typically returns to the physician who typically only reaffirms the initial negative findings. The frustrated patient and employer enter a sustained phase of anger and tension; employers feel trapped by laws protecting disabled patients, and the patient feels all symptoms result from the resistance of the employer to accept the organic cause of the problem. If terminated, patients invariably seek legal redress, and are often successful. However, the legal process may drag on for years as the patient's health worsens, in cases that easily could have been resolved with a few months of understanding therapy and minor accommodations.

When the appropriately treated patient begins to stabilize, it is imperative for the patient and family to devise with the therapist a comprehensive rehabilitation program. This is always difficult. Family members remain both suspicious and stressed, as therapists desire to end their role in therapy. At this juncture, patients harbor well-founded suspicions of their own. Physical and mental disorders render career plans difficult to formulate and impossible to realize in the absence of support or when future support, be it habitual, emotional, or economic is uncertain. If the patient sustained frontal lobe damage, apathy leads to loss of drive rendering a productive career impossible even when physical and cognitive problems have been overcome. Hormone changes resulting from blood pooling at the hippocampus lessens the patients' ability to deal with stress, challenge or to "rise to the occasion", even if the patient is otherwise able to resume his prior role in society. As Drs. Straub and Black aptly conclude, "Because of his multiple handicaps, the patient with severe head trauma must rely on family resources and family counseling is a critical component of the rehabilitative program. The family must understand the patient's deficits and capabilities in order to work effectively with the patient after discharge. Without family support, the patient will flounder. Social workers are necessary to prepare the family and the therapist for sustained, successful therapy, in arranging resources and in providing continuing support" [70].

STEM CELLS AND ORGANIC DISEASES OF THE BRAIN

The Raisman hypothesis appears flawed, and if so, casts doubt on the extent of endogenous neural repair mediated by stem cells. As mentioned above, even effects of mild brain injury are not entirely reversible. Stem cell-mediated tissue regeneration would result in complete functional recovery. Rather, it is likely that the clinical improvement observed in individuals who sustained severe neural trauma results from potentiation of function in non-damaged areas of the brain. Adaptive neural potentiation afforded by potentiation of the contralateral hemisphere has been well defined in neonates born with congenital hemiparesis [71] and results in complete absence of symptoms. Recent investigations implicate contralateral potentiation as well as potentiation of surrounding areas of the damaged tissue to recovery from trauma and stroke some patient's experience. In contrast, contralateral hemispheres often results in decreased function as assessed by fMRI after stroke for reasons that remain unclear. Spontaneous recovery has been attributed to stem cells and growth factors, but no evidence yet supports these attractive hypotheses. Largely overlooked is the fact that avid determination of patients to re-acquire lost functions by educating non-damaged brain areas to replace the functional abilities lost to trauma plays a major role in recovery from the effects of traumatic brain injury.

As mentioned above, "higher" intellectual functions are curiously spared in many brain damaged patients. Prior to the onset of delayed symptoms, patients may enter a period of enhanced productivity and euphoria that they later cannot recall due to a process referred to as anteriograde amnesia. Paradoxically, as symptoms develop, higher intellectual functions are often enhanced. Thus, a good writer may become an excellent one, as the patient regains motor, language and coordination abilities. This enhancement may be a side effect of potentiation. It may result from regeneration of neural structures from tissue-specific endogenous stem cells or mesenchymal (bone marrow) stem cells, resulting in activity of neural patterns new to the patient; patterns which may elicit talents not previously realized as areas of the brain responsible for them were left untapped. The results may lead the patient to believe recovery was total and endogenous. But the patient inevitably soon realizes that this conclusion is but another example of wishful thinking, as he glides his car through a glaring red light, argues with supportive friends, sits at airport terminals and watches his flight depart, failing to recall the connection between possession of a boarding pass and the act of boarding, the color red and the act of stopping, or the consequences of adversity. The behavior of recovering patients is often affected in other ways that we fail to understand, owing to our lack of appreciation of just how the brain works.

A recovering patient may see a car approach as he waits at an intersection, but not connect that sight with the consequences that result as he resumes movement into the path of the oncoming vehicle. We *think* that stopping at a red light, not moving into the path of a 3 ton tri-axle truck or acknowledging the call of our name are "instinctual" processes. In fact, they are not. These acts and others result from learned behavior that has become so deeply embedded into the neural circuitry that we think the behavior results from the process we refer to as "instinct". This explains the fact that new drivers have many more accidents that experienced ones, regardless of the age they learned to drive. "Instinct" is nothing more than learned behavior. As a result, loss of the ability to perform functions we reg.ard as both basic and instinctual often are the first, and always are the most obvious, result of traumatic brain injury. Explaining later to authorities that the driver saw the car coming but proceeded anyway leads inevitably to suspicions of substance use and intoxication, as individuals do not understand that what we often take as instinctual behavior is actually learned behavior involving interconnected neural networks that are readily disconnected by trauma in an manner that inconsistently affects different areas of the brain. Some functions remain intact while others are lost. Traumatic brain injured patients often report an ability to recall some memories of their youth, but others are completely lost, even if they were experienced at the same age. We learn to apply the brakes when we see a stop sign or red light; we learn not to proceed into the path of an oncoming car; we learn how to speak, walk, and respond to environmental clues. We learn how to tie our shoe laces early in life, and how to initiate and finish simple tasks. What we fail to realize is the fact that we learn these and other functions we attribute to "lower intellect" over a period of many years while we are very young.

Many are stunned by the ability of individuals who claim they had sustained a brain injury to adeptly carry out neural functions considered to result from "higher intellect". Thus, a brain damaged patient may not be very good at driving, yet be able to recall the laws of physics flawlessly. This inevitably reinforces the concept that the patient is "faking it", as the result is not consistent with the concept of neural function most individuals hold. In fact, the failure to meet expectations the patient's acquaintances expect frustrates the patient and aggravates symptoms Few realize that "higher" intellectual functions are acquired more quickly than basic processes. A well-educated individual easily grasps basic aspects of aerodynamics in a few months, but required years to learn how to talk. Be that as it may, it is often the case that the patient's ability to recall complex facts yet fail to navigate a car enhances suspicion of fraud. Patients are not aware of the doubt surrounding them. To the patient, everything appears normal; except for the fact that they often get lost driving home, can't find their car in the parking lot at the mall, or forget to arrive at important appointments. However, most patients' remain in denial, unaware of the gossip surrounding them, and unaware of their diagnosis, even if test results (WAIF Scores, e.g.) indicate substantial injury.

Patients whose symptoms develop late typically do not realize they sustained any brain damage; the affected neural tissue is not capable of communicating that defect and intact neural circuits are unaware of it. When an individual sustains a leg injury, for example, the intact brain senses the damage and quickly designs plans to deal with it. Only when injury is so severe that the brain is overwhelmed with fear, or influenced by shock, hypothermia, blood loss, hyperthermia, toxemia, or other factors does its function diminish, often with fatal consequences. However, when the circuitry of the brain is damaged, even in a small area, that damage is always total. Either the circuit functions or it does not; there is no middle ground. When a damaged circuit ceases to function, the effects eventually encompass all the neural networks it was once integrated with. These intact circuits are eventually and progressively disrupted as a result of altered inputs from damaged neurons as well as from their consistent inability to elicit responses previously processed when messages they compose are delivered to disrupted neurons. The results are variable, unpredictable and confusing. Complicating the confusion this disruption engenders, patients with traumatic brain injury never think they sustained any brain injury, especially in cases where symptoms development is delayed, and when the dermal barrier is not breached. The simple fact of the matter is that absent bleeding, patients may be initially confused, but often soon regain composure. Happy to be alive, the individual insists he or she is "OK"; often they appear to be. More often, they do not. Most fail to recall the day of the week, the name of the President, the month of the year. Failure to recall the day of their birth indicates severe damage that is typically fatal. The patient may stumble and fall walking from the site, or revert to behavior characterized as "childlike" or "goofy" when they become aware of their limitations, but do not understand them. These individuals face a limited time for any therapy to be effective. Presently, well within an hour after the injury, the patient's fate is sealed. If the injury is severe enough to cause frank blood release into the neural cavity, cerebral swelling or ischemia, death is imminent. If the injury is minor, fully functional capability resumes quickly, often leaving the patient with a concussion and a very bad headache. Between these two endpoints, patients emerge with irreversible organic brain disease, which is a rare but devastating consequence of traumatic brain injury that changes the equation that once defined the life of the injured person in ways that are difficult to understand.

Problems the brain injured patient faces are further amplified when minor distractions lead to major disruptions, as the patient loses ability to perform more that a single task at any given time. Patients lose their sense of timing, as well as their ability to gate information based on significance or to perform acts based on consequences. Thus, a recovering patient may persist indefinitely in the most insignificant task he faces, abandoning matters that are far more important. Patients recovering from severe traumatic brain injury that is associated with frontal lobe defects cannot discern important facts from trivial ones and tend to communicate aimlessly in a pattern termed to result from "tangential thought". Disruption of the efferent aspect of the frontal-temporal circuit often leads the patient to forget exactly what he is talking about while he is talking. These patients often "ramble on incessantly" as their hopelessly confused audience quickly learns not to listen to anything said. Aware of the importance of the message he is attempting to deliver, but completely unaware of the fact that his inability to do so results from disrupted afferent and efferent hippocampal connections to a dysfunctional prefrontal lobe, the patient quickly concludes that more information is necessary to convey his point. Additional information is ignored, even disdained, and the process leads to an auto-amplifying cycle that ends in devastation. The inability of such patients to thrive without assistance results from similar problems that impinge upon the patient in a similar, self - amplifying manner, resulting in total confusion and bewilderment. Eventually, the patient "gives up". The results are often drastic. A vivid example is found in patients who find they are consistently unable to follow directions they receive from individuals who don't understand where exactly the patient wants go. As a result, the patient stops asking, and instead wanders about aimlessly seeking his destination.

Unlike patients with Alzheimer's disease, the disoriented brain injured patient retains skills and thought patterns necessary for survival. The results have provided the basis of plots of humorous popular movies (Peter Segal's and Adam Sandler's, "*50 First Dates*") as well as tragic cinema (Star Trek's episode, "*Twilight*").

In progressive disease, retrograde amnesia extends to events that occurred prior to the injury as anteriograde amnesia renders the patient unable to recall yesterday's activities. As the patient's world closes into a sliver of time; desperation becomes the major issue the patient faces. The patient then becomes particularly vulnerable to any hope of complete recovery and often seeks the well-aired promise of stem cell therapy, with consistently negative results.

THE DECISION TO TRANSPLANT BASED ON CURRENT KNOWLEDGE

Recently, the United Kingdom has approved the transplantation of neural stem cells into stroke patients that have been paralyzed for at least 6 months. The genetically engineered stem cells produced by ReNeuron *Inc* were derived from the cell line CTX0E03, a line of fetal neural stem cells developed by this group for the treatment of stable ischemic stroke. Regulatory agencies granted approval for phase I trials. This raises an important issue about how to define the stem cell one uses for the purposes of investigations and transplantation as this will predict its properties after transplantation. For example, there are Neuronal restricted precursors which do not form oligodendrocytes or astrocytes isolated from spinal cord and may be useful for spinal cord injury [72]. Although adult stem cells hold promise, a side by side comparison between embryonic stem cells and adult stem cells is required for each disease before transplantation potential could be fully evaluated. Interestingly, neural stem cells are known to be present at different stages of development starting from 8.5 days in case of mice to 5 weeks in case of human embryos [73]. Not all the stem cells possess EGFR, some have no detectable levels of EGFR called the neuroepithelial stem cell and only respond to FGF and yet have stem cell properties such as self renewal and differentiation. These cells therefore co-exist together in various regions of brain. The compromises between biological utility and molecular specificity of stem cells will determine the translational pace of biotherapeutics. Cell therapy for stroke is a relatively new area of translational and clinical research with preliminary studies showing safety and some measurable benefit in small numbers of subjects [74].

Ironically, the advancements in stroke have been faster than those in Parkinson's Disease (PD) given the fact that PD presents a more localized target for stem cell therapy. The teratoma cell line NT2/D1, able to be differentiate into neurons by the addition of 10 μM retinoic acid (termed LBS-Neurons developed by Layton BioScience), has entered clinical trials. In a phase I study these neurons were stereotactically transplanted to the basal ganglia of 12 patients with basal ganglia stroke and fixed motor deficits [75]. No toxicities or tumor formation were seen with this approach and there was a statistically significant improvement in patients as assessed by the European Stroke Scale (ESS). Subsequently, a phase II randomized study of LBS neurons for patients with sub-cortical motor stroke was reported by Kondziolka *et al.* [76]. In this study 18 patients with fixed motor deficits stable for at least 2 months were randomized at two different centers to receive two different doses of LBS neurons (7 patients per dose level) with non-surgical controls (4 patients). Although there was no overall improvement at 6 months in the treatment groups (assessed by the ESS), the Action Research Arm Test gross hand movement scores improved compared with the control group (p = 0.017) and baseline (p = 0.01).There were no surgical complications in the 14 patients who underwent cell transplantation. Several statistically significant improvements were observed for gross hand movement scores from baseline and compared with controls. As discussed above, adult stem cells were once considered a viable alternative to ES cells to avoid ethical problems. However the hopes once held by these stem cells have not been realized.

NEURAL STEM CELLS FOR PARKINSON'S DISEASE THERAPY

Neural Stem Cells possess characteristics which enhance the hope of targeting delivery of biochemical reagents to specific areas of the brain. In this respect, neural stem cells have been evaluated for degenerative disorders due to a specific defect, particularly Parkinson's disease. Parkinson's disease has been alleviated to some by transplantation of intact fetal tissue that fed L-DOPA to the systemic circulation. Studies carried out in the 1980'used fetal cells that were thought to act like "dopamine pumps" in Parkinson's patients with limited but widely heralded successes. These studies have since been abandoned. However, at that time, several investigators suggested that similar implants may produce factors such as VEGF needed to maintain surviving dopaminergic neurons. As a result, several investigators explored the role of VEGF- expressing NSCs in animal's models. NSCs have also been used in attempts to target delivery of growth factors in several disease models of neurological disorders, including ALS, Parkinson's disease and cancer.

So far, such approaches have been largely ineffective. Further, reactions to the transplanted cells often enhance the symptoms of the recipient such that they typically refuse further experimental approaches. Efficient cell replacement is more demanding than cursory thought would lead one to believe. Precise restoration of connectivity is required to restore both motor and sensory pathways in all cases. Re-establishment of original connection patterns with both local and distant host partners is both required and elusive. As a consequence, all behavioral benefits reported to date likely result from non-specific effects and cannot be attributed to the re-establishment of disrupted circuits in the neural system.

Åkerud *et al.* [77] have studied the ability of NSCs to stably express transgenes and locally deliver soluble molecules with neuroprotective activity, such as glial cell line-derived neurotrophic factor (GDNF). NSCs engineered to release GDNF engrafted well in the host striatum, integrated and gave rise to neurons, astrocytes, and oligodendrocytes as they maintained stable high levels of GDNF expression for at least 4 months. The therapeutic potential of intrastriatal GDNF-NSCs grafts was tested in a mouse 6-hydroxydopamine model of Parkinson's disease with promising results. However, no therapeutic benefit of this approach has been established.

In an study never published in a peer reviewed Journal but well covered by the local media, Williams *et al.* of the University of South Florida implanted genetically marked "fetal" stem cells along with intact neural tissues taken from the brain of a recent accident victim which was to be used to provide dopanergic neurons into the brain of a patient with Parkinson's disease. Absent stem cells, the tissue implantation technique developed by Dr Williams, the Medical Director of the University of South Florida's Center for Aging and Brain Repair Research, had attained some credibility as a therapeutic modality to lessen the symptoms of Parkinson's disease, if only transiently. The technique is neither widely available nor widely hailed as effective. Dr. Williams and colleagues implanted "fetal" stem cells from an unidentified source along with a neural "plug" in a single patient 5 years ago. It is not clear if the study was evaluated by any committee. The patient recently died. Stem cells were isolated from the brain of the corpse based on the genetic marker used. Unsurprisingly, all had transformed into cells with a Parkinson's – like phenotype. Still the investigators involved suggested the approach somehow rendered therapeutic improvement. As stated, the results have not passed peer review, and are not likely to anytime soon. After the stem cells were implanted, along with the neural tissue of the accident victim, the physicians involved in the study continued to assert that she (the patient) was "doing better than expected" in this highly unscientific study. They didn't assert this when she died and the "stem cells" were found to have not produced any neural recovery, new cells or decreased pathology. It is possible that the environment that causes the disease prevents effective cell therapy despite the source of cells used. Further, it is extremely likely that matrix alterations or environmental conditions that elicit the development of Parkinson's or other chronic diseases of aging cannot be easily overcome. Such alterations seem to transform both mature neural tissue and stem cells to cells which exhibit the pathologic changes.

EMBRYONIC STEM CELLS (ES CELLS)

Adult stem cells were once considered a viable alternative to ES cells to avoid ethical problems. The ban on ES cell research no longer exists, but the hopes once held for embryonic stem cells still have not been realized. In the progressive country of India, several multicenter clinical trials have been initiated in patients with ischemic stroke with limited success. Many argue that the failure results from deficient training. The fact is that the failure of embryonic stem cells to regenerate adult tissues is readily obvious. Embryonic stem cells generate embryonic tissue. It is incredible that individuals cannot appreciate the limitations imposed by that simple and irrefutable fact. If one wishes to derive a neonatal brain, then transplantation of embryonic stem cells would be appropriate. If one wishes to restore function to an adult brain, there exists a large and well documented gap between the progeny embryonic stem cells initially produce and the emergence of functional adult neural tissue. Meanwhile, investigators managed to "duck the bullet" by insisting that that the governmental ban on ES cell research precluded advance. These individuals now instead incessantly hail the characteristics of cells termed iPS cells (induced pluripotential cells) that are generated from non-embryonic tissues and are advertised to hold characteristics equivalent to those of ES cells. The question addressed by several groups of investigators is whether these cells replicate functions of bona fide ES cells, and if they can be generated so as to be safely administered, since techniques to generate them use various viruses to alter the genome of the cells used to induce their pluripotentiality. In an era where embryonic stem cells can be used for research without restriction, this question is debated needlessly, since tissue regeneration has not been achieved using bona fide ES cells. The focus on iPS cells deflects that more important question; can ES cells regenerate adult tissues? Studies currently underway should reveal the utility of ES cells for neural regeneration in the near future.

CONCLUSIONS

Several investigations indicate that neural stem cells exist in the brain and perhaps the bone marrow and studies have been initiated to assess the ability of these cells to regenerate neural tissue after transplantation. Abundant data in experimental models support the use of stem cells for neural diseases. However, despite extensive study, no clinically applicable therapy utilizing neural stem cells has emerged. The situation of patients facing the effects of severe brain injury or disease render them compromised in their ability to decide if such therapy is worthwhile as they address a question scientists cannot answer. Scientists should be quite conservative in their public pronouncements of the potential they feel neural stem cells hold until that potential is realized. In this respect, science has been negligent in its responsibility to keep the public informed and in many instances this negligence can be traced to agenda motivated by profit. It is time for the scientific community to rise to the occasion and tell it like it is. It is time to reassess reports of stunning neural stem cell successes and to temper the enthusiasm of this extremely desperate audience until key questions are answered. Studies of neural stem cells shall certainly reveal secrets held tightly by nature and increase our understanding of the processes that maintain life. For that reason, these studies should continue and expand. Exploration of regenerative capacity of primitive vertebrate brains exposed to prolonged intervals of hypoxia or hypothermia may yield new and exciting approaches to regeneration of elements of the human brain. However, pronouncements of miraculous cures for neural disorders are counterproductive, non-scientific, unethical and premature. They represent everything that science was designed to avoid. Future reports shall pay appropriate consideration to the damage that false hope engenders and shall take proactive steps to avoid it while focusing on excellent scientific evidence that ultimately will lead to successful therapy.

ACKNOWLEDGEMENT

We greatly appreciate the input of Dr. Mahendra Rao in several important aspects of this review.

This work was made possible by the support of NIH Grant RO-1-61751 awarded to Professor English.

REFERENCES

[1]   Filip S, Mokry J, English D, *et al.* Stem cell plasticity and issues of stem cell therapy. Folia Biol [Praha]   2005; 51: 180-187. Review.
[2]   Alvarez-Buylla A, Garcia-Verdugo JM, Tramontin AD. A unified hypothesis on the lineage of neural stem cells. Nat Rev 2001; 2: 287-293.
[3]   Hong-jun Song, Stevens CF, Gage FH. Neural stem cells from adult hippocampus develop essential properties of functional CNS neurons, Nat Neurosci 2002; 5: 438-445.
[4]   Alvarez-Buylla A, Lim DA. For the long run: maintaining germinal niches in the adult brain. Neuron 2004; 41: 683-686.

[5] Lennington JB, Yang Z, Conover JC. Neural stem cells and the regulation of adult neurogenesis. Reprod Biol Endocrinol 2003; 1: 99-103.

[6] Aboody, KS. Neural stem cells display extensive tropism for pathology in adult brain: evidence from intracranial gliomas. Proc Natl Acad Sci (US) 2000; 97: 12846-12851.

[7] Tang J, Xu H, Fan X, *et al.* Embryonic stem cell-derived neural precursor cells improve memory dysfunction in Ab [1-40] injured rats. Neurosci Res 2008; 62: 86-96.

[8] Gao J, Prough DS, McAdoo DJ, *et al.* Transplantation of primed human fetal neural stem cells improves cognitive function in rats after traumatic brain injury. Exptl Neurol 2006; 201: 281-292.

[9] Yamasaki TR, Blurton-Jones M, Morrissette DA, *et al.* Neural Stem Cells Improve Memory in an Inducible Mouse Model of Neuronal Loss. J Neurosci 2007; 27: 11925-11933.

[10] English D, Klasko SK, Sanberg R. Elusive mechanisms of stem cell-mediated repair of cerebral damage. Exp Neurol 2006; 199: 10-15.

[11] Barry FP. Biology and clinical applications of mesenchymal stem cells. Birth Defects Res. Embryo Today 2003; 69 :250-256. Review.

[12] Habich A, Jurga M, Markiewicz I, *et al.* Early appearance of stem/progenitor cells with neural-like characteristics in human cord blood mononuclear fraction cultured in vitro. Exp Hematol 2006; 34: 914-925.

[13] Li Y, Chopp M. Marrow stromal cell transplantation in stroke and traumatic brain injury. Neurosci Lett 2009;456:120-123. Review.

[14] Kitada M, Dezawa M. Induction system of neural and muscle lineage cells from bone marrow stromal cells; a new strateg.y for tissue reconstruction in degenerative diseases. Histol Histopathol 2009; 24 :631-642. Review.

[15] Kassis I, Grigoriadis N, Gowda-Kurkalli B, *et al.* Neuroprotection and immunomodulation with mesenchymal stem cells in chronic experimental autoimmune encephalomyelitis.. Arch Neurol 2008; 65:753-761.

[16] Alexanian AR, Maiman DJ, Kurpad SN, *et al.* In vitro and in vivo characterization of neurally modified mesenchymal stem cells induced by epigenetic modifiers and neural stem cell environment. Stem Cells Dev 2008; 17:1123-1130.

[17] Karussis D, Kassis I, Kurkalli BG, *et al.* Immunomodulation and neuroprotection with mesenchymal bone marrow stem cells (MSCs): a proposed treatment for multiple sclerosis and other neuroimmunological/neurodegen- erative diseases. J Neurol Sci 2008 ;265 :131-135. Review.

[18] Parr AM, Tator CH, Keating A. Bone marrow-derived mesenchymal stromal cells for the repair of central nervous system injury. Bone Marrow Transplant 2007;40: 609-619. Review.

[19] Chen X, Wang XD, Chen G, *et al.* Study of in vivo differentiation of rat bone marrow stromal cells into Schwann cell-like cells. Microsurgery 2006;26:111-115.

[20] Zhang P, He X, Liu K, *et al.* Bone marrow stromal cells differentiated into functional Schwann cells in injured rats sciatic nerve. Artif Cells Blood Substit Immobil Biotechnol. 2004; 32 :509-518.

[21] Dezawa M. Central and peripheral nerve regeneration by transplantation of Schwann cells and transdifferentiated bone marrow stromal cells. Anat Sci Int 2002; 77:12-25. Review.

[22] Caplan-AI. Mesenchymal stem cells. Orthop Res 1991; 9: 64-650.

[23] Lange C, Schroeder J, Lioznov M., *et al.* High – potential human mesenchymal stem cells. Stem Cells Develop 2005; 14: 70-80.

[24] Liu Y, Rao MS. Transdifferentiation--fact or artifact. J Cell Biochem 2003; 88 : 29-40.

[25] Wells WA. Is transdifferentiation in trouble? J Cell Biol 2002 ;157:15-18. Review.

[26] English D. Transdifferentiation wars. Stem Cells Develop 2005; 14l: 605-607: 2005 [editorial].

[27] Jang YK, Park JJ, Lee MC, *et al.* Retinoic acid-mediated induction of neurons and glial cells from human umbilical cord-derived hematopoietic stem cells. J Neurosci Res. 2004 ;75: 573-584.

[28] Sergent-Tanguy S, Michel DC, Neveu I, *et al.* Long-lasting coexpression of nestin and glial fibrillary acidic protein in primary cultures of astroglial cells with a major participation of nestin(+)/GFAP(-) cells in cell proliferation. J Neurosci Res 2006; 83 :1515-1524.

[29] Hao HN, Zhao J, Thomas RL, *et al.* Fetal human hematopoietic stem cells can differentiate sequentially into neural stem cells and then astrocytes in vitro. J Hematother Stem Cell Res 2003;12: 23-32.

[30] Filip S, Mokrý J, Karbanová J, *et al.* The transplantation of neural stem cells and predictive factors in hematopoietic recovery in irradiated mice. Transfus Apher Sci 2005;32:157-166.

[31] Mokrý J, Karbanová J, Filip S, *et al.* Phenotypic and morphological characterization of in vitro oligodendrogliogenesis. Stem Cells Dev 2008; 17: 333-341.

[32] Mokrý J, Cízková D, Filip S, *et al.* Nestin expression by newly formed human blood vessels. Stem Cells Dev 2004; 13:658-664.

[33] Filip S, Mokrý J, Karbanová J, *et al*. Local environmental factors determine hematopoietic differentiation of neural stem cells. Stem Cells Dev. 2004; 13:113-120.

[34] English D. The hope and hype of nonembryonic stem cells. J Hematother Stem Cell Res 2003 ;12 : 253-254.

[35] Goldman SA, Nottebohm F. Neuronal production, migration, and differentiation in a vocal control nucleus of the adult female canary brain. Proc Natl Acad Sci U S A 1983; 80:2390-2394.

[36] Kesaraju S, Milton SL. Preliminary evidence of neuronal regeneration in the anoxia tolerant vertebrate brain. Exp Neurol 2009; 215: 401-403.

[37] Panchision DM. The role of oxygen in regulating neural stem cells in development and disease. J Cell Physiol. 2009 220:562-568.

[38] Zhu LL, Wu LY, Yew DT, *et al*. Effects of hypoxia on the proliferation and differentiation of NSCs. Mol Neurobiol. 2005; 31:231-242.

[39] He MC, Li J, Zhao CH. Effect of hypoxia on mesenchymal stem cells – review. Zhongguo Shi Yan Xue Ye Xue Za Zhi. 2007; 15: 433-436.

[40] Levison SW, Goldman, JE. Multipotential and lineage restricted precursors coexist in the mammalian perinatal subventricular zone. J Neurosci Res 1997; 48: 83-94.

[41] Luskin, MB, Zigova CT., Sotheres, BJ, *et al*. Neuronal progenitor cells derived from the anterior subventricular zone of the neonatal rat forebrain continue to proliferate in vitro and express a neuronal phenotype. Mol Cell Neurosci 1997; 8: 351-366.

[42] Huang AH, Snyder EY, Cheng PH, *et al*. Putative dental pulp-derived stem/stromal cells promote proliferation and differentiation of endogenous neural cells in the hippocampus of mice. Stem Cells 2008; 26:2654-2663.

[43] Marmur R, Mabie PC, Gokhan S, *et al*. Isolation and developmental characterization of cerebral cortical multipotent progenitors. Dev Biol 1998; 204, 577-591.

[44] Roy NS, Wang S, Jiang L, *et al*. In vitro neurogenesis by progenitor cells isolated from the adult human hippocampus. Nat Med 2000; 6: 271-277.

[45] Chang Q, Hanks S, Akard L, *et al*. Maturation of mobilized peripheral blood progenitor cells: Preclinical and phase I clinical studies. J. Hematotherapy 1995; 4: 289-297.

[46] Glück S, Chadderton T, Porter K, *et al*. Characterization and transfusion of *in vitro* cultivated haematopoietic progenitor Cells. Transfus Sci 1995; 16:273-281.

[47] Svetlov SI, Ignatova TN, Wang KK, *et al*. Lysophosphatidic acid induces clonal generation of mouse neurospheres via proliferation of Sca-1- and AC133-positive neural progenitors. Stem Cells Dev. 2004; 13: 685-693.

[48]. Pierret C, Spears K, Maruniak JA, *et al*.Neural crest as the source of adult stem cells. Stem Cells Dev 2006 ;15:286-291.

[49] Teng L, Labosky PA. Neural crest stem cells. Adv Exp Med Biol. 2006;589:206-212.

[50] English D, Williams MA. Stem cells and development. Stem Cells Dev 2004; 13: 223- 224.

[51] Parker GC, Anastassova-Kristeva M, Broxmeyer HE, *et al*.(for the Editorial Board of Stem Cells and Development). Stem cells: Shibboleths of development. Stem Cells Dev 2004;13:579-584.

[52] Parker GC, Anastassova-Kristeva M, Eisenberg LM, *et al*.(for the Editorial Board of Stem Cells and Development). Stem cells: Shibboleths of development, part II: Toward a functional definition. Stem Cells Dev 2005; 14: 463-469.

[53] English D, Williams MA. The therapeutic promise of non embryonic stem cells. Where's the beef? J. Hematothr Stem Cell Res 2003;12: 465-466 (editorial).

[54] Li Calzi S, Kent DL, Chang KH, *et al*. Labeling of stem cells with monocrystalline iron oxide for tracking and localization by]magnetic resonance imaging. Microvasc Res 2009;78:132-139.

[55] Harvey K, Higgins N, Akard L, *et al*. Lineage commitment of HLA-DR/CD38-defined progenitor cell subpopulations in bone marrow and mobilized peripheral blood assessed by four-color immunofluorescence. J Hematother. 1997; 6:243-252.

[56] Scheltens P. Imaging in Alzheimer's disease. Dialogues Clin Neurosci. 2009;11:191-199. Review

[57] Jansen J, Hanks S, Akard LP, et al. Immunomagnetic CD4+ and CD8+ cell depletion for patients at high risk for severe acute GVHD. Bone Marrow Transplant 1996;17: 377-382.

[58] S. Glück S, Ross AA, Layton TJ, *et al*. Decrease in tumour cell contamination and progenitor cell yield in leukapheresis products after consecutive cycles of chemotherapy for breast cancer. Biol Blood Marrow Transp 1997; 3:316-323.

[59] Jansen J, Hanks S, English D, *et al*. Immunomagnetic depletion of CD8+ lymphocytes from marrow grafts. Prog Clin Biol Res 1992; 377:405-410.

[60] Broxmeyer HE, Douglas GW, Hangoc G, *et al*. Human umbilical cord blood as a source of transplantable hematopoietic stem/progenitor cells. Proc Natl Acad Sci. USA 1989; 86: 3828-3838.

[61] Gluckman E, Broxmeyer HE, Auerbach, A, *et al*. Hematopoietic reconstitution in a patient with Fanconi's anemia by means of umbilical-cord blood from an HLA-identical sibling. N. Engl. J. Med. 1989; 321: 1174-1178.

[62]   English, D , Lamberson, R, Graves V, *et al*. Semi-automated processing of bone marrow grafts for transplantation. Transfusion 1989; 29: 12-16.

[63]   Yang AX, Mejido J, Luo Y, *et al*. Development of a focused microarray to assess human embryonic stem cell differentiation. Stem Cells Dev 2005; 14: 270-284.

[64]   English D, Sanberg PR. Neural specification of stem cell differentiation. Stem Cells Dev. 2006; 15:139-140. [Editorial].

[65]   Nakayama T, Sai T, Otsu M, *et al*. Astrocytogenesis of embryonic stem-cell-derived neural stem cells: Default differentiation. Neuroreport. 2006; 17:1519-1523.

[66]   Kratchmarova I, Blagoev B , Haack-Sorensen M, *et al*. Mechanism of divergent growth factor effects in mesenchymal stem cell differentiation. Science 2005; 308:1472-1477.

[67]   Yamasaki TR, Blurton-Jones M, Morrissette DA, *et al*. Neural stem cells improve memory in an inducible mouse model of neuronal loss. J. Neurosci 2007; 27 :11925-11933.

[68]   Russell, WR. Recovery after minor head injury. Lancet 1977; 2: 1-6.

[69]   Raisman, A. What hope for repair of the brain? Annals Neuro 1978; 3: 101-110.

[70]   Strub EL, Black FW. Organic brain syndromes: An introduction to neurobehavioral disorders. Philadelphia: FA Davis Co 1981.

[71]   Lotze M, Sauseng P, Staudt M. Functional relevance of ipsilateral motor activation in congenital hemiparesis as tested by fMRI-navigated TMS. Exp Neuro 2009; (in press).

[72]   Piper DR, Mujtaba T, Rao MS, *et al*. Immunocytochemical and physiological characterization of a population of cultured human neural precursors. J. Neurophysiol 2000; 84, 534-548.

[73]   Kalyani A, Hobsin K, Roa, MS. Neuroepithelial stem cells from the embryonic spinal cord: isolation, characterization, and clonal analysis. Dev. Biol. 1997; 186: 202-223.

[74]   Williams BA, Keating, A. Cell therapy for age-related disorders: myocardial infarction and stroke. A mini-Review. Gerontology 2008; 54:300-311.

[75]   Kondziolka D, Wechsler L, Goldstein S, *et al*. Bynum L: Transplantation of cultured human neuronal cells for patients with stroke. Neurology 2000; 55: 565-569.

[76]   Kondziolka D, Steinberg GK, Wechsler L *et al*. Neurotransplantation for patients with subcortical motor stroke: a phase 2 randomized trial. J Neurosurg 2005; 103: 38–45.

[77]   Åkerud, P, Canals J.M, Snyder EY, *et al*. Neuroprotection through delivery of glial cell line-derived neurotrophic factor by neural stem cells in a mouse model of Parkinson's disease. J Neurosci 2001, 21: 8108-8118.

CHAPTER 9

Diabetes and Stem Cells

Juan Domínguez-Bendala* and Camillo Ricordi

Diabetes Research Institute, University of Miami Leonard M. Miller School of Medicine, 1450 NW 10th Avenue, Miami, FL 33136, USA

Abstract: The existence of clinically successful cell therapies (islet transplantation) for type 1 diabetes has stoked a keen interest in developing alternative, inexhaustible sources of insulin-producing cells. In this chapter we will broadly cover the state of the art regenerative therapies for the endocrine component of the pancreas, from stem cells to transdifferentiation. In particular, we will review the basics of pancreatic development, whose recapitulation remains the subject of a plethora of *in vitro* differentiation strategies using both embryonic and adult stem cells. Then we will examine the leading theories about the cellular and molecular mechanisms behind the *in vivo* regeneration of the organ that is observed under specific circumstances, as well as the purported ability of some tissues to turn into pancreatic endocrine cells when subjected to specific interventions (transdifferentiation). Finally, we will conclude with a general overview of the remaining challenges and clinical perspectives of all the above strategies, with a special emphasis on the immunological hurdles to be overcome for these approaches to find their way to standard clinical practice.

INTRODUCTION

Type 1 diabetes is an autoimmune condition in which the insulin-producing cells within the pancreatic islets are targeted and eventually destroyed by the immune system of the patient. The disease can only be managed by means of chronic exogenous insulin administration. However, even intensive regimens with several daily insulin injections cannot replicate the physiologic glycemic regulation exerted by native islets. As a consequence, the long term use of this therapy is often associated with the development of debilitating and sometimes life-threatening complications. While whole pancreas or islet transplantation are effective at restoring normoglycemia, they are very rarely indicated as a treatment for the disease unless the patient is already immunosuppressed because of a previous or simultaneous kidney transplant [1-3].

The identification of type 1 diabetes as an ideal target of future stem cell/regenerative therapies is based on several objective criteria: (a) there is only one cell type destroyed (unlike other conditions in which replacement would require complex tissue engineering involving several cell types); (b) replacement can be ectopic, as long as the transplanted cells are properly vascularized; and, most importantly, (c) there is already a cell-based therapy (islet transplantation) successfully used in humans [4-7]. This therapy is considered a safer and easier procedure than whole pancreas transplantation, offering most of the advantages of the latter without some of the drawbacks [4]. In short, pancreatic tissue from either a deceased or a living-related donor [8-12] is processed in a semi-automated fashion through a continuous digestion process that makes use of a continuous flow of an enzymatic solution through a digestion chamber, to evenly mix the progressively disassembled pancreatic tissue. The process results in the separation of the endocrine cell clusters (islets) from the exocrine and ductal components [13]. Fractions highly enriched for islets are obtained by gradient centrifugation, and the final islet cell product can be cultured for days –and pre-conditioned, if necessary [4]– prior to infusion into the recipient (generally through percutaneous catheterization of the portal vein). Upon lodging at different pre-sinusoidal levels in the liver (depending on the individual cell cluster sizes), graft neovascularization occurs within two to four weeks [3, 4, 14-16]. This outpatient, minimally invasive procedure has generally little or no complications if performed by expert teams, especially when compared to the alternative of whole organ transplantation.

The development of a steroid-free immunosuppressive regime in 2000 [7] improved very significantly the long-term survival and function of transplanted islets, with most of the treated patients who remained insulin-free for

---

*Address Correspondence to this Author Juan Domínguez-Bendala: Diabetes Research Institute, University of Miami Leonard M. Miller School of Medicine, 1450 NW 10th Avenue, Miami, FL 33136, USA; Tel: 305-243-4092; E-mail: j.dominguezbendala@miami.edu

Herman S. Cheung (Ed)

over one year after the procedure [17] reporting a much better quality of life [18]. However, as only a sufficiently large number of islets can sustain full metabolic control, many patients still have required two or even three islet infusions [7, 19, 20]. Also, despite the persistence of C-peptide secretion –resulting in near-normalization of metabolic control in the absence of severe hypoglycemic episodes– only 10-50% of the patients remain insulin-free over five years after the transplant [17, 21]. The observation that only a small percentage of islets survive the combined insults of enzymatic/mechanical isolation and post-transplantation inflammatory processes [22] prompted renewed efforts to minimize islet losses before and after transplantation by selected cytoprotective strategies, including gene therapy [23-27], protein transduction [28-34] and the pharmacologic inhibition of apoptosis [35-43]. A recently reported technique by which islets can be experimentally engrafted in the eye [44] allows now for the real-time study of the mechanisms responsible for islet engraftment and function after transplantation, with the aim of optimizing cytoprotection, post-transplant vascularization, immunomodulation and long-term survival of the transplanted islets.

At any rate, even in a best case scenario in which we made every islet count by protecting them from apoptosis before and after transplantation, organ donation alone would be clearly insufficient to make this therapy available to the millions of subjects affected by type 1 diabetes who could benefit from the procedure. In addition, the requirement for life-long recipient immunosuppression would still limit the applicability of the procedure to the most severe cases of type 1 diabetes. However, as successful strategies for tolerance induction are developed [3] - thus overcoming the risks associated with systemic immunosuppression–, every insulin-requiring patient will become eligible for a transplant of insulin-producing cells. At this point, the demand will clearly become overwhelming compared to the potential offered by pancreata coming from either deceased or living-related donors.

The rest of this chapter will review how stem cells may be used to effectively tackle the two critical issues (supply and immunity) that need to be addressed in order to develop a cure.

SUPPLY

Introduction

In general, stem cells can be defined by their capacity to proliferate in an undifferentiated state (self-renewal) while maintaining the ability to give rise to several differentiated cell types (potency). From a therapeutic perspective, these two unique properties make stem cells an ideal substrate for the replacement of damaged/lost tissues. As mentioned earlier, type 1 diabetes is the pathological manifestation of the selective ablation of insulin-producing beta cells. Islet transplantation has proven effective at treating the disease, but it is not realistic to expect that organ donation alone will ever be sufficient to satisfy the demand. In this section, we will discuss the most updated progress on the use of both embryonic and adult stem cells for the directed differentiation into pancreatic beta cells, as well as other replacement options such as transdifferentiation and endogenous regeneration. An introduction on pancreatic beta cell development is provided as background, as it is our belief that only from a clear understanding of the molecular "roadmap" leading to the generation of beta cells *in vivo*, will we be able to recapitulate the process *in vitro*.

Pancreatic Development

The advent of gene targeting/knockout techniques more than two decades ago [45] has allowed us to dissect with great precision the molecular determinants of pancreatic development in the mouse. Despite some slight differences between the two species [46-48], most of our findings in the mouse model have thus far been confirmed in humans. Thus, for the sake of simplicity, throughout this chapter we will refer by default to the former.

The pancreas originates around e8.5 from a region of the foregut epithelium where sonic hedgehog (*Shh*[41]) is down-regulated through a complex series of events mediated by the interaction between the epithelium and the surrounding mesenchyme. This *Shh*-excluded area is characterized by the almost simultaneous onset of expression of Pdx1 [49, 50] and Ptf1a/p48 [51-53], two of the earlier master regulators of pancreatic fate [54, 55]. Endothelial signals from the developing aorta have been demonstrated to play an important role in these early specification events [53, 56, 57].

Around e9.5, the pancreas can be identified as two distinct evaginations from the epithelium, termed the dorsal and the ventral anlages [58]. These compartments will develop independently until their fusion later in development. At this point, each primordium is composed of virtually equipotent Pdx1+ progenitor cells. The first fate decisions will take place shortly thereafter through a complex molecular interplay choreographed by Notch. In short, neighboring cells at this stage have an active cross-talk in which they both secrete and receive the Notch ligand. Upon activation, the Notch receptor triggers a cascade of events resulting in the up-regulation of HES-1 (Hairy Enhancer of Split-1), which represses, among other genes, the pro-endocrine factor neurogenin 3 (Ngn3). Persistent Notch signaling precludes any further differentiation. However, the system is highly unstable: even minute differences in the levels of secretion of Notch have proportional effects on the activation of HES-1. A feedback mechanism ensures that cells with strong up-regulation of HES-1 also secrete less ligand, which in turn leads to additional down-regulation of HES-1 in the adjacent cells. At the end of the process, cells without Notch signaling completely de-repress HES-1, which results in the expression of Ngn3 and the adoption of a pro-endocrine fate. In contrast, surrounding cells maintain active Notch signaling and endocrine differentiation is blocked [59-62]. Ngn3+ cells will respond differentially to evolving molecular microenvironments during development: thus, they will chiefly differentiate into α (glucagon-producing) cells from e9.5; β (insulin-producing) cells from e10.5-e11.5; δ (somatostatin-producing) cells from e14.5; and PP (pancreatic polypeptide-producing) cells from e18.5. As for the exocrine and ductal lineages, they are believed to arise from Notch-active, Pdx1+ /Ptf1a/p48+ and Pdx1+/Ngn3- progenitors, respectively [63, 64]. After the initial specification of the first endocrine and exocrine cell types, around e13.5 a phase termed "secondary transition" takes over proliferation and differentiation [65, 66]. The markers found in the progenitor cells responsible for the expansion of the pancreatic tissue during this secondary wave might be different than those characterizing earlier stages, which some consider largely to be developmental *cul-de-sacs* [67]. Table 1 offers a brief description of the major molecular players involved in pancreatic development.

Embryonic Stem Cells

Embryonic stem (ES) cells are derived from the inner cell mass (ICM) of the early blastocyst, and they are known to give rise to all cell types of the organism [68-70]. Under defined *in vitro* conditions, ES cells can be expanded very rapidly [71] without loss of pluripotency, which makes them the gold standard of stem cells for replacement purposes. Critical genes involved in the maintenance of their undifferentiated phenotype are Oct3/4, Nanog and Sox2 [72-74], which in fact have been recently used to reprogram somatic cells into ES-like induced pluripotent stem (IPS) cells [75-81]. After a number of groundbreaking reports in mouse ES cells (some of which eventually turned out to be dead ends) [75-81], the first proof of concept that human ES cells could differentiate into insulin-producing cells was established by Assady and colleagues in 2001 in a model of spontaneous differentiation [82]. Many of the ensuing attempts at generating beta cells were based on the adaptation of protocols originally designed for neural differentiation [83, 84], but the first reports on "canonical" beta cell specification (i.e., devised upon the blueprint of native pancreatic development) did not appear until the conditions for the formation of definitive endoderm were first elucidated by D'Amour and colleagues [85]. Indeed, it did not take long for this team to follow up the original study with the first report on true beta cell differentiation *in vitro* [86], a protocol that is still considered the state of the art. In short, definitive endoderm generated by exposure to Activin A (an analog of Nodal [87-91]) in the presence of low concentrations of serum (which is known to interfere with endodermal differentiation [92, 93]) was sequentially forced along the foregut and pancreatic lineages by treatment with Notch activators/*Shh* inhibitors and retinoic acid, respectively. The final maturation of these Pdx1+ cells, however, was arguably the weakest point of the method, as the efficiency was very low (7% of insulin-producing cells) and insulin was not secreted in a glucose-regulated manner. Another method described shortly thereafter [94] resulted in the formation of cells with high amounts of insulin and some degree of glucose responsiveness, but similarly low beta cell generation efficiency. At this point, the authors of the original study decided to abandon their efforts at completing differentiation *in vitro* and implanted Pdx1+ progenitors into immunodeficient mice. Several weeks later, human C-peptide could be detected in the circulation of these animals, which became resistant to streptozotocin-induced diabetes [95]. The caveat of these studies was that up to 15% of the transplanted mice developed teratomas, perhaps due to the higher incidence of carry-over undifferentiated cells at the progenitor stage [96]. The direction the field will take now is uncertain, as we are witnessing the development of two schools of thought: those who claim that beta cell maturation is too complex a process to be mimicked *in vitro*, favoring instead an *in vivo* microenvironment for the last stages; and those who will avoid transplantation of anything but a completely differentiated product, so as to minimize the occurrence of tumoral lesions –which could set the entire field back many years if ever detected in clinical trials. The preliminary success reported by the first camp makes the *in vivo* approach the one to beat. However, the emergence of new culture techniques based on the replication of the extracellular matrix [97-102]and physiological oxygenation [103, 104] of the developing islet, as well as novel differentiation tools such as microRNAs [105, 106] and protein transduction [107-113] might still tip the balance towards terminal *in vitro* differentiation.

Adult Stem Cells

Adult stem cells can be found in most tissues, where they are thought to support their regular turnover and regeneration. Their definition is still imprecise, because they are extremely difficult to study in their native niches. There is a growing consensus that what we see *in vitro* might just be an artifact induced by our inadvertent selection of cells that will expand in regular culture conditions. This would explain why the phenotype of most adult-derived stem cells almost invariably ends up resembling that of fibroblastic-like mesenchymal stem cells (MSCs). Originally identified in the bone marrow, MSCs can now be cultured from virtually any tissue of the body, with the possible exception of peripheral blood [114]. According to the criteria recently established by the International Society for Cellular Therapy (ISCT), MSCs must adhere to plastic; express CD73, CD90 and CD105; be negative for hematopoietic markers and HLA-DR; and differentiate into a range of connective tissues (osteoblasts, adipocytes and chrondroblasts) [115, 116]. Many attempts at inducing MSC specification into islet cell types have already been reported, but their ability to differentiate into definitive endoderm remains to be demonstrated. This is perhaps not surprising, since MSCs are already committed along the mesodermal lineage –with the possible exception of the elusive multipotent adult progenitor cells described earlier this decade by Verfaillie and colleagues [117-122]. Although insulin production has been shown following a variety of soluble factor-driven [123, 124,125-129] and genetic manipulation [130-135] approaches, their ability to sustain long-term normoglycemia upon transplantation tends to be limited. Studies in which undifferentiated MSCs are transplanted into diabetic animals without any pre-conditioning have yielded some intriguing results [126, 136-138], but no mechanistic studies have been conducted yet. Interestingly, these cells may end up contributing to a cure for diabetes not as a substrate for differentiation, but rather as immunomodulatory [139-142] and angiogenic [143,144] adjuvants. There is already substantive evidence that MSCs, when co-cultured or co-transplanted with other cells (including islets) can significantly enhance their function and survival [145-149]. This is still a largely untapped field, but one that may prove crucial for the effective translation of stem cell research into therapies for type 1 diabetes.

Other adult stem cells that have been considered for directed beta cell differentiation are hematopoietic bone marrow and cord blood cells. Many studies have already established that both the bone marrow and the cord blood contain multipotent cells [150, 151]. For the reasons previously explained, it can be expected that MSCs constitute the main cellular component of cultured hematopoietic tissues, and as such can undergo differentiation procedures similar to those already described [152, 153]. Ongoing studies on other mesenchymal-like cells derived from the amniotic fluid [154] and endometrial tissue [155, 156] may offer additional insights on the potential of these cells. As for the hematopoietic cells proper, they have been primarily used to modify the immunity of the recipient (see last section), rather than as building blocks for beta cell neogenesis.

Transdifferentiation

An alternative to the use of stem cells for the differentiation of beta cells is that of reprogramming adult tissues. The liver, in particular, has been shown to be greatly amenable to this "transdifferentiation" approach, perhaps due to its close developmental relationship with the pancreas [53,157-166]. Normally, this process requires the transfection of recipient liver cells with a constitutively active version of the master pancreatic regulator Pdx1, either *in vitro* or *in vivo* [167-171]. Transgenic experiments have also established that transdifferentiation can occur earlier in development [172]. More recently, other factors such as Ngn3, Beta2/NeuroD or MafA have been shown to potentiate the effects of Pdx1, both in the liver [173-179] and in the exocrine pancreas [180].

A general caveat of this approach is that the use of viruses for gene delivery is almost invariably required (with some studies even suggesting that the adenoviral-elicited response is actually necessary for the desired effect [173]). An encouraging observation, however, is that the ectopic cassette is not necessary beyond an initial push that will prime self-sustaining endogenous regulatory networks [170]. Since adenoviruses are short-lived and do not induce permanent integration in the genome, a therapy can be conceived in which, by the time the patient's own *ex vivo* transdifferentiated hepatocytes are re-infused, there would be no traces of the viral vehicle.

Regeneration

The endocrine component of the pancreas is known to undergo regeneration under specific conditions, both physiological (e.g., pregnancy [181-190]) and pathological/experimental (e.g., high glucose [191, 192], obesity [193-196], partial pancreatectomy [197-199], duct ligation [200, 201], cellophane wrapping [202-205] and chemical ablation [206-208]). However, the origin of newly created islets remains highly controversial, with emphatic proponents of the ductal/acinar tissue [209-217], the islet itself [218-221] or the bone marrow [222]. As for the molecular mechanisms behind the process, early suggestions that it could be mediated through reversible epithelial-to-mesenchymal transition [223] were disproven shortly thereafter [224-226] and abandoned in favor of two competing –but not necessarily exclusive of each other– theories: self-duplication (which appears to be the default mechanism of beta cell turnover and replenishment in the mouse [221, 227, 228]) and the reactivation of embryonic-like pancreatic progenitors (which has also been conclusively demonstrated in at least one model of regeneration, namely partial duct ligation [229]). Be it as it may, the observation that beta cells can be regenerated is now established beyond any doubt, and the study of the molecular determinants involved in the process might help develop new strategies either to induce beta cell neogenesis *in vivo* or for the expansion of beta cells *in vitro*. In this context, recent clinical trials of intrapancreatic autologous stem cell infusions and hyperbaric oxygen therapy indicate a potential regenerative effect *in vivo* [230]. Ongoing randomized prospective trials are in progress to determine the effectiveness of this strategy in patients with type 2 diabetes –with obvious implications for type 1 diabetes.

IMMUNITY

General Considerations

Unfortunately, most immunosuppresants not only have serious systemic side effects [231], but also are intrinsically diabetogenic [232-234]. The recent development of biocompatible devices that can be implanted subcutaneously and act as recipients of islets upon vascularization may help address the first problem, as immunosuppressive agents is small doses would prevent rejection if delivered locally [235]. The second problem, however, is more difficult to tackle. Indeed, it could be argued that, unless we reeducate the immune system of the recipient to recognize the donor cells as "self", the success of any cell-based therapy will be just temporary. Many groups are currently pursuing this "reeducation" by interfering with the co-stimulatory pathways involved in the activation of autoreactive T cells [236, 237]. A caveat of these efforts is that such blockade has also a negative effect on T regulatory (Treg) cells, which are known to exert a counterbalance on autoreactive T cells, imparting protection against autoimmune diabetes [238, 239]. A promising alternative is that of identifying key co-inhibitory molecules that will prevent the activation of the autoreactive T cells without interfering with Treg function [240].

Other strategies to tolerize the grafts include the induction of bone marrow chimaerism [241-249], as well as the auto-infusion of hematopoietic stem cells after a strong immunosuppresion regimen (a treatment that was initially reported to turn the clock of the immune system back to a time prior to the onset of the disease) [250-256].

Finally, encapsulation techniques aim at providing the transplanted cells with a physical barrier that will prevent both humoral and cell-mediated rejection while allowing the free transit of nutrients, glucose and insulin [257-263]. If successful, this "brute force" tactic might actually open the door to the transplantation of non-human tissues. However, conventional encapsulation exacerbates the problem of oxygen and nutrient deprivation, which is a prime cause of islet demise after transplantation [264-271]. Hence the recent emphasis on *nanoencapsulation*, an alternative strategy based on the design of thin conformal polymeric layers that can be coated upon the surface of the islets [272, 273]. By significantly reducing the diffusion distance between the islets and their microenvironment, their chances of survival are greatly enhanced.

Immunology of Stem Cells: In Search of a Comprehensive Approach

The definition of a universal strategy for the treatment of type 1 diabetes with stem cells is complicated by the fact that there is no clear "winner" yet among the many options that we have discussed in previous sections. We can safely assume, however, that the practice of cell banking will greatly aid in the clinical applicability of many of these potential therapies. While the collection of adult stem cells representing a wide range of common HLA haplotypes is obviously easier than the generation of genetically diverse human ES cell lines, progress in the latter field has been nothing short of unprecedented. Thus, HLA homozygous huES cells have already been generated by parthenogenesis, with one cell line carrying the most widespread HLA haplotype in the United States [274, 275]. Alternatively, secondary rejection mechanisms could be eliminated altogether by creating patient-tailored iPS cells [77, 79-81, 276, 277], a burgeoning area of research that has made somatic cell nuclear transfer (SCNT) practically obsolete. Although there are still significant hurdles (the use of retroviruses for reprogramming is incompatible with clinical applications), progress in defining non-viral alternatives is steadfast [278, 279].

At any rate, few would argue that the harvest, expansion and differentiation of the patient's own stem cells would be a faster and preferable option, provided that beta cell differentiation can be effectively attained. However, both with custom-made iPS cells and self-derived stem cells, the issue of autoimmunity would still stand in the way of a cure. Therefore, a comprehensive approach to treat the disease will require not only an exogenous boost of insulin-producing cells, but also a permanent reeducation of the immune system. Embryonic stem cells might actually help address both problems in a theoretical co-transplantation setting in which the patient would receive both hematopoietic and islet cells derived from the same huES cell line. A mirror strategy would be one in which cord blood or bone marrow hematopoietic cells, upon differentiation into insulin-producing cells, were co-transplanted with undifferentiated ones. Provided that effective chimaerism could be induced in a safe manner [241-249], the stem cells would act both as a replacement and a tolerizing tool. In a different experimental design, it is conceivable that incomplete transdifferentiation might yield insulin-producing surrogates that are in a better position than true beta cells to evade the immune response. Finally, if nothing else because of their ability to favor engraftment, vascularization and even local immunosuppresion, it is likely that MSCs will find their way to virtually any cell replacement therapy. The take home message is that, contrary to the widespread perception that the many cell sources and methods discussed above are exclusive of each other, an open-minded view of the problem may lead to the realization that a subjacent synergy is just waiting to be unveiled.

Gene	*Described function*	*References*
Pdx1	Pancreatic and duodenal homeobox 1, also known as Insulin Promoter Factor 1 (Ipf1) or islet/duodenum homeobox 1 (IDX1). Expressed as early as e8.5 in the foregut epithelium; de-regulated subsequently and expressed again in newly developing β cells. Pdx1 mutants are born without pancreas. Also essential for β cell function in the adult pancreas	[49, 54, 55, 280-282]
Ptf1a	Also known as p48. Knockouts lack exocrine tissue (endocrine cells are not affected but relocate in the spleen). Also critically involved in the earlier stages of pancreatic development together with Pdx1.	[51-53, 283-285]
HNF6	Hepatocyte nuclear factor 6, also known as Onecut-1. Precedes expression of Pdx1 in the foregut. However, pancreatic development, even if severely impaired, is not arrested in knockouts. Essential regulator of Ngn3. Expression excluded from islets at e18.5.	[221, 227, 286-288] [229, 288, 289]
TCF2	Transcription factor 2, also known as hepatocyte nuclear factor (HNF1β). Mutations associated with maturity-onset diabetes of the young (MODY). Co-localizes in early development with Pdx1 and Ptf1a, and may possibly regulate the latter. Indispensable for Ngn3 expression.	[284, 288, 290-293]
Hlxb9	Human homeobox gene 9. Expression precedes that of Pdx1 in the dorsal anlagen, and knockouts display a selective ablation of the dorsal pancreas.	[294-297]
Ngn3	Neurogenin 3. Knockouts lack endocrine pancreas. Essential for the development of all endocrine cell types within the islet.	[59-61, 63, 64] [59, 298]
Isl1	Islet-1. Detected immediately after maturation of endocrine cell types. Knockouts lack endocrine cell types and dorsal pancreatic mesenchyme.	[299-301]
Beta2/NeuroD	Beta cell E-box transactivator 2. Knockouts show a dramatic reduction in the number of β cells, imperfect islet morphogenesis and defects in the exocrine component. Effected by Ngn3.	[302-304]
Brn-4	Brain-4. First marker of α cells, preceding Pax6 and Isl1. However, mutants do not exhibit any noticeable abnormality in endocrine development.	[305-307]
Nkx2.2	NK2 homeobox 2. First expressded during pancreatic specification and then restricted to islets. Mutants lack beta cells and have lower numbers of other islet cells. Might be essential for the terminal differentiation of β cells.	[308, 309]
Nkx6.1	NK6 homeobox 1. Downstream of Nkx2.2 First observed in pancreatic epithelium as early as e10.5, but later restricted to β cells. Knockouts have few beta cells, perhaps due to defects during the secondary transition	[310, 311]

Pax6	Paired box-containing gene 6. Expressed in several endocrine cell types throughout development. Knockouts have very few islet cells, with an almost complete depletion of α cells. May interact with Pax4 in the specification of α and β cells.	[312-319]
Pax4	Paired box-containing gene 4. First detected around e9.5 and later restricted to β cells. Knockouts lack both β and δ cells, whose disappearance is compensated by a higher number of α cells. Pax4 is a direct target of Ngn3. Its interplay with Arx and Pax6 may regulate α and β cell differentiation.	[320-327]
Arx	aristaless-related homeobox gene. First detected around e9.5 and later restricted to endocrine cells. Downstream of Ngn3, mutants lack α cells (which is compensated by an excess of δ cells). Believed to promote α cell differentiation at the expense of β cells.	[325, 326, 328]
MafA/B	MafA is preferentially found in β cells as opposed to MafB, which is more abundant in α cells. A switch from MafB to MafA might be important for appropriate beta cell maturation, although MafA knockouts (which are diabetic) have no developmental effects.	[329-334]
Foxa2	Also known as hepatocyte nuclear factor (HNF) 3β. Controls Pdx1 expression in mature β cells, but pancreatic specification is not affected in conditional knockouts.	[335-338] [339]
Prox1	Prospero-related homeobox 1. Detected from e9.5 in endocrine tissue. Knockouts exhibit pancreatic development arrest from e11.5. May repress exocrine differentiation.	[340-342]
Sox4	Broadly expressed in the epithelium, later restricted to hormone-producing cells. Knockouts have impared secondary transition	[343, 344]
Sox9	Expressed from e10.5 together with Pdx1. Known to regulate the Ngn3 promoter and believed to regulate the maintenance of the pancreatic progenitor pool	[67, 343]

REFERENCES

[1]   White SA, Manas DW. Pancreas transplantation. Ann R Coll Surg Engl 2008;90(5):368-370.

[2]   Burke GW, Ciancio G, Sollinger HW. Advances in pancreas transplantation. Transplantation 2004;77(9 Suppl):S62-67.

[3]   Ricordi C, Strom TB. Clinical islet transplantation: advances and immunological challenges. Nat Rev Immunol 2004;4(4):259-268.

[4]   Pileggi A, Alejandro R, Ricordi C. Clinical islet transplantation. Minerva Endocrinol 2006;31(3):219-232.

[5]   Tzakis AG, Ricordi C, Alejandro R, *et al.* Pancreatic islet transplantation after upper abdominal exenteration and liver replacement. Lancet 1990;336(8712):402-405.

[6]   Fontes PA, Rilo HL, Carroll PB, *et al.* Human islet isolation and transplantation in chronic pancreatitis using the automated method. Transplant Proc 1992;24(6):2809.

[7]   Shapiro AM, Lakey JR, Ryan EA, *et al.* Islet transplantation in seven patients with type 1 diabetes mellitus using a glucocorticoid-free immunosuppressive regimen. N Engl J Med 2000;343(4):230-238.

[8]   Iwanaga Y, Matsumoto S, Okitsu T, *et al.* Living donor islet transplantation, the alternative approach to overcome the obstacles limiting transplant. Ann N Y Acad Sci 2006;1079:335-339.

[9]   Matsumoto S, Okitsu T, Iwanaga Y, *et al.* Follow-up study of the first successful living donor islet transplantation. Transplantation 2006;82(12):1629-1633.

[10]   Matsumoto S, Okitsu T, Iwanaga Y, *et al.* Insulin independence after living-donor distal pancreatectomy and islet allotransplantation. Lancet 2005;365(9471):1642-1644.

[11]   Matsumoto S, Okitsu T, Iwanaga Y, *et al.* Insulin independence of unstable diabetic patient after single living donor islet transplantation. Transplant Proc 2005;37(8):3427-3429.

[12]   Jung HS, Choi SH, Kim SJ, *et al.* A better yield of islet cell mass from living pancreatic donors compared with cadaveric donors. Clin Transplant 2007;21(6):738-743.

[13]   Ricordi C, Lacy PE, Finke EH, *et al.* Automated method for isolation of human pancreatic islets. Diabetes 1988;37(4):413-420.

[14]   Merani S, Shapiro AM. Current status of pancreatic islet transplantation. Clin Sci (Lond) 2006;110(6):611-625.

[15]   Ricordi C. Islet transplantation: a brave new world. Diabetes 2003;52(7):1595-1603.

[16]   Sakuma Y, Ricordi C, Miki A, *et al.* Factors that affect human islet isolation. Transplant Proc 2008;40(2):343-345.

[17]   Ryan EA, Paty BW, Senior PA, *et al.* Five-year follow-up after clinical islet transplantation. Diabetes 2005;54(7):2060-2069.

[18]   Poggioli R, Faradji RN, Ponte G, *et al.* Quality of life after islet transplantation. Am J Transplant 2006;6(2):371-378.

[19]   Froud T, Ricordi C, Baidal DA, *et al.* Islet transplantation in type 1 diabetes mellitus using cultured islets and steroid-free immunosuppression: Miami experience. Am J Transplant 2005;5(8):2037-2046.

[20]   Markmann JF, Deng S, Huang X, *et al.* Insulin independence following isolated islet transplantation and single islet infusions. Ann Surg 2003;237(6):741-749; discussion 749-750.

[21]   Bellin MD, Kandaswamy R, Parkey J, *et al.* Prolonged insulin independence after islet allotransplants in recipients with type 1 diabetes. Am J Transplant 2008;8(11):2463-2470.

[22]   Barshes NR, Wyllie S, Goss JA. Inflammation-mediated dysfunction and apoptosis in pancreatic islet transplantation: implications for intrahepatic grafts. J Leukoc Biol 2005;77(5):587-597.

[23]   McCabe C, O'Brien T. The rational design of beta cell cytoprotective gene transfer strategies: targeting deleterious iNOS expression. Mol Biotechnol 2007;37(1):38-47.

[24]   Flotte T, Agarwal A, Wang J, *et al.* Efficient *ex vivo* transduction of pancreatic islet cells with recombinant adeno-associated virus vectors. Diabetes 2001;50(3):515-520.

[25]   Curran MA, Ochoa MS, Molano RD, *et al.* Efficient transduction of pancreatic islets by feline immunodeficiency virus vectors1. Transplantation 2002;74(3):299-306.

[26]   Fenjves ES, Ochoa MS, Cechin S, *et al.* Protection of human pancreatic islets using a lentiviral vector expressing two genes: cFLIP and GFP. Cell Transplant 2008;17(7):793-802.

[27]   Kapturczak MH, Flotte T, Atkinson MA. Adeno-associated virus (AAV) as a vehicle for therapeutic gene delivery: improvements in vector design and viral production enhance potential to prolong graft survival in pancreatic islet cell transplantation for the reversal of type 1 diabetes. Curr Mol Med 2001;1(2):245-258.

[28]   Embury J, Klein D, Pileggi A, *et al.* Proteins linked to a protein transduction domain efficiently transduce pancreatic islets. Diabetes 2001;50(8):1706-1713.

[29]   Klein D, Mendoza V, Pileggi A, *et al.* Delivery of TAT/PTD-fused proteins/peptides to islets via pancreatic duct. Cell Transplant 2005;14(5):241-248.

[30]   Klein D, Ribeiro MM, Mendoza V, *et al.* Delivery of Bcl-XL or its BH4 domain by protein transduction inhibits apoptosis in human islets. Biochem Biophys Res Commun 2004;323(2):473-478.

[31]   Mendoza V, Klein D, Ichii H, *et al.* Protection of islets in culture by delivery of oxygen binding neuroglobin via protein transduction. Transplant Proc 2005;37(1):237-240.

[32]   Pastori RL, Klein D, Ribeiro MM, *et al.* Delivery of proteins and peptides into live cells by means of protein transduction domains: potential application to organ and cell transplantation. Transplantation 2004;77(11):1627-1631.

[33]   Pileggi A, Molano RD, Berney T, *et al.* Heme oxygenase-1 induction in islet cells results in protection from apoptosis and improved *in vivo* function after transplantation. Diabetes 2001;50(9):1983-1991.

[34]   Ribeiro MM, Klein D, Pileggi A, *et al.* Heme oxygenase-1 fused to a TAT peptide transduces and protects pancreatic beta-cells. Biochem Biophys Res Commun 2003;305(4):876-881.

[35]   Cobianchi L, Fornoni A, Pileggi A, *et al.* Riboflavin inhibits IL-6 expression and p38 activation in islet cells. Cell Transplant 2008;17(5):559-566.

[36]   Fornoni A, Cobianchi L, Sanabria NY, *et al.* The l-isoform but not d-isoforms of a JNK inhibitory peptide protects pancreatic beta-cells. Biochem Biophys Res Commun 2007;354(1):227-233.

[37]   Coppola T, Beraud-Dufour S, Antoine A, *et al.* Neurotensin protects pancreatic beta cells from apoptosis. Int J Biochem Cell Biol 2008;40(10):2296-2302.

[38]   Ollinger R, Wang H, Yamashita K, *et al.* Therapeutic applications of bilirubin and biliverdin in transplantation. Antioxid Redox Signal 2007;9(12):2175-2185.

[39]   Wang H, Lee SS, Gao W, *et al.* Donor treatment with carbon monoxide can yield islet allograft survival and tolerance. Diabetes 2005;54(5):1400-1406.

[40]   Fornoni A, Pileggi A, Molano RD, *et al.* Inhibition of c-jun N terminal kinase (JNK) improves functional beta cell mass in human islets and leads to AKT and glycogen synthase kinase-3 (GSK-3) phosphorylation. Diabetologia 2008;51(2):298-308.

[41]   Ijaz A, Tejada T, Catanuto P, *et al.* Inhibition of C-jun N-terminal kinase improves insulin sensitivity but worsens albuminuria in experimental diabetes. Kidney Int 2008.

[42]   Varona-Santos JL, Pileggi A, Molano RD, *et al.* c-Jun N-terminal kinase 1 is deleterious to the function and survival of murine pancreatic islets. Diabetologia 2008;51(12):2271-2280.

[43]   Yamamoto T, Ricordi C, Mita A, *et al.* beta-Cell specific cytoprotection by prolactin on human islets. Transplant Proc 2008;40(2):382-383.

[44]   Speier S, Nyqvist D, Cabrera O, *et al.* Noninvasive *in vivo* imaging of pancreatic islet cell biology. Nat Med 2008 May;14(5):574-578.

[45]   Capecchi MR. Altering the genome by homologous recombination. Science 1989;244(4910):1288-1292.

[46]   Falin LI. The development and cytodifferentiation of the islets of Langerhans in human embryos and foetuses. Acta Anat (Basel) 1967;68(1):147-168.

[47]　Slack JM. Developmental biology of the pancreas. Development 1995;121(6):1569-1580.

[48]　Piper K, Brickwood S, Turnpenny LW, *et al.* Beta cell differentiation during early human pancreas development. J Endocrinol 2004;181(1):11-23.

[49]　Jonsson J, Carlsson L, Edlund T, *et al.* Insulin-promoter-factor 1 is required for pancreas development in mice. Nature 1994;371(6498):606-609.

[50]　Sellick GS, Barker KT, Stolte-Dijkstra I, *et al.* Mutations in PTF1A cause pancreatic and cerebellar agenesis. Nat Genet 2004;36(12):1301-1305.

[51]　Kawaguchi Y, Cooper B, Gannon M, *et al.* The role of the transcriptional regulator Ptf1a in converting intestinal to pancreatic progenitors. Nat Genet 2002;32(1):128-134.

[52]　Kumar M, Melton D. Pancreas specification: a budding question. Curr Opin Genet Dev 2003;13(4):401-407.

[53]　Yoshitomi H, Zaret KS. Endothelial cell interactions initiate dorsal pancreas development by selectively inducing the transcription factor Ptf1a. Development 2004;131(4):807-817.

[54]　Kim SK, Melton DA. Pancreas development is promoted by cyclopamine, a hedgehog signaling inhibitor. Proc Natl Acad Sci U S A 1998;95(22):13036-13041.

[55]　Apelqvist A, Ahlgren U, Edlund H. Sonic hedgehog directs specialised mesoderm differentiation in the intestine and pancreas. Curr Biol 1997;7(10):801-804.

[56]　Lammert E, Cleaver O, Melton D. Role of endothelial cells in early pancreas and liver development. Mech Dev 2003;120(1):59-64.

[57]　Lammert E, Cleaver O, Melton D. Induction of pancreatic differentiation by signals from blood vessels. Science 2001;294(5542):564-567.

[58]　Wessells NK, Cohen, J. H. Early pancreas organogenesis: Morphogenesis, tissue interactions and mass effects. Dev Biol 1967;15:237.

[59]　Apelqvist A, Li H, Sommer L, *et al.* Notch signalling controls pancreatic cell differentiation. Nature 1999;400(6747):877-881.

[60]　Gradwohl G, Dierich A, LeMeur M, *et al.* Nneurogenin3 is required for the development of the four endocrine cell lineages of the pancreas. Proc Natl Acad Sci U S A 2000;97(4):1607-1611.

[61]　Jensen J, Pedersen EE, Galante P, *et al.* Control of endodermal endocrine development by Hes-1. Nat Genet 2000;24(1):36-44.

[62]　Edlund H. Factors controlling pancreatic cell differentiation and function. Diabetologia 2001;44(9):1071-1079.

[63]　Gu G, Dubauskaite J, Melton DA. Direct evidence for the pancreatic lineage: NGN3+ cells are islet progenitors and are distinct from duct progenitors. Development 2002;129(10):2447-2457.

[64]　Gu G, Brown JR, Melton DA. Direct lineage tracing reveals the ontogeny of pancreatic cell fates during mouse embryogenesis. Mech Dev 2003;120(1):35-43.

[65]　Pictet R, Rutter, W. J. Development of the embryonic endocrine pancreas in Handbook of Physiology. Baltimore: Williams & Wilkins; 1972.

[66]　Pictet RL, Clark WR, Williams RH, *et al.* An ultrastructural analysis of the developing embryonic pancreas. Dev Biol 1972;29(4):436-467.

[67]　Lynn FC, Smith SB, Wilson ME, *et al.* Sox9 coordinates a transcriptional network in pancreatic progenitor cells. Proc Natl Acad Sci U S A 2007;104(25):10500-10505.

[68]　Evans MJ, Kaufman MH. Establishment in culture of pluripotential cells from mouse embryos. Nature 1981;292(5819):154-156.

[69]　Martin GR. Isolation of a pluripotent cell line from early mouse embryos cultured in medium conditioned by teratocarcinoma stem cells. Proc Natl Acad Sci U S A 1981;78(12):7634-7638.

[70]　Thomson JA, Itskovitz-Eldor J, Shapiro SS, *et al.* Embryonic stem cell lines derived from human blastocysts. Science 1998;282(5391):1145-1147.

[71]　Cowan CA, Klimanskaya I, McMahon J, *et al.* Derivation of embryonic stem-cell lines from human blastocysts. N Engl J Med 2004;350(13):1353-1356.

[72]　Bhattacharya B, Miura T, Brandenberger R, *et al.*Gene expression in human embryonic stem cell lines: unique molecular signature. Blood 2004;103(8):2956-2964.

[73]　Boiani M, Scholer HR. Regulatory networks in embryo-derived pluripotent stem cells. Nat Rev Mol Cell Biol 2005;6(11):872-884.

[74]　Boyer LA, Lee TI, Cole MF, *et al.* Core transcriptional regulatory circuitry in human embryonic stem cells. Cell 2005;122(6):947-956.

[75]　Yu J, Vodyanik MA, Smuga-Otto K, *et al.* Induced pluripotent stem cell lines derived from human somatic cells. Science 2007;318(5858):1917-1920.

[76]   Lewitzky M, Yamanaka S. Reprogramming somatic cells towards pluripotency by defined factors. Curr Opin Biotechnol 2007;18(5):467-473.

[77]   Nakagawa M, Koyanagi M, Tanabe K, *et al.* Generation of induced pluripotent stem cells without Myc from mouse and human fibroblasts. Nat Biotechnol 2007.

[78]   Okita K, Ichisaka T, Yamanaka S. Generation of germline-competent induced pluripotent stem cells. Nature 2007;448(7151):313-317.

[79]   Takahashi K, Okita K, Nakagawa M, *et al.* Induction of pluripotent stem cells from fibroblast cultures. Nat Protoc 2007;2(12):3081-3089.

[80]   Takahashi K, Tanabe K, Ohnuki M, *et al.* Induction of pluripotent stem cells from adult human fibroblasts by defined factors. Cell 2007;131(5):861-872.

[81]   Takahashi K, Yamanaka S. Induction of pluripotent stem cells from mouse embryonic and adult fibroblast cultures by defined factors. Cell 2006;126(4):663-676.

[82]   Assady S, Maor G, Amit M, *et al.* Insulin production by human embryonic stem cells. Diabetes 2001;50(8):1691-1697.

[83]   Lumelsky N, Blondel O, Laeng P, *et al.* Differentiation of embryonic stem cells to insulin-secreting structures similar to pancreatic islets. Science 2001;292(5520):1389-1394.

[84]   Baharvand H, Jafary H, Massumi M, *et al.* Generation of insulin-secreting cells from human embryonic stem cells. Dev Growth Differ 2006;48(5):323-332.

[85]   D'Amour KA, Agulnick AD, Eliazer S, *et al.* Efficient differentiation of human embryonic stem cells to definitive endoderm. Nat Biotechnol 2005;23(12):1534-1541.

[86]   D'Amour KA, Bang AG, Eliazer S, *et al.* Production of pancreatic hormone-expressing endocrine cells from human embryonic stem cells. Nat Biotechnol 2006.

[87]   Beck S, Le Good JA, Guzman M, *et al.* Extraembryonic proteases regulate Nodal signalling during gastrulation. Nat Cell Biol 2002;4(12):981-985.

[88]   McLean AB, D'Amour KA, Jones KL, *et al.* Activin a efficiently specifies definitive endoderm from human embryonic stem cells only when phosphatidylinositol 3-kinase signaling is suppressed. Stem Cells 2007;25(1):29-38.

[89]   Perea-Gomez A, Vella FD, Shawlot W, *et al.* Nodal antagonists in the anterior visceral endoderm prevent the formation of multiple primitive streaks. Dev Cell 2002;3(5):745-756.

[90]   Tada S, Era T, Furusawa C, *et al.* Characterization of mesendoderm: a diverging point of the definitive endoderm and mesoderm in embryonic stem cell differentiation culture. Development 2005;132(19):4363-4374.

[91]   Yamamoto M, Saijoh Y, Perea-Gomez A, *et al.* Nodal antagonists regulate formation of the anteroposterior axis of the mouse embryo. Nature 2004;428(6981):387-392.

[92]   Ying QL, Nichols J, Chambers I, *et al.* BMP induction of Id proteins suppresses differentiation and sustains embryonic stem cell self-renewal in collaboration with STAT3. Cell 2003;115(3):281-292.

[93]   Xu RH, Peck RM, Li DS, *et al.* Basic FGF and suppression of BMP signaling sustain undifferentiated proliferation of human ES cells. Nat Methods 2005;2(3):185-190.

[94]   Jiang J, Au M, Lu K, *et al.* Generation of Insulin-producing Islet-like Clusters from Human Embryonic Stem Cells. Stem Cells 2007 Aug;25(8):1940-1953.

[95]   Kroon E, Martinson LA, Kadoya K, *et al.* Pancreatic endoderm derived from human embryonic stem cells generates glucose-responsive insulin-secreting cells *in vivo*. Nat Biotechnol 2008;26(4):443-452.

[96]   Ricordi C, Edlund H. Toward a renewable source of pancreatic beta-cells. Nat Biotechnol 2008;26(4):397-398.

[97]   Jiang FX, Harrison LC. Extracellular signals and pancreatic beta-cell development: a brief review. Mol Med 2002;8(12):763-770.

[98]   Jiang FX, Cram DS, DeAizpurua HJ, *et al.* Laminin-1 promotes differentiation of fetal mouse pancreatic beta-cells. Diabetes 1999;48(4):722-730.

[99]   Jiang FX, Georges-Labouesse E, Harrison LC. Regulation of laminin 1-induced pancreatic beta-cell differentiation by alpha6 integrin and alpha-dystroglycan. Mol Med 2001;7(2):107-114.

[100]   Dedhar S, Hannigan GE. Integrin cytoplasmic interactions and bidirectional transmembrane signalling. Curr Opin Cell Biol 1996;8(5):657-669.

[101]   Hannigan GE, Dedhar S. Protein kinase mediators of integrin signal transduction. J Mol Med 1997;75(1):35-44.

[102]   Newham P, Humphries MJ. Integrin adhesion receptors: structure, function and implications for biomedicine. Mol Med Today 1996;2(7):304-313.

[103]   Fraker C, Ricordi, C, Inverardi, L, *et al.* Culture in perfluorinated platforms results in enhanced human islet function. In: XIV International Society for Cellular Therapy meeting, May 17-20; 2008 May 17-20; Miami; 2008. p. 81.

[104]   Fraker CA, Alvarez S, Papadopoulos P, *et al.* Enhanced oxygenation promotes beta-cell differentiation in vitro. Stem Cells 2007;25(12):3155-164.

[105] Bravo-Egana V, Rosero S, Molano RD, P *et al.* Quantitative differential expression analysis reveals miR-7 as major islet microRNA. Biochem Biophys Res Commun 2008;366(4):922-926.

[106] Poy MN, Eliasson L, Krutzfeldt J, *et al.* A pancreatic islet-specific microRNA regulates insulin secretion. Nature 2004;432(7014):226-230.

[107] Kwon YD, Oh SK, Kim HS, *et al.* Cellular manipulation of human embryonic stem cells by TAT-PDX1 protein transduction. Mol Ther 2005;12(1):28-32.

[108] Domínguez-Bendala J, Klein D, Ribeiro M, *et al.* TAT-mediated neurogenin 3 protein transduction stimulates pancreatic endocrine differentiation in vitro. Diabetes 2005;54(3):720-726.

[109] Spitere K, Toulouse A, O'Sullivan DB, *et al.* TAT-PAX6 protein transduction in neural progenitor cells: A novel approach for generation of dopaminergic neurones in vitro. Brain Res 2008;1208:25-34.

[110] Noguchi H, Kaneto H, Weir GC, *et al.* PDX-1 protein containing its own antennapedia-like protein transduction domain can transduce pancreatic duct and islet cells. Diabetes 2003;52(7):1732-1737.

[111] Noguchi H, Matsushita M, Matsumoto S, *et al.* Mechanism of PDX-1 protein transduction. Biochem Biophys Res Commun 2005;332(1):68-74.

[112] Noda T, Kawamura R, Funabashi H, *et al.* Transduction of NeuroD2 protein induced neural cell differentiation. J Biotechnol 2006.

[113] Noguchi H, Ueda M, Matsumoto S, *et al.* BETA2/NeuroD protein transduction requires cell surface heparan sulfate proteoglycans. Hum Gene Ther 2007;18(1):10-17.

[114] da Silva Meirelles L, Chagastelles PC, Nardi NB. Mesenchymal stem cells reside in virtually all post-natal organs and tissues. J Cell Sci 2006;119(Pt 11):2204-2213.

[115] Dominici M, Le Blanc K, Mueller I, *et al.* Minimal criteria for defining multipotent mesenchymal stromal cells. The International Society for Cellular Therapy position statement. Cytotherapy 2006;8(4):315-317.

[116] Horwitz EM, Le Blanc K, Dominici M, *et al.* Clarification of the nomenclature for MSC: The International Society for Cellular Therapy position statement. Cytotherapy 2005;7(5):393-395.

[117] Jiang Y, Jahagirdar BN, Reinhardt RL, *et al.* Pluripotency of mesenchymal stem cells derived from adult marrow. Nature 2002;418(6893):41-49.

[118] Jiang Y, Vaessen B, Lenvik T, *et al.* Multipotent progenitor cells can be isolated from postnatal murine bone marrow, muscle, and brain. Exp Hematol 2002;30(8):896-904.

[119] Schwartz RE, Reyes M, Koodie L, J *et al.* Multipotent adult progenitor cells from bone marrow differentiate into functional hepatocyte-like cells. J Clin Invest 2002;109(10):1291-1302.

[120] Verfaillie CM. Multipotent adult progenitor cells: an update. Novartis Found Symp 2005;265:55-61; discussion 61-5, 92-97.

[121] Luttun A, Ross JJ, Verfaillie C, *et al.* Differentiation of multipotent adult progenitor cells into functional endothelial and smooth muscle cells. Curr Protoc Immunol 2006;Chapter 22:Unit 22F 9.

[122] Pelacho B, Nakamura Y, Zhang J, *et al.* Multipotent adult progenitor cell transplantation increases vascularity and improves left ventricular function after myocardial infarction. J Tissue Eng Regen Med 2007;1(1):51-59.

[123] Chen LB, Jiang XB, Yang L. Differentiation of rat marrow mesenchymal stem cells into pancreatic islet beta-cells. World J Gastroenterol 2004;10(20):3016-3020.

[124] Choi KS, Shin JS, Lee JJ, *et al.* In vitro trans-differentiation of rat mesenchymal cells into insulin-producing cells by rat pancreatic extract. Biochem Biophys Res Commun 2005;330(4):1299-1305.

[125] Baertschiger RM, Bosco D, Morel P, *et al.* Mesenchymal stem cells derived from human exocrine pancreas express transcription factors implicated in beta-cell development. Pancreas 2008;37(1):75-84.

[126] Chang CF, Hsu KH, Chiou SH, *et al.* Fibronectin and pellet suspension culture promote differentiation of human mesenchymal stem cells into insulin producing cells. J Biomed Mater Res A 2008;86(4):1097-1105.

[127] Chang C, Niu D, Zhou H, *et al.* Mesenchymal stem cells contribute to insulin-producing cells upon microenvironmental manipulation in vitro. Transplant Proc 2007;39(10):3363-3368.

[128] Hisanaga E, Park KY, Yamada S, *et al.* A simple method to induce differentiation of murine bone marrow mesenchymal cells to insulin-producing cells using conophylline and betacellulin-delta4. Endocr J 2008;55(3):535-543.

[129] Wu XH, Liu CP, Xu KF, *et al.*Reversal of hyperglycemia in diabetic rats by portal vein transplantation of islet-like cells generated from bone marrow mesenchymal stem cells. World J Gastroenterol 2007;13(24):3342-3349.

[130] Sun J, Yang Y, Wang X, *et al.*Expression of Pdx-1 in bone marrow mesenchymal stem cells promotes differentiation of islet-like cells in vitro. Sci China C Life Sci 2006;49(5):480-489.

[131] Li Y, Zhang R, Qiao H, *et al.* Generation of insulin-producing cells from PDX-1 gene-modified human mesenchymal stem cells. J Cell Physiol 2007;211(1):36-44.

[132] Moriscot C, de Fraipont F, Richard MJ, *et al.* Human bone marrow mesenchymal stem cells can express insulin and key transcription factors of the endocrine pancreas developmental pathway upon genetic and/or microenvironmental manipulation in vitro. Stem Cells 2005;23(4):594-603.

[133] Karnieli O, Izhar-Prato Y, Bulvik S, *et al.* Generation of insulin-producing cells from human bone marrow mesenchymal stem cells by genetic manipulation. Stem Cells 2007;25(11):2837-2844.

[134] Xu J, Lu Y, Ding F, *et al.* Reversal of diabetes in mice by intrahepatic injection of bone-derived GFP-murine mesenchymal stem cells infected with the recombinant retrovirus-carrying human insulin gene. World J Surg 2007;31(9):1872-1882.

[135] Masaka T, Miyazaki M, Du G, *et al.* Derivation of hepato-pancreatic intermediate progenitor cells from a clonal mesenchymal stem cell line of rat bone marrow origin. Int J Mol Med 2008;22(4):447-452.

[136] Dong QY, Chen L, Gao GQ, *et al.* Allogeneic diabetic mesenchymal stem cells transplantation in streptozotocin-induced diabetic rat. Clin Invest Med 2008;31(6):E328-37.

[137] Ezquer FE, Ezquer ME, Parrau DB, *et al.* Systemic administration of multipotent mesenchymal stromal cells reverts hyperglycemia and prevents nephropathy in type 1 diabetic mice. Biol Blood Marrow Transplant 2008;14(6):631-640.

[138] Chang C, Wang X, Niu D, *et al.* Mesenchymal Stem Cells Adopt beta-Cell Fate Upon Diabetic Pancreatic Microenvironment. Pancreas 2008 Apr;38(3):275-281.

[139] Abdi R, Fiorina P, Adra CN, *et al.* Immunomodulation by mesenchymal stem cells: a potential therapeutic strategy for type 1 diabetes. Diabetes 2008;57(7):1759-1767.

[140] Mishra PK. Bone marrow-derived mesenchymal stem cells for treatment of heart failure: is it all paracrine actions and immunomodulation? J Cardiovasc Med (Hagerstown) 2008;9(2):122-128.

[141] Le Blanc K, Ringden O. Immunomodulation by mesenchymal stem cells and clinical experience. J Intern Med 2007;262(5):509-525.

[142] Ozaki K, Sato K, Oh I, *et al.* Mechanisms of immunomodulation by mesenchymal stem cells. Int J Hematol 2007;86(1):5-7.

[143] Wu Y, Chen L, Scott PG, *et al.* Mesenchymal stem cells enhance wound healing through differentiation and angiogenesis. Stem Cells 2007;25(10):2648-2659.

[144] Ball SG, Shuttleworth CA, Kielty CM. Mesenchymal stem cells and neovascularization: role of platelet-derived growth factor receptors. J Cell Mol Med 2007;11(5):1012-1030.

[145] Johansson U, Rasmusson I, Niclou SP, *et al.* Formation of composite endothelial cell-mesenchymal stem cell islets: a novel approach to promote islet revascularization. Diabetes 2008;57(9):2393-2401.

[146] Fang B, Li N, Song Y, *et al.* Cotransplantation of haploidentical mesenchymal stem cells to enhance engraftment of hematopoietic stem cells and to reduce the risk of graft failure in two children with severe aplastic anemia. Pediatr Transplant 2008 Jun;13(4):499-502.

[147] Lee ST, Maeng H, Chwae YJ, *et al.* Effect of mesenchymal stem cell transplantation on the engraftment of human hematopoietic stem cells and leukemic cells in mice model. Int J Hematol 2008;87(3):327-337.

[148] Ball LM, Bernardo ME, Roelofs H, *et al.* Cotransplantation of *ex vivo* expanded mesenchymal stem cells accelerates lymphocyte recovery and may reduce the risk of graft failure in haploidentical hematopoietic stem-cell transplantation. Blood 2007;110(7):2764-2767.

[149] Noort WA, Kruisselbrink AB, in't Anker PS, *et al.* Mesenchymal stem cells promote engraftment of human umbilical cord blood-derived CD34(+) cells in NOD/SCID mice. Exp Hematol 2002;30(8):870-878.

[150] Harris DT, Badowski M, Ahmad N, *et al.* The potential of cord blood stem cells for use in regenerative medicine. Expert Opin Biol Ther 2007;7(9):1311-1322.

[151] Harris DT, Rogers I. Umbilical cord blood: a unique source of pluripotent stem cells for regenerative medicine. Curr Stem Cell Res Ther 2007;2(4):301-309.

[152] Gao F, Wu DQ, Hu YH, *et al.* In vitro cultivation of islet-like cell clusters from human umbilical cord blood-derived mesenchymal stem cells. Transl Res 2008;151(6):293-302.

[153] Chao KC, Chao KF, Fu YS, *et al.* Islet-like clusters derived from mesenchymal stem cells in Wharton's Jelly of the human umbilical cord for transplantation to control type 1 diabetes. PLoS ONE 2008;3(1):e1451.

[154] De Coppi P, Bartsch G, Jr., Siddiqui MM, *et al.* Isolation of amniotic stem cell lines with potential for therapy. Nat Biotechnol 2007;25(1):100-106.

[155] Dimitrov R, Timeva T, Kyurkchiev D, *et al.* Characterization of clonogenic stromal cells isolated from human endometrium. Reproduction 2008;135(4):551-558.

[156] Wolff EF, Wolff AB, Hongling D, *et al.* Demonstration of multipotent stem cells in the adult human endometrium by in vitro chondrogenesis. Reprod Sci 2007;14(6):524-533.

[157] Deutsch G, Jung J, Zheng M, *et al.* A bipotential precursor population for pancreas and liver within the embryonic endoderm. Development 2001;128(6):871-881.

[158] Melton D. Signals for tissue induction and organ formation in vertebrate embryos. Harvey Lect 1997;93:49-64.

[159] Jung J, Zheng M, Goldfarb M, *et al.* Initiation of mammalian liver development from endoderm by fibroblast growth factors. Science 1999;284(5422):1998-2003.

[160] Lemaigre F, Zaret KS. Liver development update: new embryo models, cell lineage control, and morphogenesis. Curr Opin Genet Dev 2004;14(5):582-590.

[161] Tremblay KD, Zaret KS. Distinct populations of endoderm cells converge to generate the embryonic liver bud and ventral foregut tissues. Dev Biol 2005;280(1):87-99.

[162] Zaret KS. Hepatocyte differentiation: from the endoderm and beyond. Curr Opin Genet Dev 2001;11(5):568-574.

[163] Zaret KS. Liver specification and early morphogenesis. Mech Dev 2000;92(1):83-8.

[164] Wells JM, Melton DA. Vertebrate endoderm development. Annu Rev Cell Dev Biol 1999;15:393-410.

[165] Gualdi R, Bossard P, Zheng M, *et al.* Hepatic specification of the gut endoderm in vitro: cell signaling and transcriptional control. Genes Dev 1996;10(13):1670-1682.

[166] Douarin NM. An experimental analysis of liver development. Med Biol 1975;53(6):427-455.

[167] Ferber S, Halkin A, Cohen H, *et al.* Pancreatic and duodenal homeobox gene 1 induces expression of insulin genes in liver and ameliorates streptozotocin-induced hyperglycemia. Nat Med 2000;6(5):568-572.

[168] Ber I, Shternhall K, Perl S, *et al.* Functional, persistent, and extended liver to pancreas transdifferentiation. J Biol Chem 2003;278(34):31950-1957.

[169] Meivar-Levy I, Sapir T, Gefen-Halevi S, *et al.* Pancreatic and duodenal homeobox gene 1 induces hepatic dedifferentiation by suppressing the expression of CCAAT/enhancer-binding protein beta. Hepatology 2007;46(3):898-905.

[170] Li WC, Horb ME, Tosh D, *et al. In vitro* transdifferentiation of hepatoma cells into functional pancreatic cells. Mech Dev 2005;122(6):835-847.

[171] Tang DQ, Lu S, Sun YP, *et al.* Reprogramming liver-stem WB cells into functional insulin-producing cells by persistent expression of Pdx1- and Pdx1-VP16 mediated by lentiviral vectors. Lab Invest 2006;86(1):83-93.

[172] Horb ME, Shen CN, Tosh D, *et al.* Experimental conversion of liver to pancreas. Curr Biol 2003;13(2):105-115.

[173] Wang AY, Ehrhardt A, Xu H, *et al.* Adenovirus transduction is required for the correction of diabetes using Pdx-1 or Neurogenin-3 in the liver. Mol Ther 2007;15(2):255-263.

[174] Kaneto H, Matsuoka TA, Nakatani Y, *et al.*A crucial role of MafA as a novel therapeutic target for diabetes. J Biol Chem 2005;280(15):15047-15052.

[175] Kaneto H, Miyatsuka T, Fujitani Y, *et al.* Role of PDX-1 and MafA as a potential therapeutic target for diabetes. Diabetes Res Clin Pract 2007;77 Suppl 1:S127-137.

[176] Kaneto H, Miyatsuka T, Shiraiwa T, *et al.* Crucial role of PDX-1 in pancreas development, beta-cell differentiation, and induction of surrogate beta-cells. Curr Med Chem 2007;14(16):1745-1752.

[177] Matsuoka TA, Kaneto H, Stein R, *et al.*MafA regulates expression of genes important to islet beta-cell function. Mol Endocrinol 2007;21(11):2764-2774.

[178] Miyatsuka T, Kaneto H, Kajimoto Y, *et al.* Ectopically expressed PDX-1 in liver initiates endocrine and exocrine pancreas differentiation but causes dysmorphogenesis. Biochem Biophys Res Commun 2003;310(3):1017-1025.

[179] Kojima H, Fujimiya M, Matsumura K, *et al.* NeuroD-betacellulin gene therapy induces islet neogenesis in the liver and reverses diabetes in mice. Nat Med 2003;9(5):596-603.

[180] Zhou Q, Brown J, Kanarek A, *et al. In vivo* reprogramming of adult pancreatic exocrine cells to beta-cells. Nature 2008 Oct 2;455(7213):627-632.

[181] Buchanan TA, Kjos SL. Gestational diabetes: risk or myth? J Clin Endocrinol Metab 1999;84(6):1854-1857.

[182] Kjos SL, Buchanan TA. Gestational diabetes mellitus. N Engl J Med 1999;341(23):1749-1756.

[183] Van Assche FA, Aerts L, De Prins F. A morphological study of the endocrine pancreas in human pregnancy. Br J Obstet Gynaecol 1978;85(11):818-820.

[184] Hellerstrom C, Swenne I. Functional maturation and proliferation of fetal pancreatic beta-cells. Diabetes 1991;40 Suppl 2:89-93.

[185] Brelje TC, Bhagroo NV, Stout LE, *et al.* Beneficial effects of lipids and prolactin on insulin secretion and beta-cell proliferation: a role for lipids in the adaptation of islets to pregnancy. J Endocrinol 2008;197(2):265-276.

[186] Brelje TC, Scharp DW, Lacy PE, *et al.* Effect of homologous placental lactogens, prolactins, and growth hormones on islet B-cell division and insulin secretion in rat, mouse, and human islets: implication for placental lactogen regulation of islet function during pregnancy. Endocrinology 1993;132(2):879-887.

[187] Brelje TC, Sorenson RL. Role of prolactin versus growth hormone on islet B-cell proliferation in vitro: implications for pregnancy. Endocrinology 1991;128(1):45-57.

[188] Sorenson RL, Brelje TC. Adaptation of islets of Langerhans to pregnancy: beta-cell growth, enhanced insulin secretion and the role of lactogenic hormones. Horm Metab Res 1997;29(6):301-307.

[189] Sorenson RL, Brelje TC, Roth C. Effects of steroid and lactogenic hormones on islets of Langerhans: a new hypothesis for the role of pregnancy steroids in the adaptation of islets to pregnancy. Endocrinology 1993;133(5):2227-2234.

[190] Parsons JA, Brelje TC, Sorenson RL. Adaptation of islets of Langerhans to pregnancy: increased islet cell proliferation and insulin secretion correlates with the onset of placental lactogen secretion. Endocrinology 1992;130(3):1459-1466.

[191] Bonner-Weir S, Deery D, Leahy JL, et al. Compensatory growth of pancreatic beta-cells in adult rats after short-term glucose infusion. Diabetes 1989;38(1):49-53.

[192] Schuppin GT, Bonner-Weir S, Montana E, Kaiser N, Weir GC. Replication of adult pancreatic-beta cells cultured on bovine corneal endothelial cell extracellular matrix. In Vitro Cell Dev Biol Anim 1993;29A(4):339-344.

[193] Butler AE, Janson J, Soeller WC, et al. Increased beta-cell apoptosis prevents adaptive increase in beta-cell mass in mouse model of type 2 diabetes: evidence for role of islet amyloid formation rather than direct action of amyloid. Diabetes 2003;52(9):2304-2314.

[194] Milburn JL, Jr., Hirose H, Lee YH, et al. Pancreatic beta-cells in obesity. Evidence for induction of functional, morphologic, and metabolic abnormalities by increased long chain fatty acids. J Biol Chem 1995;270(3):1295-1299.

[195] Butler PC, Meier JJ, Butler AE, Bhushan A. The replication of beta cells in normal physiology, in disease and for therapy. Nat Clin Pract Endocrinol Metab 2007;3(11):758-768.

[196] Butler AE, Janson J, Bonner-Weir S, Ritzel R, Rizza RA, Butler PC. Beta-cell deficit and increased beta-cell apoptosis in humans with type 2 diabetes. Diabetes 2003;52(1):102-110.

[197] Allen FM. Experimental studies in diabetes. Series III. The pathology of diabetes 1. Hydropic degteneration of islands of Langerhans after partial pancreatectomy. J. Metab. Res. 1922;1:5-41.

[198] Bonner-Weir S, Trent DF, Weir GC. Partial pancreatectomy in the rat and subsequent defect in glucose-induced insulin release. J Clin Invest 1983;71(6):1544-1553.

[199] Brockenbrough JS, Weir GC, Bonner-Weir S. Discordance of exocrine and endocrine growth after 90% pancreatectomy in rats. Diabetes 1988;37(2):232-236.

[200] Wang RN, Kloppel G, Bouwens L. Duct- to islet-cell differentiation and islet growth in the pancreas of duct-ligated adult rats. Diabetologia 1995;38(12):1405-1411.

[201] Peters K, Panienka R, Li J, Kloppel G, Wang R. Expression of stem cell markers and transcription factors during the remodeling of the rat pancreas after duct ligation. Virchows Arch 2005;446(1):56-63.

[202] Rosenberg L, Brown RA, Duguid WP. A new approach to the induction of duct epithelial hyperplasia and nesidioblastosis by cellophane wrapping of the hamster pancreas. J Surg Res 1983;35(1):63-72.

[203] Rosenberg L, Vinik AI. Induction of endocrine cell differentiation: a new approach to management of diabetes. J Lab Clin Med 1989;114(1):75-83.

[204] Rosenberg L, Duguid WP, Brown RA, Vinik AI. Induction of nesidioblastosis will reverse diabetes in Syrian golden hamster. Diabetes 1988;37(3):334-341.

[205] Rosenberg L, Vinik AI, Pittenger GL, Rafaeloff R, Duguid WP. Islet-cell regeneration in the diabetic hamster pancreas with restoration of normoglycaemia can be induced by a local growth factor(s). Diabetologia 1996;39(3):256-262.

[206] Ferber S, BeltrandelRio H, Johnson JH, Noel RJ, Cassidy LE, Clark S, et al. GLUT-2 gene transfer into insulinoma cells confers both low and high affinity glucose-stimulated insulin release. Relationship to glucokinase activity. J Biol Chem 1994;269(15):11523-11529.

[207] Schnedl WJ, Ferber S, Johnson JH, Newgard CB. STZ transport and cytotoxicity. Specific enhancement in GLUT2-expressing cells. Diabetes 1994;43(11):1326-1333.

[208] Lenzen S. The mechanisms of alloxan- and streptozotocin-induced diabetes. Diabetologia 2008;51(2):216-226.

[209] Rosenberg L, Vinik AI. Trophic stimulation of the ductular-islet cell axis: a new approach to the treatment of diabetes. Adv Exp Med Biol 1992;321:95-104; discussion 105-109.

[210] Gepts W. Pathologic anatomy of the pancreas in juvenile diabetes mellitus. Diabetes 1965;14(10):619-633.

[211] Weaver CV, Sorenson RL, Kaung HC. Immunocytochemical localization of insulin-immunoreactive cells in the pancreatic ducts of rats treated with trypsin inhibitor. Diabetologia 1985;28(10):781-785.

[212] Bonner-Weir S, Baxter LA, Schuppin GT, Smith FE. A second pathway for regeneration of adult exocrine and endocrine pancreas. A possible recapitulation of embryonic development. Diabetes 1993;42(12):1715-1720.

[213] Sharma A, Zangen DH, Reitz P, Taneja M, Lissauer ME, Miller CP, et al. The homeodomain protein IDX-1 increases after an early burst of proliferation during pancreatic regeneration. Diabetes 1999;48(3):507-513.

[214] Bonner-Weir S, Taneja M, Weir GC, Tatarkiewicz K, Song KH, Sharma A, et al. In vitro cultivation of human islets from expanded ductal tissue. Proc Natl Acad Sci U S A 2000;97(14):7999-8004.

[215] Bonner-Weir S, Inada A, Yatoh S, Li WC, Aye T, Toschi E, et al. Transdifferentiation of pancreatic ductal cells to endocrine beta-cells. Biochem Soc Trans 2008;36(Pt 3):353-356.

[216] Martin-Pagola A, Sisino G, Allende G, Dominguez-Bendala J, Gianani R, Reijonen H, et al. Insulin protein and proliferation in ductal cells in the transplanted pancreas of patients with type 1 diabetes and recurrence of autoimmunity. Diabetologia 2008;51(10):1803-1813.

[217] Hao E, Tyrberg B, Itkin-Ansari P, Lakey JR, Geron I, Monosov EZ, et al. Beta-cell differentiation from nonendocrine epithelial cells of the adult human pancreas. Nat Med 2006;12(3):310-316.

[218] Fernandes A, King LC, Guz Y, Stein R, Wright CV, Teitelman G. Differentiation of new insulin-producing cells is induced by injury in adult pancreatic islets. Endocrinology 1997;138(4):1750-1762.

[219] Guz Y, Nasir I, Teitelman G. Regeneration of pancreatic beta cells from intra-islet precursor cells in an experimental model of diabetes. Endocrinology 2001;142(11):4956-4968.

[220] Kodama S, Toyonaga T, Kondo T, Matsumoto K, Tsuruzoe K, Kawashima J, et al. Enhanced expression of PDX-1 and Ngn3 by exendin-4 during beta cell regeneration in STZ-treated mice. Biochem Biophys Res Commun 2005;327(4):1170-1178.

[221] Dor Y, Brown J, Martinez OI, Melton DA. Adult pancreatic beta-cells are formed by self-duplication rather than stem-cell differentiation. Nature 2004;429(6987):41-46.

[222] Ianus A, Holz GG, Theise ND, Hussain MA. *In vivo* derivation of glucose-competent pancreatic endocrine cells from bone marrow without evidence of cell fusion. J Clin Invest 2003;111(6):843-850.

[223] Gershengorn MC, Hardikar AA, Wei C, Geras-Raaka E, Marcus-Samuels B, Raaka BM. Epithelial-to-mesenchymal transition generates proliferative human islet precursor cells. Science 2004;306(5705):2261-2264.

[224] Chase LG, Ulloa-Montoya F, Kidder BL, Verfaillie CM. Islet-derived fibroblast-like cells are not derived via epithelial-mesenchymal transition from Pdx-1 or insulin-positive cells. Diabetes 2007;56(1):3-7.

[225] Kayali AG, Flores LE, Lopez AD, Kutlu B, Baetge E, Kitamura R, et al. Limited capacity of human adult islets expanded in vitro to redifferentiate into insulin-producing beta-cells. Diabetes 2007;56(3):703-708.

[226] Atouf F, Park CH, Pechhold K, Ta M, Choi Y, Lumelsky NL. No evidence for mouse pancreatic beta-cell epithelial-mesenchymal transition in vitro. Diabetes 2007;56(3):699-702.

[227] Nir T, Melton DA, Dor Y. Recovery from diabetes in mice by beta cell regeneration. J Clin Invest 2007;117(9):2553-2561.

[228] Teta M, Rankin MM, Long SY, Stein GM, Kushner JA. Growth and regeneration of adult beta cells does not involve specialized progenitors. Dev Cell 2007;12(5):817-826.

[229] Xu X, D'Hoker J, Stange G, Bonne S, De Leu N, Xiao X, et al. Beta cells can be generated from endogenous progenitors in injured adult mouse pancreas. Cell 2008;132(2):197-207.

[230] Estrada E, Valacchi F., Nicora E, Brieva, S., Esteve, C., Echevarria, L., Froud, T., Bernetti, K., Messinger Cayetano, S., Velazquez, O., Alejandro, R., Ricordi, C. Combined treatment of intrapancreatic autologous bone marrow stem cells and hyperbaric oxygen in type 2 diabetes mellitus. Cell Transplant 2008;17(12):1295-1304.

[231] Soulillou JP, Giral M. Controlling the incidence of infection and malignancy by modifying immunosuppression. Transplantation 2001;72(12 Suppl):S89-93.

[232] Zahr E, Molano RD, Pileggi A, Ichii H, Jose SS, Bocca N, et al. Rapamycin impairs *in vivo* proliferation of islet beta-cells. Transplantation 2007;84(12):1576-1583.

[233] Zahr E, Molano RD, Pileggi A, Ichii H, San Jose S, Bocca N, et al. Rapamycin impairs beta-cell proliferation *in vivo*. Transplant Proc 2008;40(2):436-437.

[234] Seung E, Mordes JP, Greiner DL, Rossini AA. Induction of tolerance for islet transplantation for type 1 diabetes. Curr Diab Rep 2003;3(4):329-335.

[235] Pileggi A, Molano RD, Ricordi C, Zahr E, Collins J, Valdes R, et al. Reversal of diabetes by pancreatic islet transplantation into a subcutaneous, neovascularized device. Transplantation 2006;81(9):1318-1324.

[236] Balasa B, Krahl T, Patstone G, Lee J, Tisch R, McDevitt HO, et al. CD40 ligand-CD40 interactions are necessary for the initiation of insulitis and diabetes in nonobese diabetic mice. J Immunol 1997;159(9):4620-4627.

[237] Lenschow DJ, Ho SC, Sattar H, Rhee L, Gray G, Nabavi N, et al. Differential effects of anti-B7-1 and anti-B7-2 monoclonal antibody treatment on the development of diabetes in the nonobese diabetic mouse. J Exp Med 1995;181(3):1145-1155.

[238] Fontenot JD, Gavin MA, Rudensky AY. Foxp3 programs the development and function of CD4+CD25+ regulatory T cells. Nat Immunol 2003;4(4):330-336.

[239] Salomon B, Lenschow DJ, Rhee L, Ashourian N, Singh B, Sharpe A, et al. B7/CD28 costimulation is essential for the homeostasis of the CD4+CD25+ immunoregulatory T cells that control autoimmune diabetes. Immunity 2000;12(4):431-440.

[240] Truong W, Hancock WW, Anderson CC, Merani S, Shapiro AM. Coinhibitory T-cell signaling in islet allograft rejection and tolerance. Cell Transplant 2006;15(2):105-119.

[241] Inverardi L, Linetsky E, Pileggi A, Molano RD, Serafini A, Paganelli G, et al. Targeted bone marrow radioablation with 153Samarium-lexidronam promotes allogeneic hematopoietic chimerism and donor-specific immunologic hyporesponsiveness. Transplantation 2004;77(5):647-655.

[242] Li H, Inverardi L, Molano RD, Pileggi A, Ricordi C. Nonlethal conditioning for the induction of allogeneic chimerism and tolerance to islet allografts. Transplantation 2003;75(7):966-970.

[243] Mineo D, Ricordi C, Xu X, Pileggi A, Garcia-Morales R, Khan A, et al. Combined islet and hematopoietic stem cell allotransplantation: a clinical pilot trial to induce chimerism and graft tolerance. Am J Transplant 2008;8(6):1262-1274.

[244] Neto AB, DeFaria W, Berho M, Carreno M, Misiakos EP, Ruiz P, et al. Mixed allogeneic chimerism by combined use of nonlethal radiation and antilymphocyte serum in a rat small bowel transplantation model. Transplant Proc 2000;32(6):1311-1312.

[245] Han D, Ricordi C, Kenyon NS. Establishment of a method for analysis of chimerism in a baboon model (Papio hamadryas) of islet/bone marrow transplantation. Transplant Proc 1998;30(2):554-555.

[246] Bakonyi A, Berho M, Ruiz P, Misiakos EP, Carreno M, de Faria W, et al. Donor and recipient pretransplant conditioning with nonlethal radiation and antilymphocyte serum improves the graft survival in a rat small bowel transplant model. Transplantation 2001;72(6):983-988.

[247] Sharabi Y, Abraham VS, Sykes M, Sachs DH. Mixed allogeneic chimeras prepared by a non-myeloablative regimen: requirement for chimerism to maintain tolerance. Bone Marrow Transplant 1992;9(3):191-197.

[248] Sharabi Y, Sachs DH. Mixed chimerism and permanent specific transplantation tolerance induced by a nonlethal preparative regimen. J Exp Med 1989;169(2):493-502.

[249] Sykes M, Sharabi Y, Sachs DH. Achieving alloengraftment without graft-versus-host disease: approaches using mixed allogeneic bone marrow transplantation. Bone Marrow Transplant 1988;3(5):379-386.

[250] Burt RK, Cohen B, Rose J, Petersen F, Oyama Y, Stefoski D, et al. Hematopoietic stem cell transplantation for multiple sclerosis. Arch Neurol 2005;62(6):860-864.

[251] Burt RK, Marmont A, Oyama Y, Slavin S, Arnold R, Hiepe F, et al. Randomized controlled trials of autologous hematopoietic stem cell transplantation for autoimmune diseases: the evolution from myeloablative to lymphoablative transplant regimens. Arthritis Rheum 2006;54(12):3750-3760.

[252] Couri CE, Foss MC, Voltarelli JC. Secondary prevention of type 1 diabetes mellitus: stopping immune destruction and promoting beta-cell regeneration. Braz J Med Biol Res 2006;39(10):1271-1280.

[253] Couri CE, Voltarelli JC. Autologous stem cell transplantation for early type 1 diabetes mellitus. Autoimmunity 2008:1.

[254] Couri CE, Voltarelli JC. Potential role of stem cell therapy in type 1 diabetes mellitus. Arq Bras Endocrinol Metabol 2008;52(2):407-415.

[255] Rosa SB, Voltarelli JC, Chies JA, Pranke P. The use of stem cells for the treatment of autoimmune diseases. Braz J Med Biol Res 2007;40(12):1579-1597.

[256] Voltarelli JC, Couri CE, Stracieri AB, Oliveira MC, Moraes DA, Pieroni F, et al. Autologous nonmyeloablative hematopoietic stem cell transplantation in newly diagnosed type 1 diabetes mellitus. JAMA 2007;297(14):1568-1576.

[257] Orive G, Bartkowiak A, Lisiecki S, De Castro M, Hernandez RM, Gascon AR, et al. Biocompatible oligochitosans as cationic modifiers of alginate/Ca microcapsules. J Biomed Mater Res B Appl Biomater 2005;74(1):429-439.

[258] Orive G, Carcaboso AM, Hernandez RM, Gascon AR, Pedraz JL. Biocompatibility evaluation of different alginates and alginate-based microcapsules. Biomacromolecules 2005;6(2):927-931.

[259] Orive G, Gascon AR, Hernandez RM, Dominguez-Gil A, Pedraz JL. Techniques: new approaches to the delivery of biopharmaceuticals. Trends Pharmacol Sci 2004;25(7):382-387.

[260] Orive G, Hernandez RM, Gascon AR, Igartua M, Pedraz JL. Survival of different cell lines in alginate-agarose microcapsules. Eur J Pharm Sci 2003;18(1):23-30.

[261] Orive G, Hernandez RM, Gascon AR, Igartua M, Pedraz JL. Development and optimisation of alginate-PMCG-alginate microcapsules for cell immobilisation. Int J Pharm 2003;259(1-2):57-68.

[262] Orive G, Hernandez RM, Rodriguez Gascon A, Calafiore R, Chang TM, de Vos P, et al. History, challenges and perspectives of cell microencapsulation. Trends Biotechnol 2004;22(2):87-92.

[263] Orive G, Ponce S, Hernandez RM, Gascon AR, Igartua M, Pedraz JL. Biocompatibility of microcapsules for cell immobilization elaborated with different type of alginates. Biomaterials 2002;23(18):3825-3831.

[264] Avgoustiniatos ES, Colton CK. Effect of external oxygen mass transfer resistances on viability of immunoisolated tissue. Ann N Y Acad Sci 1997;831:145-167.

[265] Dionne KE, Colton CK, Yarmush ML. Effect of hypoxia on insulin secretion by isolated rat and canine islets of Langerhans. Diabetes 1993;42(1):12-21.

[266] Dionne KE, Colton CK, Yarmush ML. Effect of oxygen on isolated pancreatic tissue. ASAIO Trans 1989;35(3):739-741.

[267] Papas KK, Avgoustiniatos ES, Tempelman LA, Weir GC, Colton CK, Pisania A, et al. High-density culture of human islets on top of silicone rubber membranes. Transplant Proc 2005;37(8):3412-3414.

[268] Giuliani M, Moritz W, Bodmer E, Dindo D, Kugelmeier P, Lehmann R, et al. Central necrosis in isolated hypoxic human pancreatic islets: evidence for postisolation ischemia. Cell Transplant 2005;14(1):67-76.

[269] Moritz W, Meier F, Stroka DM, Giuliani M, Kugelmeier P, Nett PC, et al. Apoptosis in hypoxic human pancreatic islets correlates with HIF-1alpha expression. FASEB J 2002;16(7):745-747.

[270] Clayton HA, London NJ. Survival and function of islets during culture. Cell Transplant 1996;5(1):1-12; discussion 13-7, 19.

[271] London NJ, Swift SM, Clayton HA. Isolation, culture and functional evaluation of islets of Langerhans. Diabetes Metab 1998;24(3):200-207.

[272] Krol S, del Guerra S, Grupillo M, Diaspro A, Gliozzi A, Marchetti P. Multilayer nanoencapsulation. New approach for immune protection of human pancreatic islets. Nano Lett 2006;6(9):1933-1939.

[273] Nolan K, Millet Y, Ricordi C, Stabler CL. Tissue engineering and biomaterials in regenerative medicine. Cell Transplant 2008;17(3):241-243.

[274] Lin G, OuYang Q, Zhou X, Gu Y, Yuan D, Li W, et al. A highly homozygous and parthenogenetic human embryonic stem cell line derived from a one-pronuclear oocyte following in vitro fertilization procedure. Cell Res 2007;17(12):999-1007.

[275] Revazova ES, Turovets NA, Kochetkova OD, Agapova LS, Sebastian JL, Pryzhkova MV, et al. HLA homozygous stem cell lines derived from human parthenogenetic blastocysts. Cloning Stem Cells 2008;10(1):11-24.

[276] Park IH, Zhao R, West JA, Yabuuchi A, Huo H, Ince TA, et al. Reprogramming of human somatic cells to pluripotency with defined factors. Nature 2008;451(7175):141-146.

[277] Tateishi K, He J, Taranova O, Liang G, D'Alessio AC, Zhang Y. Generation of insulin-secreting islet-like clusters from human skin fibroblasts. J Biol Chem 2008 Nov 14;283(46):31601-31607.

[278] Okita K, Nakagawa M, Hyenjong H, Ichisaka T, Yamanaka S. Generation of Mouse Induced Pluripotent Stem Cells Without Viral Vectors. Science 2008 Nov 7;322(5903):949-953.

[279] Bosnali M, Edenhofer F. Generation of transducible versions of transcription factors Oct4 and Sox2. Biol Chem 2008;389(7):851-861.

[280] Ohlsson H, Karlsson K, Edlund T. IPF1, a homeodomain-containing transactivator of the insulin gene. EMBO J 1993;12(11):4251-4259.

[281] Jonsson J, Ahlgren U, Edlund T, Edlund H. IPF1, a homeodomain protein with a dual function in pancreas development. Int J Dev Biol 1995;39(5):789-798.

[282] Ahlgren U, Jonsson J, Jonsson L, Simu K, Edlund H. beta-cell-specific inactivation of the mouse Ipf1/Pdx1 gene results in loss of the beta-cell phenotype and maturity onset diabetes. Genes Dev 1998;12(12):1763-1768.

[283] Cockell M, Stevenson BJ, Strubin M, Hagenbuchle O, Wellauer PK. Identification of a cell-specific DNA-binding activity that interacts with a transcriptional activator of genes expressed in the acinar pancreas. Mol Cell Biol 1989;9(6):2464-2476.

[284] Krapp A, Knofler M, Ledermann B, Burki K, Berney C, Zoerkler N, et al. The bHLH protein PTF1-p48 is essential for the formation of the exocrine and the correct spatial organization of the endocrine pancreas. Genes Dev 1998;12(23):3752-3763.

[285] Afelik S, Chen Y, Pieler T. Combined ectopic expression of Pdx1 and Ptf1a/p48 results in the stable conversion of posterior endoderm into endocrine and exocrine pancreatic tissue. Genes Dev 2006;20(11):1441-1446.

[286] Lemaigre FP, Durviaux SM, Truong O, Lannoy VJ, Hsuan JJ, Rousseau GG. Hepatocyte nuclear factor 6, a transcription factor that contains a novel type of homeodomain and a single cut domain. Proc Natl Acad Sci U S A 1996;93(18):9460-9464.

[287] Landry C, Clotman F, Hioki T, Oda H, Picard JJ, Lemaigre FP, et al. HNF-6 is expressed in endoderm derivatives and nervous system of the mouse embryo and participates to the cross-regulatory network of liver-enriched transcription factors. Dev Biol 1997;192(2):247-257.

[288] Jacquemin P, Durviaux SM, Jensen J, Godfraind C, Gradwohl G, Guillemot F, et al. Transcription factor hepatocyte nuclear factor 6 regulates pancreatic endocrine cell differentiation and controls expression of the proendocrine gene ngn3. Mol Cell Biol 2000;20(12):4445-4454.

[289] Jacquemin P, Lemaigre FP, Rousseau GG. The Onecut transcription factor HNF-6 (OC-1) is required for timely specification of the pancreas and acts upstream of Pdx-1 in the specification cascade. Dev Biol 2003;258(1):105-116.

[290] Barbacci E, Chalkiadaki A, Masdeu C, Haumaitre C, Lokmane L, Loirat C, et al. HNF1beta/TCF2 mutations impair transactivation potential through altered co-regulator recruitment. Hum Mol Genet 2004;13(24):3139-3149.

[291] Barbacci E, Reber M, Ott MO, Breillat C, Huetz F, Cereghini S. Variant hepatocyte nuclear factor 1 is required for visceral endoderm specification. Development 1999;126(21):4795-4805.

[292] Haumaitre C, Barbacci E, Jenny M, Ott MO, Gradwohl G, Cereghini S. Lack of TCF2/vHNF1 in mice leads to pancreas agenesis. Proc Natl Acad Sci U S A 2005;102(5):1490-1495.

[293] Maestro MA, Boj SF, Luco RF, Pierreux CE, Cabedo J, Servitja JM, et al. Hnf6 and Tcf2 (MODY5) are linked in a gene network operating in a precursor cell domain of the embryonic pancreas. Hum Mol Genet 2003;12(24):3307-3314.

[294] Harrison KA, Druey KM, Deguchi Y, Tuscano JM, Kehrl JH. A novel human homeobox gene distantly related to proboscipedia is expressed in lymphoid and pancreatic tissues. J Biol Chem 1994;269(31):19968-19975.

[295] Li H, Arber S, Jessell TM, Edlund H. Selective agenesis of the dorsal pancreas in mice lacking homeobox gene Hlxb9. Nat Genet 1999;23(1):67-70.

[296] Li H, Edlund H. Persistent expression of Hlxb9 in the pancreatic epithelium impairs pancreatic development. Dev Biol 2001;240(1):247-253.

[297] Harrison KA, Thaler J, Pfaff SL, Gu H, Kehrl JH. Pancreas dorsal lobe agenesis and abnormal islets of Langerhans in Hlxb9-deficient mice. Nat Genet 1999;23(1):71-75.

[298] Grapin-Botton A, Majithia AR, Melton DA. Key events of pancreas formation are triggered in gut endoderm by ectopic expression of pancreatic regulatory genes. Genes Dev 2001;15(4):444-454.

[299] Dawid IB, Toyama R, Taira M. LIM domain proteins. C R Acad Sci III 1995;318(3):295-306.

[300] Karlsson O, Thor S, Norberg T, Ohlsson H, Edlund T. Insulin gene enhancer binding protein Isl-1 is a member of a novel class of proteins containing both a homeo- and a Cys-His domain. Nature 1990;344(6269):879-882.

[301] Ahlgren U, Pfaff SL, Jessell TM, Edlund T, Edlund H. Independent requirement for ISL1 in formation of pancreatic mesenchyme and islet cells. Nature 1997;385(6613):257-260.

[302] Naya FJ, Stellrecht CM, Tsai MJ. Tissue-specific regulation of the insulin gene by a novel basic helix-loop-helix transcription factor. Genes Dev 1995;9(8):1009-1019.

[303] Huang HP, Liu M, El-Hodiri HM, Chu K, Jamrich M, Tsai MJ. Regulation of the pancreatic islet-specific gene BETA2 (neuroD) by neurogenin 3. Mol Cell Biol 2000;20(9):3292-3307.

[304] Naya FJ, Huang HP, Qiu Y, Mutoh H, DeMayo FJ, Leiter AB, et al. Diabetes, defective pancreatic morphogenesis, and abnormal enteroendocrine differentiation in BETA2/neuroD-deficient mice. Genes Dev 1997;11(18):2323-2334.

[305] Hussain MA, Lee J, Miller CP, Habener JF. POU domain transcription factor brain 4 confers pancreatic alpha-cell-specific expression of the proglucagon gene through interaction with a novel proximal promoter G1 element. Mol Cell Biol 1997;17(12):7186-7194.

[306] Hussain MA, Miller CP, Habener JF. Brn-4 transcription factor expression targeted to the early developing mouse pancreas induces ectopic glucagon gene expression in insulin-producing beta cells. J Biol Chem 2002;277(18):16028-16032.

[307] Heller RS, Stoffers DA, Liu A, Schedl A, Crenshaw EB, 3rd, Madsen OD, et al. The role of Brn4/Pou3f4 and Pax6 in forming the pancreatic glucagon cell identity. Dev Biol 2004;268(1):123-1234.

[308] Sussel L, Kalamaras J, Hartigan-O'Connor DJ, Meneses JJ, Pedersen RA, Rubenstein JL, et al. Mice lacking the homeodomain transcription factor Nkx2.2 have diabetes due to arrested differentiation of pancreatic beta cells. Development 1998;125(12):2213-2221.

[309] Price M. Members of the Dlx- and Nkx2-gene families are regionally expressed in the developing forebrain. J Neurobiol 1993;24(10):1385-1399.

[310] Sander M, Sussel L, Conners J, Scheel D, Kalamaras J, Dela Cruz F, et al. Homeobox gene Nkx6.1 lies downstream of Nkx2.2 in the major pathway of beta-cell formation in the pancreas. Development 2000;127(24):5533-5540.

[311] Rudnick A, Ling TY, Odagiri H, Rutter WJ, German MS. Pancreatic beta cells express a diverse set of homeobox genes. Proc Natl Acad Sci U S A 1994;91(25):12203-12207.

[312] Cvekl A, Kashanchi F, Sax CM, Brady JN, Piatigorsky J. Transcriptional regulation of the mouse alpha A-crystallin gene: activation dependent on a cyclic AMP-responsive element (DE1/CRE) and a Pax-6-binding site. Mol Cell Biol 1995;15(2):653-660.

[313] Cvekl A, Sax CM, Li X, McDermott JB, Piatigorsky J. Pax-6 and lens-specific transcription of the chicken delta 1-crystallin gene. Proc Natl Acad Sci U S A 1995;92(10):4681-4685.

[314] Richardson J, Cvekl A, Wistow G. Pax-6 is essential for lens-specific expression of zeta-crystallin. Proc Natl Acad Sci U S A 1995;92(10):4676-4680.

[315] Hill RE, Favor J, Hogan BL, Ton CC, Saunders GF, Hanson IM, et al. Mouse small eye results from mutations in a paired-like homeobox-containing gene. Nature 1991;354(6354):522-525.

[316] Turque N, Plaza S, Radvanyi F, Carriere C, Saule S. Pax-QNR/Pax-6, a paired box- and homeobox-containing gene expressed in neurons, is also expressed in pancreatic endocrine cells. Mol Endocrinol 1994;8(7):929-938.

[317] St-Onge L, Sosa-Pineda B, Chowdhury K, Mansouri A, Gruss P. Pax6 is required for differentiation of glucagon-producing alpha-cells in mouse pancreas. Nature 1997;387(6631):406-409.

[318] Sander M, Neubuser A, Kalamaras J, Ee HC, Martin GR, German MS. Genetic analysis reveals that PAX6 is required for normal transcription of pancreatic hormone genes and islet development. Genes Dev 1997;11(13):1662-1673.

[319] Dohrmann C, Gruss P, Lemaire L. Pax genes and the differentiation of hormone-producing endocrine cells in the pancreas. Mech Dev 2000;92(1):47-54.

[320] Walther C, Guenet JL, Simon D, Deutsch U, Jostes B, Goulding MD, et al. Pax: a murine multigene family of paired box-containing genes. Genomics 1991;11(2):424-434.

[321] Heremans Y, Van De Casteele M, in't Veld P, Gradwohl G, Serup P, Madsen O, et al. Recapitulation of embryonic neuroendocrine differentiation in adult human pancreatic duct cells expressing neurogenin 3. J Cell Biol 2002;159(2):303-312.

[322] Sosa-Pineda B. The gene Pax4 is an essential regulator of pancreatic beta-cell development. Mol Cells 2004;18(3):289-294.

[323] Smith SB, Gasa R, Watada H, Wang J, Griffen SC, German MS. Neurogenin3 and hepatic nuclear factor 1 cooperate in activating pancreatic expression of Pax4. J Biol Chem 2003;278(40):38254-38259.

[324] Wang J, Elghazi L, Parker SE, Kizilocak H, Asano M, Sussel L, et al. The concerted activities of Pax4 and Nkx2.2 are essential to initiate pancreatic beta-cell differentiation. Dev Biol 2004;266(1):178-189.

[325] Collombat P, Hecksher-Sorensen J, Broccoli V, Krull J, Ponte I, Mundiger T, et al. The simultaneous loss of Arx and Pax4 genes promotes a somatostatin-producing cell fate specification at the expense of the alpha- and beta-cell lineages in the mouse endocrine pancreas. Development 2005;132(13):2969-2980.

[326] Collombat P, Mansouri A, Hecksher-Sorensen J, Serup P, Krull J, Gradwohl G, et al. Opposing actions of Arx and Pax4 in endocrine pancreas development. Genes Dev 2003;17(20):2591-2603.

[327] Heller RS, Jenny M, Collombat P, Mansouri A, Tomasetto C, Madsen OD, et al. Genetic determinants of pancreatic epsilon-cell development. Dev Biol 2005;286(1):217-224.

[328] Miura H, Yanazawa M, Kato K, Kitamura K. Expression of a novel aristaless related homeobox gene 'Arx' in the vertebrate telencephalon, diencephalon and floor plate. Mech Dev 1997;65(1-2):99-109.

[329] Zhang C, Moriguchi T, Kajihara M, Esaki R, Harada A, Shimohata H, et al. MafA is a key regulator of glucose-stimulated insulin secretion. Mol Cell Biol 2005;25(12):4969-4976.

[330] Nishimura W, Kondo T, Salameh T, El Khattabi I, Dodge R, Bonner-Weir S, et al. A switch from MafB to MafA expression accompanies differentiation to pancreatic beta-cells. Dev Biol 2006;293(2):526-539.

[331] Kawauchi S, Takahashi S, Nakajima O, Ogino H, Morita M, Nishizawa M, et al. Regulation of lens fiber cell differentiation by transcription factor c-Maf. J Biol Chem 1999;274(27):19254-19260.

[332] Ochi H, Sakagami K, Ishii A, Morita N, Nishiuchi M, Ogino H, et al. Temporal expression of L-Maf and RaxL in developing chicken retina are arranged into mosaic pattern. Gene Expr Patterns 2004;4(5):489-494.

[333] Ogino H, Yasuda K. Induction of lens differentiation by activation of a bZIP transcription factor, L-Maf. Science 1998;280(5360):115-118.

[334] Reza HM, Ogino H, Yasuda K. L-Maf, a downstream target of Pax6, is essential for chick lens development. Mech Dev 2002;116(1-2):61-73.

[335] Ang SL, Rossant J. HNF-3 beta is essential for node and notochord formation in mouse development. Cell 1994;78(4):561-574.

[336] Weinstein DC, Ruiz i Altaba A, Chen WS, Hoodless P, Prezioso VR, Jessell TM, et al. The winged-helix transcription factor HNF-3 beta is required for notochord development in the mouse embryo. Cell 1994;78(4):575-588.

[337] Lee CS, Sund NJ, Behr R, Herrera PL, Kaestner KH. Foxa2 is required for the differentiation of pancreatic alpha-cells. Dev Biol 2005;278(2):484-495.

[338] Ben-Shushan E, Marshak S, Shoshkes M, Cerasi E, Melloul D. A pancreatic beta -cell-specific enhancer in the human PDX-1 gene is regulated by hepatocyte nuclear factor 3beta (HNF-3beta), HNF-1alpha, and SPs transcription factors. J Biol Chem 2001;276(20):17533-17540.

[339] Sund NJ, Vatamaniuk MZ, Casey M, Ang SL, Magnuson MA, Stoffers DA, et al. Tissue-specific deletion of Foxa2 in pancreatic beta cells results in hyperinsulinemic hypoglycemia. Genes Dev 2001;15(13):1706-1715.

[340] Oliver G, Sosa-Pineda B, Geisendorf S, Spana EP, Doe CQ, Gruss P. Prox 1, a prospero-related homeobox gene expressed during mouse development. Mech Dev 1993;44(1):3-16.

[341] Wang J, Kilic G, Aydin M, Burke Z, Oliver G, Sosa-Pineda B. Prox1 activity controls pancreas morphogenesis and participates in the production of "secondary transition" pancreatic endocrine cells. Dev Biol 2005;286(1):182-194.

[342] Burke Z, Oliver G. Prox1 is an early specific marker for the developing liver and pancreas in the mammalian foregut endoderm. Mech Dev 2002;118(1-2):147-155.

[343] Wilson ME, Yang KY, Kalousova A, Lau J, Kosaka Y, Lynn FC, *et al.* The HMG Box Transcription Factor Sox4 Contributes to the Development of the Endocrine Pancreas. Diabetes 2005;54(12):3402-3409.

[344] Ya J, Schilham MW, de Boer PA, Moorman AF, Clevers H, Lamers WH. Sox4-deficiency syndrome in mice is an animal model for common trunk. Circ Res 1998;83(10):986-994.

CHAPTER 10

Stem Cells in Dentistry

Li Wu Zheng and Lim Kwong Cheung*

Discipline of Oral & Maxillofacial Surgery, Faculty of Dentistry, The University of Hong Kong, China

Abstract: Stem cells have been isolated and characterized from embryonic, fetal, and adult tissues. The therapeutic and clinical application of embryonic stem cells and fetal stem cells is challenging to the many ethical and political controversies concerning their use. Adult stem cells have been isolated and characterized from a wide variety of tissues including bone marrow, brain, skin, hair follicles, skeletal muscle, adipose tissue, cord blood, dental tissue, and their differentiation potential may reflect their local environment. To date, several sources of dental stem cells have been isolated and being characterized as dental epithelial stem cells, dental pulp stem cells, dental follicle precursor cells, stem cells from human exfoliated deciduous teeth, stem cells from apical papilla, and periodontal ligament stem cellsDental stem cells have been shown to have multi-potential by their ability to differentiate into neuronal, adipogenic, myogenic, chondrogenic, osteogenic and dentinogenic cells when cultured under specific conditions. These facilitated studies to address an important property of stem cells, that is, the capacity of a given stem cell population to regenerate an organized, functional tissue following transplantation *in vivo*. Furthermore, the ready availability of tooth tissues from redundant teeth such as third molars can provide a good supply of dental stem cells that may be utilized for regenerating other body parts or organs.

INTRODUCTION

The human body has an endogenous system of regeneration and repair through stem cells, where stem cells can be found almost in every type of tissue [1]. Two properties, self-renewable and capable of multi-lineage differentiation, must both be satisfied for a cell to be defined as a stem cell. Self-renewal denotes that undifferentiated daughter cells are a precise replica and can further replicate many generations without losing their original characteristics. Multi-lineage differentiation refers to the capacity of a single population of stem cells to differentiate into at least two distinctively different cell types [2, 3].

Stem cells have been isolated and characterized from embryonic, fetal, and adult tissues. Embryonic stem cells are pluripotent (able to give rise to cell types and tissues of all three germ layers of the body), and are capable of unlimited proliferation in an undifferentiated state [4]. Fetal stem cells isolated from a wide range of developing organs have great proliferative potential and a wide range of differentiation, and are an intermediate between embryonic stem cells (totally uncommitted cells that need entire reprogramming to become differentiated tissue) and adult progenitor or stem cells (highly committed cells that might require some reprogramming) [5, 6]. The therapeutic and clinical application of embryonic stem cells and fetal stem cells is challenging due to the many ethical and political controversies concerning their use. Consequently, progenitor cells harbored by the adult organism have been examined. These postnatal stem cells, known as adult stem cells, have been isolated and characterized from a wide variety of tissues including bone marrow, brain, skin, hair follicles, skeletal muscle, adipose tissue, cord blood, dental tissue, and their differentiation potential may reflect their local environment [7-21]. Historically, adult stem cells were thought to be developmentally restricted to specific cell lineages that are related to the tissue in which the cells reside. The extraordinary plasticity of postnatal stem cells was explored, neural stem cells was found able to differentiate to blood and skeletal muscle [22, 23], whereas bone marrow stem cells (BMSCs) was found to differentiate to muscle, liver, and neuronal tissue [10, 19, 24, 25]. Recent emerging evidence implies that cell-fusion events may account for some of these observations [26, 27].

To date, several sources of dental stem cells have been isolated (Fig. **1**) and being characterized as follows: dental

---

***Address Correspondence to this Author Prof. Lim Kwong Cheung:** Oral & Maxillofacial Surgery, The Prince Philip Dental Hospital, 34 Hospital Road, Hong Kong SAR, China; Tel: (852)2859-0267, Fax: (852) 2559-9014, E-mail: lkcheung@hkucc.hku.hk

epithelial stem cells [28], dental pulp stem cells (DPSCs) [29], dental follicle precursor cells (DFPCs) [30, 31], stem cells from human exfoliated deciduous teeth (SHED) [32], stem cells from apical papilla (SCAP) [33, 34], and periodontal ligament stem cells (PDLSCs) [35]

STEM CELLS DERIVED FROM DENTAL TISSUE

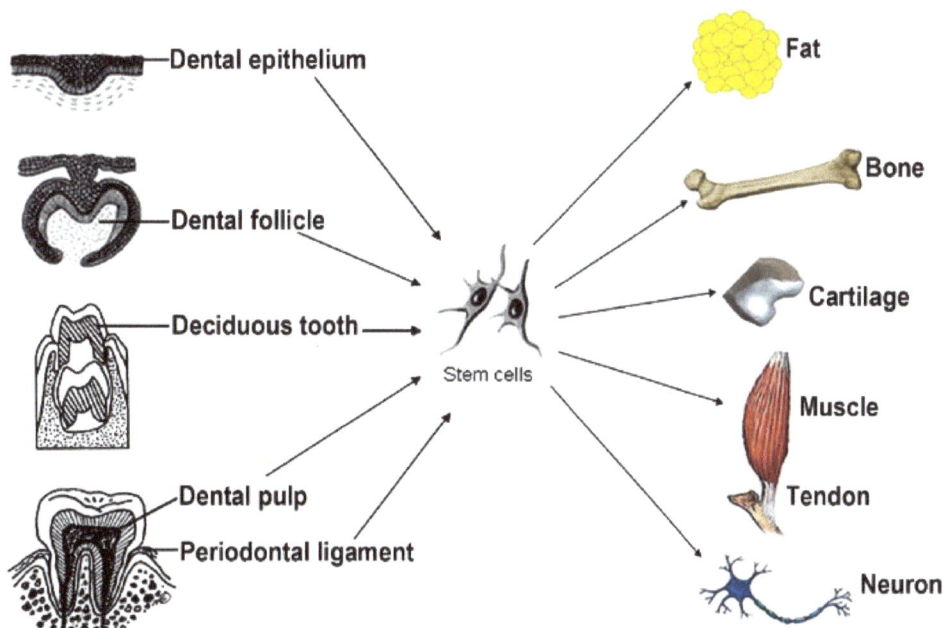

Figure 1: Sources of dental stem cells and potential tissue regeneration

DENTAL EPITHELIAL STEM CELLS

Tooth development is based on interactions between the ectodermal and the ectomesenchymal (neural crest) germ layers. The development of a tooth begins at the mandibular arch of embryo. The oral ectoderm is in close vicinity with the underlying ectomesenchymal tissue and builds the surface of the mandibular arch. It is accepted that dental development is initiated in the oral ectoderm. Previous study demonstrated that embryonic dental epithelial tissues were capable of inducing the development of a tooth germ in combination with non-dental ectomesenchymal tissues [36].

Although it is evident that epithelial stem cells or progenitor cells are involved in dental development, the identification of these cells was not easy. BrdU-labelled stem cells enabled a detailed examination of cell migration and ameloblast development in human dental explants, and these dental epithelial stem cells are lost after tooth eruption, therefore, they are not available for studies on dental development. In some mammalian species, continuously growing incisors and molars show replenishing populations of enamel organs composed of a core of stellate reticulum, stratum intermedium and surrounding enamel epithelial cells [37]. Irma Thesleff's group identified these dental ectodermal stem cells in tissue explants of adult mouse incisors for the first time [28]. Today the murine incisors become an ideal model to study epithelial stem cells, tooth development and dental diseases.

DENTAL PULP STEM CELLS (DPSCs)

Although the regenerative capacity of the human dentin/pulp complex is not well-understood, it is known that, upon injury, reparative dentin is formed as a protective barrier for the pulp [38]. Accordingly, it has been anticipated that dental pulp could contain the dentinogenic progenitors that are responsible for dentin repair. Previous work showed that dental pulp contained proliferating cells that were analogous to bone cells, because they expressed osteogenic markers and responded to many growth factors for osteo/odontogenic differentiation [39-41]. In addition, dental pulp cells were capable of forming mineral deposits with distinctive dentin-like crystalline structures [29, 42, 43].

It has become possible to isolate precursor cells from the dental pulp since 1990' [44]. Later, DPSCs were isolated from the dental pulp of extracted wisdom teeth [29, 45]. These ectomesenchymal stem cells display similar features as BMSCs. For example, both cell types adhere to plastic and are colony-forming cells. In contrast to BMSCs, DPSCs were found to differentiate into odontoblast-like cells. A DNA microarray study distinguishes DPSCs from BMSCs that DPSCs differentially express cell-cycle-associated genes [45]. This result is in accordance to findings of a high proliferation rate in DFPCs when compared to mesenchymal stem cells [29].

Stem cells derived from the dental pulp are often mentioned in regenerative endodontics [46, 47]. When DPSCs were transplanted into immunocompromised mice, they generated a dentin-like structure lined with human odontoblast-like cells that surround a pulp-like interstitial tissue. Under chemically defined culture conditions, DPSCs can also be induced to undergo uniform differentiation into myogenic, neurogenic, adipogenic, chondrogenic and osteogenic cells [29, 39-41, 48-52].

Dental Follicle Precursor Cells (DFPCs)

The dental follicle is separated from developing dentin by epithelial cell layers (Hertwig's epithelial root sheath) during early steps of periodontal development [53, 54]. For this reason, this tissue should contain progenitor cells, capable of forming osteoblasts of the alveolar bone, periodontal ligament fibroblasts or cementoblasts. Bovine DFPCs formed spheroid-like cell clusters under *in vitro* conditions [31]. The human dental follicle can be easily isolated after wisdom tooth extraction.

Human DFPCs have multipotential mesenchymal precursor cell properties. This is confirmed by the expression of mesenchymal stem cell marker Stro-1 [30]. DFPCs are plastic adherent and colony forming cells, and they can differentiate into osteoblast like cells under *in vitro* conditions. Similar to PDLSCs, DFPCs can also differentiate, form robust connective tissues and produce clusters of mineralized tissues [31, 55, 56].

STEM CELLS FROM HUMAN EXFOLIATED DECIDUOUS TEETH (SHED)

The transition from deciduous teeth to adult permanent teeth is a very unique and dynamic process in which the development and eruption of permanent teeth coordinate with the root resorption of deciduous teeth [57]. The remnant dental pulp derived from exfoliated deciduous teeth contains a stem-cell population capable of extensive proliferation and multipotential differentiation.

Deciduous teeth are significantly different from permanent teeth with regards to their developmental processes, tissue structure and function. Therefore, it is not a surprise to find that SHED are distinct from DPSCs with respect to their higher proliferation rate, increased cell-population doublings, sphere-like cell-cluster formation, osteoinductive capacity *in vivo*, and failure to reconstitute a dentin–pulp-like complex [32, 49]. *Ex vivo*-expanded SHED expressed STRO-1 and CD146 (MUC18), two early cell-surface markers for BMSCs [58]. SHED apparently represent a population of multipotent stem cells that are perhaps more immature than postnatal stromal stem-cell populations. SHED demonstrated a strong capacity to induce recipient cell-mediated bone formation *in vivo*. These stem cells can not differentiate directly into osteoblasts but capable of inducing new bone formation by forming an osteoinductive template to recruit murine host osteogenic cells. These data imply that deciduous teeth may not only provide guidance for the eruption of permanent teeth, as generally assumed, but may also be involved in inducing bone formation during the eruption of permanent teeth. It is notable that SHED expressed neuronal and glial cell markers, which may be related to the neural crest-cell origin of the dental pulp [59].

SHED can be isolated and expanded *ex vivo*, thereby providing a unique and accessible population of stem cells from an unexpected tissue resource. Similar in some ways to umbilical cord containing stem cells that may offer a unique stem-cell resource for potential clinical applications, deciduous teeth may be an potentially non-invasive source of stem cells to repair damaged tooth structures, induce bone regeneration, and possibly to treat neural tissue injury or degenerative diseases.

Stem Cells from the Apical Papilla (SCAP)

Dental stem cells have also been isolated from the dental papilla of developing wisdom teeth or incisors [33, 60]. The dental papilla is an embryonic-like tissue that becomes also the dental pulp during maturation and formation of the roots. Moreover, SCAPs can only be isolated at a certain stage of tooth development. SCAPs are likely to be less differentiated than DPSCs, as they originate from an embryonic-like tissue. Therefore, SCAPs have a greater capacity for dentin regeneration than DPSCs because the dental papilla contains a higher number of adult stem cells compared to the mature dental pulp. A combination of SCAPs and PDLSCs induced the formation of a dental connective tissue providing stability for the teeth [33].

PERIODONTAL LIGAMENT STEM CELLS (PDLSCs)

The periodontal ligament connects the cementum to alveolar bone, and functions primarily to support the tooth in the alveolar socket. Studies showed that only the periodontal ligament, but not gingival connective tissue or bone, contains cells capable of establishing new attachment fibers between cementum and bone [61, 62]. The ability of periodontal ligament cell populations to achieve regeneration has implied that progenitor cells, and possibly stem cells, exist within the periodontal ligament.

Today, PDLSCs are successfully isolated from periodontal ligament and show the potential for forming periodontal structures [35, 63]. The implantation of human PDLSCs into nude mice generated the cementum/periodontal ligament like structures that resemble the native periodontal ligament as a thin layer of cementum that interfaced with dense collagen fibers, similar to Sharpey's fibers [35]. Under chemically defined culture conditions, PDLSCs can also differentiated toward Oil-red-O-positive, lipid-laden adipogenic and osteo/odontogenic direction, similar to BMSCs and DPSCs [35, 63]. Thus, PDLSCs have the potential for forming periodontal structures, including the cementum and periodontal ligament. The clinical potential for the use of PDLSCs has been further enhanced by the demonstration that these cells can be isolated from cryopreserved periodontal ligaments, thus providing a ready source of mesenchymal stem cells [64].

Clinical Potentials of Dental Stem Cell-Based Tissue Engineering

Mesenchymal stem cells provide an ideal cell source for cell-based tissue engineering for the following reasons: 1) they possess extensive self-renewal or expansion capability, 2) they have the capacity to differentiate readily into various cell types, 3), their use is not complicated by ethical and legal controversies, 4) they are easily accessible and readily available, and 5) they possess little to no immunogenic or tumorigenic ability [65]. All of these characteristics are also well suited to the dental mesenchymal stem cells for cell-based tissue engineering.

Under the same culture conditions, DPSCs and SHED showed a higher proliferation rate than BMSCs [32, 45]. In addition, the life-span of post-natal mesenchymal stem cell populations is finite due to a decline in their developmental potential as the cells begin to exhaust their growth potential *in vitro*. In contrast, the embryonic stem cells which are virtually immortal show the high expression of telomerase, the enzyme complex responsible for maintaining telomere lengths and chromosomal stability during cellular division [66]. Telomerase appears to be a critical factor for prolonging cellular senescence by up-regulating cell cycle regulators such as cyclin D3, cyclin E1, E2F-4, DP2, and inhibiting hypophosphorylated pRb to allow progression from G1 to S phase leading to an increased proliferation potential and survival rate. Telomerase activity is absent in cultured mesenchymal stem cell populations. Enforced expression of telomerase by cultured BMSCs resulted in not only an extension of the cell lifespan but also an enhanced the capacity to regenerate new bone formation [63, 67, 68]. Research efforts are continuing to unravel the mechanisms of how telomerase activity regulates the growth of mesenchymal stem cells. It is anticipated that these studies will help to develop strategies in genetically manipulating *ex vivo* expanded cells, in order to enhance and regulate the growth potential of expanded mesenchymal stem cells for clinical applications.

Recently, a practical approach to the preservation of solid-frozen human tissues for subsequent post-natal stem cell isolation further enhanced the clinical potential for the use of PDLSCs. The PDLSCs recovered from cryopreserved human periodontal ligament maintained normal PDLSC characteristics, including expression of the mesenchymal stem cell surface molecule STRO-1, single-colony-strain generation, multipotential differentiation, cementum/periodontal-ligament-like tissue regeneration, and a normal diploid karyotype, thus providing a ready source of mesenchymal stem cells [64].

Dental stem cells have been shown to have multi-potential by their ability to differentiate into neuronal, adipogenic, myogenic, chondrogenic, osteogenic and dentinogenic cells when cultured under specific conditions [29, 32, 35, 39, 40, 48-51, 59, 63, 69-71]. These studies facilitated experiments to address an important property of stem cells, that is, the capacity of a given stem cell population to regenerate an organized, functional tissue following transplantation *in vivo*. Furthermore, the ready availability of tooth tissues from redundant teeth such as third molars can provide a good supply of dental stem cells that may be utilized for regenerating other body parts or organs.

TOOTH TISSUE REGENERATION

Since the isolation and characterization of SCAP, DPSC, PDLSC and SHED, using these stem cells for dentin/pulp tissue regeneration has drawn great interest. The implantation of SHED, SCAP, DPSC, and PDLSC with the HA/TCP carrier particles generated the dentin-like structure [29, 32, 72]. Reparative dentin-like structure is deposited on the dentin surface if DPSCs are seeded onto a human dentin surface and implanted into immunocompromised mice, suggesting the possibility of forming additional new dentin on existing dentin [29]. By seeding SHED onto synthetic scaffolds seated in pulp chamber of a thin tooth slice, odontoblast-like cells can be from the stem cells and localize against existing dentin surface after implanting the tooth slice construct into immunocompromised mice [73]. These findings provide new light on the possibility of generating pulp and dentin in pulpless canals. The utilization of stem cells and an optimal scaffold system may one day be used clinically in which engineered constructs may be inserted into canals of immature teeth to allow regeneration of pulp and dentin.

Periodontal diseases are highly prevalent worldwide and the main signs are bone tissue destruction and subsequent tooth loss. Due to the complex structures of the periodontium (consisting of hard and soft tissues: cementum, bone, periodontal ligament, and gingiva), its complete regeneration would require a multipotent cell population [74, 75]. Transplantations of *ex vivo* expanded autologous mesenchymal cells have shown to significantly enhance the regeneration of new cementum, alveolar bone, and periodontal ligament in periodontal defects in animal models and clinical cases [76-78]. Recently, the stem cells from periodontal ligament, dental pulp in combination with biocompatible materials/scaffolds were used to regenerate root and periodontal ligament–like complex [72]. Attachment of human-derived periodontal ligament-like tissue to the surfaces of alveolar bone and teeth was achieved by implanting cultured human PDLSCs into surgical defects at the periodontal region of mandibular molars in immunocompromised nude rats [35]. Periodontal complex was reconstructed by the sheet culture of PDLSCs [79, 80]. These data imply a potential functional role of these dental stem cells for periodontal tissue regeneration.

To create the laboratory teeth that can be harvested and implanted into patients has been a goal in dental research [81, 82]. Studies demonstrated that the combination of dissociated dental epithelial and mesenchymal tissues led to tooth formation both *in vitro* and *in vivo* [83-85]. Recently, tooth-like structures were experimentally regenerated by mimicking the natural process of tooth regeneration from tooth-forming cells combined with or without addition of artificial scaffolds [84, 86-92]. By seeding the dissociated tooth bud cells onto polyglycolic acid fiber meshes and other biodegradable scaffolds, complex tooth-like structures were generated [88, 92-94]. Using cell pellet engineering approach, regular dentin–pulp complex and tooth-like structures was created by SCAP pellets, by DPSC pellets treated with conditioned medium, and by mixed dental epithelial/mesenchymal cell re-aggregations *in vivo* [90, 95, 96]. SCAP together with PDLSCs are able to form a root-like structure when seeded onto the hydroxyapatite-based scaffold and implanted in pig jaws. The bio-root is encircled with periodontal ligament tissue and appears to have a natural relationship with the surrounding bone. This biological approach can restore normal masticatory and aesthetic functions by creating a root supporting a crown similar to the dental implants [33].

The plausibility of a dental stem cell-based tissue engineering approach to achieve tissue regeneration is well supported by a number of studies. Among them, a recent study reveals that the periodontal ligament stem cells show similar genetic markers as neural crest and no immunological rejection following transplantation. These highlight the potential of applying dental stem cells not only for tooth replacement, but to treat spinal injuries and neurological diseases of congenital, traumatic or degenerative causes. The lack of immunological rejection of dental stem cells has more profound clinical potentials. Dental stem cells may be cultured and differentiated into other organs and transplanted to other human hosts (Fig. 1). In addition to the therapeutic potential, there are enormous economical potentials for dental stem cells. Establishment of tooth tissue banks is an important facility for people to save their SHED cells from deciduous tooth shedding or wisdom tooth extraction for future clinical use by themselves or to save life of others.

REFERENCES

[1]   Bajada S, Mazakova I, Richardson JB, Ashammakhi N. Updates on stem cells and their applications in regenerative medicine. J Tissue Eng Regen Med 2008; 2:169-183.
[2]   Caplan AI. Mesenchymal stem cells. J Orthop Res 1991; 9:641-50.
[3]   Alhadlaq A, Mao JJ. Mesenchymal stem cells: isolation and therapeutics. Stem Cells Dev 2004; 13:436-448.
[4]   Thomson JA, Itskovitz-Eldor J, Shapiro SS, et al. Embryonic stem cell lines derived from human blastocysts. Science 1998; 282:1145-1147.
[5]   Olivier V, Faucheux N, Hardouin P. Biomaterial challenges and approaches to stem cell use in bone reconstructive surgery. Drug Discov Today 2004; 9: 803-811.
[6]   Svendsen C. Stem cells: hype or hope? Drug Discov Today 2002; 7:455-456.
[7]   Hung SC, Chen NJ, Hsieh SL, Li H, Ma HL, Lo WH. Isolation and characterization of size-sieved stem cells from human bone marrow. Stem Cells 2002; 20:249-258.
[8]   Pittenger MF, Mackay AM, Beck SC, et al. Multilineage potential of adult human mesenchymal stem cells. Science 1999; 284: 143-147.
[9]   Fukushima N, Ohkawa H. Hematopoietic stem cells and microenvironment: the proliferation and differentiation of stromal cells. Crit Rev Oncol Hematol 1995; 20: 255-270.
[10] Petersen BE, Bowen WC, Patrene KD, et al. Bone marrow as a potential source of hepatic oval cells. Science 1999; 284: 1168-1170.
[11] Gussoni E, Soneoka Y, Strickland CD, et al. Dystrophin expression in the mdx mouse restored by stem cell transplantation. Nature 1999; 401: 390-394.
[12] Lansdorp PM. Developmental changes in the function of hematopoietic stem cells. Exp Hematol 1995: 187-191.
[13] Wright NA. Epithelial stem cell repertoire in the gut: clues to the origin of cell lineages, proliferative units and cancer. Int J Exp Pathol 2000; 81: 117-43.
[14] Bach SP, Renehan AG, Potten CS. Stem cells: the intestinal stem cell as a paradigm. Carcinogenesis 2000; 21: 469-476.
[15] Caterson EJ, Nesti LJ, Danielson KG, Tuan RS. Human marrow-derived mesenchymal progenitor cells: isolation, culture expansion, and analysis of differentiation. Mol Biotechnol 2002; 20: 245-256.
[16] Nakahara H, Goldberg VM, Caplan AI. Culture-expanded human periosteal-derived cells exhibit osteochondral potential *in vivo*. J Orthop Res 1991; 9: 465-476.
[17] Zuk PA, Zhu M, Mizuno H, Huang J, Futrell JW, Katz AJ, et al. Multilineage cells from human adipose tissue: implications for cell-based therapies. Tissue Eng 2001; 7: 211-228.
[18] Young HE, Steele TA, Bray RA, Hudson J, Floyd JA, Hawkins K, et al. Human reserve pluripotent mesenchymal stem cells are present in the connective tissues of skeletal muscle and dermis derived from fetal, adult, and geriatric donors. Anat Rec 2001; 264: 51-62.
[19] Ferrari G, Cusella-De Angelis G, Coletta M, Paolucci E, Stornaiuolo A, Cossu G, et al. Muscle regeneration by bone marrow-derived myogenic progenitors. Science 1998; 279: 1528-1530.
[20] Fukuda K. Molecular characterization of regenerated cardiomyocytes derived from adult mesenchymal stem cells. Congenit Anom (Kyoto) 2002; 42: 1-9.
[21] Gronthos S, Franklin DM, Leddy HA, Robey PG, Storms RW, Gimble JM. Surface protein characterization of human adipose tissue-derived stromal cells. J Cell Physiol 2001; 189: 54-63.
[22] Bjornson CR, Rietze RL, Reynolds BA, Magli MC, Vescovi AL. Turning brain into blood: a hematopoietic fate adopted by adult neural stem cells in vivo. Science 1999; 283: 534-537.
[23] Galli R, Borello U, Gritti A, et al. Skeletal myogenic potential of human and mouse neural stem cells. Nat Neurosci 2000; 3:986-991.

[24]   Mezey E, Chandross KJ, Harta G, Maki RA, McKercher SR. Turning blood into brain: cells bearing neuronal antigens generated in vivo from bone marrow. Science 2000; 290: 1779-82.

[25]   Brazelton TR, Rossi FM, Keshet GI, Blau HM. From marrow to brain: expression of neuronal phenotypes in adult mice. Science 2000; 290: 1775-1779.

[26]   Ying QL, Nichols J, Evans EP, Smith AG. Changing potency by spontaneous fusion. Nature 2002; 416: 545-548.

[27]   Terada N, Hamazaki T, Oka M, et al. Bone marrow cells adopt the phenotype of other cells by spontaneous cell fusion. Nature 2002; 416: 542-545.

[28]   Harada H, Kettunen P, Jung HS, Mustonen T, Wang YA, Thesleff I. Localization of putative stem cells in dental epithelium and their association with Notch and FGF signaling. J Cell Biol 1999; 147: 105-120.

[29]   Gronthos S, Mankani M, Brahim J, Robey PG, Shi S. Postnatal human dental pulp stem cells (DPSCs) *in vitro* and *in vivo*. Proc Natl Acad Sci USA 2000; 97: 13625-13630.

[30]   Kemoun P, Laurencin-Dalicieux S, Rue J, et al. Human dental follicle cells acquire cementoblast features under stimulation by BMP-2/-7 and enamel matrix derivatives (EMD) *in vitro*. Cell Tissue Res 2007; 329: 283-294.

[31]   Morsczeck C, Moehl C, Gotz W, et al. *In vitro* differentiation of human dental follicle cells with dexamethasone and insulin. Cell Biol Int 2005; 29: 567-575.

[32]   Miura M, Gronthos S, Zhao M, et al. SHED: stem cells from human exfoliated deciduous teeth. Proc Natl Acad Sci U S A 2003; 100: 5807-5812.

[33]   Sonoyama W, Liu Y, Fang D, et al. Mesenchymal stem cell-mediated functional tooth regeneration in swine. PLoS ONE 2006; 1: e79.

[34]   Sonoyama W, Liu Y, Yamaza T, et al. Characterization of the apical papilla and its residing stem cells from human immature permanent teeth: a pilot study. J Endod 2008; 34: 166-171.

[35]   Seo BM, Miura M, Gronthos S, et al. Investigation of multipotent postnatal stem cells from human periodontal ligament. Lancet 2004; 364: 149-155.

[36]   Ten Cate AR. The role of epithelium in the development, structure and function of the tissues of tooth support. Oral Dis 1996; 2: 55-62.

[37]   Smith CE. Cell turnover in the odontogenic organ of the rat incisor as visualized by graphic reconstructions following a single injection of 3H-thymidine. Am J Anat 1980; 158: 321-43.

[38]   Murray PE, About I, Franquin JC, Remusat M, Smith AJ. Restorative pulpal and repair responses. J Am Dent Assoc 2001; 132: 482-491.

[39]   Hanks CT, Sun ZL, Fang DN, et al. Cloned 3T6 cell line from CD-1 mouse fetal molar dental papillae. Connect Tissue Res 1998; 37: 233-249.

[40]   Unda FJ, Martin A, Hilario E, Begue-Kirn C, Ruch JV, Arechaga J. Dissection of the odontoblast differentiation process *in vitro* by a combination of FGF1, FGF2, and TGFbeta1. Dev Dyn 2000; 218: 480-489.

[41]   Ueno A, Kitase Y, Moriyama K, Inoue H. MC3T3-E1-conditioned medium-induced mineralization by clonal rat dental pulp cells. Matrix Biol 2001; 20: 347-355.

[42]   About I, Bottero MJ, de Denato P, Camps J, Franquin JC, Mitsiadis TA. Human dentin production *in vitro*. Exp Cell Res 2000; 258: 33-41.

[43]   Couble ML, Farges JC, Bleicher F, Perrat-Mabillon B, Boudeulle M, Magloire H. Odontoblast differentiation of human dental pulp cells in explant cultures. Calcif Tissue Int 2000; 66: 129-138.

[44]   Stanislawski L, Carreau JP, Pouchelet M, Chen ZH, Goldberg M. *In vitro* culture of human dental pulp cells: some aspects of cells emerging early from the explant. Clin Oral Investig 1997; 1: 131-140.

[45]   Shi S, Robey PG, Gronthos S. Comparison of human dental pulp and bone marrow stromal stem cells by cDNA microarray analysis. Bone 2001; 29: 532-539.

[46]   Murray PE, Garcia-Godoy F, Hargreaves KM. Regenerative endodontics: a review of current status and a call for action. J Endod 2007; 33: 377-390.

[47]   Sloan AJ, Smith AJ. Stem cells and the dental pulp: potential roles in dentine regeneration and repair. Oral Dis 2007; 13: 151-157.

[48]   Laino G, d'Aquino R, Graziano A, et al. A new population of human adult dental pulp stem cells: a useful source of living autologous fibrous bone tissue (LAB). J Bone Miner Res 2005; 20: 1394-1402.

[49]   Gronthos S, Brahim J, Li W, et al. Stem cell properties of human dental pulp stem cells. J Dent Res 2002; 81: 531-535.

[50]   Zhang W, Walboomers XF, Shi S, Fan M, Jansen JA. Multilineage differentiation potential of stem cells derived from human dental pulp after cryopreservation. Tissue Eng 2006; 12: 2813-2823.

[51]   d'Aquino R, Graziano A, Sampaolesi M, et al. Human postnatal dental pulp cells co-differentiate into osteoblasts and endotheliocytes: a pivotal synergy leading to adult bone tissue formation. Cell Death Differ 2007; 14: 1162-1171.

[52] Laino G, Carinci F, Graziano A, et al. *In vitro* bone production using stem cells derived from human dental pulp. J Craniofac Surg 2006; 17: 511-515.

[53] MacNeil RL, Thomas HF. Development of the murine periodontium. II. Role of the epithelial root sheath in formation of the periodontal attachment. J Periodontol 1993; 64: 285-291.

[54] Spouge JD. A new look at the rests of Malassez. A review of their embryological origin, anatomy, and possible role in periodontal health and disease. J Periodontol 1980; 51: 437-444.

[55] Morsczeck C, Gotz W, Schierholz J, et al. Isolation of precursor cells (PCs) from human dental follicle of wisdom teeth. Matrix Biol 2005; 24: 155-165.

[56] Morsczeck C. Gene expression of runx2, Osterix, c-fos, DLX-3, DLX-5, and MSX-2 in dental follicle cells during osteogenic differentiation *in vitro*. Calcif Tissue Int 2006; 78: 98-102.

[57] Parner ET, Heidmann JM, Kjaer I, Vaeth M, Poulsen S. Biological interpretation of the correlation of emergence times of permanent teeth. J Dent Res 2002; 81: 451-454.

[58] Shi S, Gronthos S. Perivascular niche of postnatal mesenchymal stem cells in human bone marrow and dental pulp. J Bone Miner Res 2003;18: 696-704.

[59] Chai Y, Jiang X, Ito Y, et al. Fate of the mammalian cranial neural crest during tooth and mandibular morphogenesis. Development 2000; 127: 1671-1679.

[60] Jo YY, Lee HJ, Kook SY, et al. Isolation and characterization of postnatal stem cells from human dental tissues. Tissue Eng 2007; 13: 767-773.

[61] Karring T, Nyman S, Lindhe J. Healing following implantation of periodontitis affected roots into bone tissue. J Clin Periodontol 1980; 7: 96-105.

[62] Nyman S, Karring T, Lindhe J, Planten S. Healing following implantation of periodontitis-affected roots into gingival connective tissue. J Clin Periodontol 1980; 7: 394-401.

[63] Shi S, Gronthos S, Chen S, et al. Bone formation by human postnatal bone marrow stromal stem cells is enhanced by telomerase expression. Nat Biotechnol 2002; 20: 587-591.

[64] Seo BM, Miura M, Sonoyama W, Coppe C, Stanyon R, Shi S. Recovery of stem cells from cryopreserved periodontal ligament. J Dent Res 2005; 84: 907-912.

[65] Song L, Baksh D, Tuan RS. Mesenchymal stem cell-based cartilage tissue engineering: cells, scaffold and biology. Cytotherapy 2004; 6: 596-601.

[66] Wright WE, Piatyszek MA, Rainey WE, Byrd W, Shay JW. Telomerase activity in human germline and embryonic tissues and cells. Dev Genet 1996; 18: 173-179.

[67] Gronthos S, Chen S, Wang CY, Robey PG, Shi S. Telomerase accelerates osteogenesis of bone marrow stromal stem cells by upregulation of CBFA1, osterix, and osteocalcin. J Bone Miner Res 2003; 18: 716-722.

[68] Simonsen JL, Rosada C, Serakinci N, et al. Telomerase expression extends the proliferative life-span and maintains the osteogenic potential of human bone marrow stromal cells. Nat Biotechnol 2002; 20: 592-596.

[69] Miura M, Chen XD, Allen MR, et al. A crucial role of caspase-3 in osteogenic differentiation of bone marrow stromal stem cells. J Clin Invest 2004; 114: 1704-1713.

[70] Batouli S, Miura M, Brahim J, et al. Comparison of stem-cell-mediated osteogenesis and dentinogenesis. J Dent Res 2003; 82: 976-981.

[71] Mikkonen M. The Nordic model: Finnish experience of the patient injury act in practice. Med Law 2001; 20: 347-353.

[72] Shi S, Bartold PM, Miura M, Seo BM, Robey PG, Gronthos S. The efficacy of mesenchymal stem cells to regenerate and repair dental structures. Orthod Craniofac Res 2005; 8: 191-199.

[73] Nor JE. Tooth regeneration in operative dentistry. Oper Dent 2006; 31: 633-642.

[74] Sanz M, Giovannoli JL. Focus on furcation defects: guided tissue regeneration. Periodontol 2000; 22: 169-189.

[75] Grzesik WJ, Narayanan AS. Cementum and periodontal wound healing and regeneration. Crit Rev Oral Biol Med 2002; 13: 474-484.

[76] Li H, Yan F, Lei L, Li Y, Xiao Y. Application of autologous cryopreserved bone marrow mesenchymal stem cells for periodontal regeneration in dogs. Cells Tissues Organs 2008. PMID: 18957835

[77] Chen YL, Chen PK, Jeng LB, et al. Periodontal regeneration using ex vivo autologous stem cells engineered to express the BMP-2 gene: an alternative to alveolaplasty. Gene Ther 2008; 15: 1469-1477.

[78] Morsczeck C, Schmalz G, Reichert TE, Vollner F, Galler K, Driemel O. Somatic stem cells for regenerative dentistry. Clin Oral Investig 2008; 12: 113-118.

[79] Flores MG, Hasegawa M, Yamato M, Takagi R, Okano T, Ishikawa I. Cementum-periodontal ligament complex regeneration using the cell sheet technique. J Periodontal Res 2008; 43: 364-371.

[80] Akizuki T, Oda S, Komaki M, et al. Application of periodontal ligament cell sheet for periodontal regeneration: a pilot study in beagle dogs. J Periodontal Res 2005; 40: 245-251.

[81] Slavkin HC, Bringas P, Jr., Bessem C, et al. Hertwig's epithelial root sheath differentiation and initial cementum and bone formation during long-term organ culture of mouse mandibular first molars using serumless, chemically-defined medium. J Periodontal Res 1989; 24: 28-40.

[82] Thomas HF, Kollar EJ. Differentiation of odontoblasts in grafted recombinants of murine epithelial root sheath and dental mesenchyme. Arch Oral Biol 1989; 34: 27-35.

[83] Amar S, Luo W, Snead ML, Ruch JV. Amelogenin gene expression in mouse incisor heterotopic recombinations. Differentiation 1989; 41: 56-561.

[84] Hu B, Unda F, Bopp-Kuchler S, et al. Bone marrow cells can give rise to ameloblast-like cells. J Dent Res 2006; 85: 416-421.

[85] Hu B, Nadiri A, Bopp-Kuchler S, Perrin-Schmitt F, Lesot H. Dental Epithelial Histomorphogenesis *in vitro*. J Dent Res 2005; 84: 521-525.

[86] Yu J, Wang Y, Deng Z, et al. Odontogenic capability: bone marrow stromal stem cells versus dental pulp stem cells. Biol Cell 2007; 99: 465-474.

[87] Ohazama A, Modino SA, Miletich I, Sharpe PT. Stem-cell-based tissue engineering of murine teeth. J Dent Res 2004; 83: 518-522.

[88] Duailibi MT, Duailibi SE, Young CS, Bartlett JD, Vacanti JP, Yelick PC. Bioengineered teeth from cultured rat tooth bud cells. J Dent Res 2004; 83: 523-528.

[89] Young CS, Terada S, Vacanti JP, Honda M, Bartlett JD, Yelick PC. Tissue engineering of complex tooth structures on biodegradable polymer scaffolds. J Dent Res 2002; 81: 695-700.

[90] Yu J, Deng Z, Shi J, et al. Differentiation of dental pulp stem cells into regular-shaped dentin-pulp complex induced by tooth germ cell conditioned medium. Tissue Eng 2006; 12: 3097-3105.

[91] Hu B, Nadiri A, Kuchler-Bopp S, Perrin-Schmitt F, Peters H, Lesot H. Tissue engineering of tooth crown, root, and periodontium. Tissue Eng 2006; 12: 2069-2075.

[92] Honda MJ, Tsuchiya S, Sumita Y, Sagara H, Ueda M. The sequential seeding of epithelial and mesenchymal cells for tissue-engineered tooth regeneration. Biomaterials 2007; 28: 680-689.

[93] Sumita Y, Honda MJ, Ohara T, et al. Performance of collagen sponge as a 3-D scaffold for tooth-tissue engineering. Biomaterials 2006; 27: 3238-3248.

[94] Iwatsuki S, Honda MJ, Harada H, Ueda M. Cell proliferation in teeth reconstructed from dispersed cells of embryonic tooth germs in a three-dimensional scaffold. Eur J Oral Sci 2006; 114: 310-317.

[95] Song Y, Zhang Z, Yu X, et al. Application of lentivirus-mediated RNAi in studying gene function in mammalian tooth development. Dev Dyn 2006; 235: 1334-1344.

[96] Yu JH, Shi JN, Deng ZH, et al. Cell pellets from dental papillae can reexhibit dental morphogenesis and dentinogenesis. Biochem Biophys Res Commun 2006; 346: 116-124.

Stem Cell and Regenerative Medicine, 2010, 149-159

CHAPTER 11

Corneal Progenitor Cells and Regenerative Potential

Gary Hin-Fai Yam, Sharon Ka-Wai Lee and Chi Pui Pang*

Department of Ophthalmology & Visual Sciences, The Chinese University of Hong Kong, Hong Kong

Abstract: The human cornea is a site of tissue-specific adult progenitor cells, residing between cornea and conjunctiva in the Palisade of Vogt of the limbus region. Advances in molecular and cell culture techniques presently provide new platforms to investigate the intrinsic biological roles and properties of cornea epithelial progenitor cells (CEPCs), which is known to maintain corneal homeostasis throughout human life. Although specific molecular markers of CEPCs are still to be discovered, results of recent research provide new information to apply them for cell replacement in damaged tissues. Cultured CEPCs, with the aid of external support, have been used for *ex vivo* cornea therapy with satisfactory clinical outcome While the niche environment, i.e., the extracellular matrix, growth factors and cytokines, provide regulatory measures in the proliferation of CEPCs. The recent discovery of CEPC specific microRNAs opens a new direction of research on the biological properties of CEPC and stem cells of other resources. This should facilitate to address important questions regarding CEPC functions and therapeutic strategies in health and diseases.

SITE OF RESIDENCE OF CORNEAL EPITHELIAL PROGENITOR CELLS

The Cornea

The cornea is the most anterior part of the eye. Beside a crucial role in refracting light through the lens to the retina, it acts as a protecting shield for inner ocular tissues. As such, normal cornea has to be transparent and avascular and has sufficient tensile strength and flexibility to resist outside pressure. It is composed of 5 layers, in the order of outermost stratified non-keratinized squamous epithelium, Bowman's membrane, corneal stroma, and the Descemet's membrane, which is the basement membrane for the innermost corneal endothelium. At the edge of the cornea is the limbus, where the corneal epithelium continues into the conjunctival epithelium and stroma into the sclera. The limbal epithelium is 10 to 12 cell layers in thickness, while there are 5 layers in the central cornea. The Bowman's membrane terminates there so that the undulated limbal basement membrane is directly above the stroma, which makes up about 80% of corneal thickness and contains regularly-spaced collagen bundles and corneal keratocytes. Here the Descemet's membrane disappears and the corneal endothelium is connected to the trabecular meshwork.

The Limbus

The limbus is an annulus of tissue approximately 1.5 mm by width located at the vascularised junction between the transparent cornea and opaque sclera (Fig. **1**). The corneal epithelial progenitor cells (CEPCs) are undifferentiated and reside in the basal layer of the limbal epithelium, sheltered in the "limbal epithelial crypts" extended from the palisades of Vogt, which are the papillae-like structures located in the region of sub-epithelial connective tissues of the limbus [1, 2]. This putative stem cell niche protects CEPCs from shear stress and provides nourishments by neighboring vasculatures.

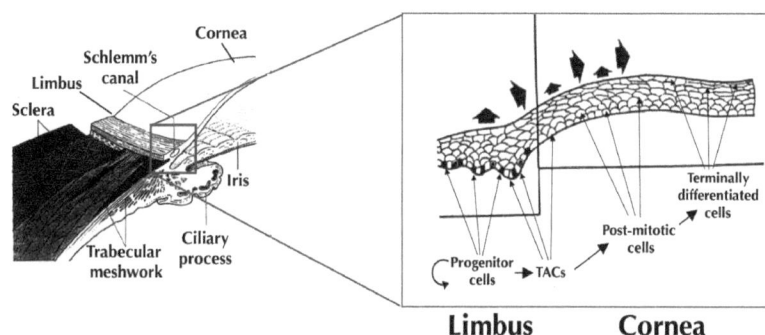

Figure 1: The location of limbus on the ocular surface. The progenitor cells CEPCs (located in the limbal basal epithelium)

***Address Correspondence to this Author C. P. Pang:** Department of Ophthalmology & Visual Sciences, The Chinese University of Hong Kong, Hong Kong Eye Hospital, 147K Argyle Street, Kowloon, Hong Kong; Email: cppang@cuhk.edu.hk

generate transient amplifying cells (TACs), which migrate upwards and centripedally towards the central cornea, eventually forming the terminally differentiated epithelium.

Since the first report in 1971 on the regenerative capacity of limbal epithelium in guinea pigs [3], accumulative evidence has confirmed limbal basal cells to have greater proliferative capacity than central corneal basal epithelial cells [4]. Normally these cells are quiescent or attain slow cell cycle as revealed by the long-term retention of labeled DNA precursors (e.g. tritiated thymidine) [5, 6]. The label retention index was about 20% in the limbal region, in contrast to less than 8% in central cornea [7]. Surgical removal of the limbus in rodents caused delayed wound healing with conjunctivalization and persistent neovascularization on the corneal surface [8]. Limbal transplantation provides long-term restoration of corneal surface in patients with limbal disruption [9]. It is noted that most corneal epithelial tumors are originated from the limbal area [10].

IDENTIFICATION OF CORNEAL EPITHELIAL PROGENITOR CELL PROPER

Cell Size and Morphology

Basal cells in the limbus and central and paracentral cornea are cuboidal in shape. Confocal microscopy showed that limbal basal cells are smaller than corneal basal cells, 10.1 ± 0.8 µm against 17.1 ± 0.8 µm in diameter [11]. They have greater nucleus/cytoplasm ratio and distinct nuclei with larger amount of heterochromatin and less defined nucleoli [12]. Putative CEPCs lie deeply in the limbal crypt structure and contain melanin pigment for protection against UV [5, 13].

High Proliferative Capacity and Clonal Expansion

CEPCs are normally slow-cycling or quiescent for long periods of time [5, 6]. When stimulated, such as during cornea wound healing, they become highly proliferative and are capable of expanding clonally with a faster rate than the cells of the central cornea [14], moving upwards and centripetally from the basal limbus towards the central corneal surface (Fig. **1**). The median distance of cell migration is approximately 17 µm per day [15]. Formation of holoclones, which are cells proliferating for 80 to 100 doublings, is a hallmark of CEPC proliferation [16]. Cells from central cornea generate mostly paraclones which are not more than 2 to 3 cell doublings.

CEPC Markers

Until now, CEPCs cannot be identified by any single specific markers. Instead, a panel of stem cell markers in combination of null expression of cornea-specific differentiation markers can be recruited to identify genuine CEPCs, although new markers with sufficient sensitivity and specificity are needed.

1. Cell Surface Transporter Protein ABCG2

ABCG2, the G subfamily of ATP binding cassette transporter protein 2, is ubiquitously expressed in stem cells of the embryo, bone marrow, skeletal muscle and epithelia [17]. Also expressed in CEPCs [18], it is a high capacity transporter for a wide range of substrates, from hydrophobic to charged molecules, including cytotoxic compounds and fluorescent dyes [19]. It actively effluxes these molecules, hence protecting stem cells from external stimuli and maintaining the undisturbed state. ABCG2 is expressed in the limbal basal epithelium but not in central corneal epithelium [12].

2. Transcription Factor p63

P53, p63, and p73 are structurally-related proteins. P53 is a tumor suppressor [20]. P63 and p73 participate in cell proliferation and morphogenesis [21]. P63 knockout ($p63^{-/-}$) mice have major defects in epithelial development with absent stratified epithelium [22], likely due to lack of stem cell capability to sustain epithelial morphogenesis [23]. Among the 6 isoforms of p63, TAp63α, β and γ and ΔNp63α, β and γ, ΔNp63α is most specific for CEPCs [24]. Expression of ΔNp63α is high in holoclones derived from the limbus, low in meroclones and absent in paraclones. ΔNp63β and γ are expressed in differentiated cells in the suprabasal layers of cornea and limbus.

3. C/EBPδ and Bmi1

Normally, a certain number of mitotically quiescent CEPCs are maintained in the limbus. They are identified by the co-expression of transcription factors ΔNp63α, C/EBPδ (CCAAT enhancer binding protein delta and Bmi1 (B-lymphoma Mo-MLV insertion region 1), which is a Polycomb ring finger gene repressor [25]. C/EBPδ induces G0/G1 cell cycle arrest in epithelial cells. Bmi1 regulates cell cycle inhibitors, the $p16^{Ink4a}$ and $p19^{Arf}$ genes from the Ink4a locus [26]. Hence it is involved in self-renewing cell divisions of embryonic and adult hematopoietic, neural and somatic stem cells [27, 28]. About 10% of limbal basal cells are positive in expressions of C/EBPδ Bmi1 and ΔNp63α (C/EBPδ+$^+$/Bmi1$^+$/ΔNp63α$^+$). During wound healing, activated CEPCs lose C/EBPδ/Bmi1 expression and ΔNp63α$^+$ cells proliferate and migrate to the repair the injury [25]. In differentiated cells, ΔNp63α expression is switched off.

4. Notch1

The transmembrane receptor Notch1 is expressed in some ABCG2$^+$ CEPCs residing in the limbal basal region [29]. It is absent in the central cornea and dividing cells. Notch1 is known to regulate cell and developmental processes through cell-cell interactions. Ligands binding to the Notch1 receptor initiate intracellular signaling cascades to modulate differentiation, proliferation and self-renewal in stem cells of various origins [30, 31].

5. SOD2 and CK15

Both manganese superoxide dismutase 2 (SOD2) and cytokeratin 15 (CK15) are expressed in clusters of cells in the limbal basal epithelium [32]. Mitochondrial SOD2 dismutates superoxide (O_2^-) to hydrogen peroxide (H_2O_2) for fur further degradation by catalase and glutathione peroxidase. This is a cellular protective mechanism against oxidative damage on DNA by H_2O_2 or UVB radiation, which is a biological role of SOD2 in CEPCs. CK15 is a known human hair follicle stem cell marker [33]. It is a cytoskeletal protein expressing in developing epidermis. Its expression in primitive limbal basal epithelium indicates the common embryonic origin of both tissues [34]. When CEPCs differentiate, CK15 expression is decreased.

6. Other Markers

Right now no single protein marker can identify genuine CEPCs. Combinations of markers have to be used. Other putative CEPC markers include vimentin, integrin α9 and cytokeratin 19, keratinocyte growth factor receptor and metallothionein [12, 35]. Lack of cornea markers such as involucrin, connexin 43 and cytokeratin 3/12, P-cadherin, nestin and integrin α2, α6 and β4 can be used to rule out non-CEPC cell populations [12, 32, 36, 37]. It is anticipated that advances in cell sorting techniques based on cell surface molecules and microarray technologies should lead to identification of specific CEPC markers.

CEPC REGULATION

Niche Environment - Extracellular Matrix

Specialized environmental niches are required, crucially, to maintain stem cells in the undifferentiated state and regulate their functions. In vitro confocal microscopy and scanning electron microscopy have revealed the limbal niche structure [13]. Putative CEPCs are found lining the edges and bases of limbal crypts (LCs) and around the tips of focal stromal projections (FSPs), which are adjacent to the highly cellularized and richly vascularized stromal regions. Cells isolated from the LC/FSP rich regions generated more holoclones and expressed higher levels of CEPC markers than corneal basal cells from non-LC/FSP regions. Patients with limbal stem cell deficiency have undetectable LC/FSP regions [13]. Besides, limbal basement membrane markedly expresses laminin α1, α2, β1 and γ3 chains, agrin, BM40/SPARC and tenascin-C. These extracellular matrix proteins co-localize with CEPCs, which exist as cell clusters of ABCG2$^+$/p63$^+$/CK19$^+$/Cx43$^-$/integrin-α2$^-$/CK3$^-$ [38].

Niche Environment - Growth Factors & Chemokines

There are complex autocrine and paracrine interactions among the epithelial cells and fibroblasts of cornea and limbus [39, 40]. Transforming growth factor alpha (TGFα), interleukin-1 beta (IL-1β) and platelet-derived growth factor BB are released from the epithelial cells to stromal fibroblasts, which produce keratinocyte growth factor

(KGF) and hepatocyte growth factor (HGF) to cause epithelial cell proliferation and migration [41]. Other cytokines, such as insulin-like growth factor-1, TGFβ1 and 2, epidermal growth factor (EGF), and basic fibroblast growth factor (bFGF) mediate both epithelial and fibroblast activities [42]. Both KGF and HGF participate in cornea wound healing. KGF is predominantly expressed in the limbal stromal fibroblasts and HGF in the corneal stromal fibroblasts. Upon injury or stress, epithelial cells release IL-1β, which stimulates the limbal fibroblasts to secrete KGF to activate CEPC division [43]. Recently it is shown that ΔNp63α is induced by KGF via the p38 pathway [44]. HGF secreted from corneal fibroblasts subsequently modulate the production and migration of transient amplifying cells (TACs) derived from CEPCs for wound repair [45]. Nerve growth factor (NGF) also participates in corneal epithelial proliferation and differentiation [46, 47]. Its high affinity receptor, TrkA, is detected in both corneal and limbal basal epithelia, but the apoptosis-related NGF receptor, p75[NTR], is absent in the limbal basal epithelium [48, 49]. This suggests that NGF signaling is involved in CEPC survival.

MICRORNA AND CEPCS

MicroRNAs are small non-coding RNAs of 20 to 25 nucleotides and act as endogenous repressor of gene activity. About 6,000 microRNA sequences have been identified across species from viruses, worms to mammals through random cloning, sequencing or computational prediction (microRNA Registry, http://www.microrna.sanger.ac.uk). They bind to the 3' untranslated region of target mRNAs for translational repression or cleavage, and mediates regulation of biological processes including cell proliferation, differentiation and death [50, 51], embryonic development, cell fate determination and patterning [52]. In human, more than 700 microRNAs, corresponding to 1% of protein coding genes, are confirmed, although many target genes remain to be identified. In eyes of human and mice, six specific microRNAs (miR-181, 182, 183, 184, 204 and 205) have been documented [53]. MiR-184 is enriched in the corneal epithelium and miR-205 in the entire corneal, limbal and conjunctival epithelia and epidermis. miR-184 antagonizes the miR-205-mediated down-regulation of SH2-containing inositol phosphatase-2 which regulates epithelial cell proliferation [54]. Other known ocular-specific microRNAs are restricted in the retinal tissues. Our laboratory has profiled microRNAs in human limbal epithelium, which is enriched with CEPCs, and central corneal epithelium without CEPCs. We used Human MicroRNA Microarray Kit (V2) (Agilent Technologies) to screen for the expression of 723 human microRNAs from Sanger database v.10.1. Two microRNAs, hsa-miR-143 and hsa-miR-145, validated by specific quantitative polymerase chain reaction, are significantly up-regulated in the limbal epithelium [Yam, manuscript in preparation] (Fig. **2**). *In situ* hybridization using locked nucleic acid-modified oligonucleotide probes on frozen human corneal sections localized both miR-143 and miR-145 specifically in the limbal epithelia but not corneal epithelia. Moreover, the expression was predominant in the winged-cell and parabasal layers, decreasing towards the superficial layers (Fig. **2**). The basal epithelium where CEPCs reside had low expression of these microRNAs. Stromal components and keratocytes were negative also. In our primary human CEPC culture, ectopic expression of miR-145, cloned in lentiviral vector driven by cytomegalovirus promoter, induced corneal differentiation markers cytokeratin 3/12 and connexin-43. By expression arrays, we detected down-regulation of markers associated with limbal basal cell maintenance (including angiopoietin-4, prostate stem cell antigen, katanin, cadherin, integrin β8 and Wnt7A) and up-regulation of corneal differentiation and inflammation markers (including interferon β1, tumor necrosis factor α, complement component, somatostatin and retinoic acid receptor α) [Yam, manuscript in preparation]. Expression of MiR-145 is low in human self-renewing ES cells but it is up-regulated during differentiation [55]. A double-negative feedback mechanism has been proposed for the core plurpotency factors (Oct4, Sox2, Klf4) and miR-145 [56]. Oct4, Sox2 and Klf4 are crucial genes in self-regulatory network to maintain self-renewal and pluripotency capacity of ES cells. Direct targeting of miR-145 to Oct4, Sox2 and Klf4 negatively controls the gene expressions and suppresses the self-renewal ability. This subsequently promotes the expression of mesoderm- and ectoderm-specific markers [55, 57-59]. In contrast, Oct4 down-regulates miR-145 expression through repressive binding to the microRNA promoter. Hence, in early ES cells, miR-145 is suppressed by Oct4 expression, and the cells are self-renewing [56]. In our study, miR-145 of CEPCs promoted the expression of corneal differentiation markers and induced early cell differentiation, resulting in a much thinner epithelium [Yam, manuscript in preparation]. In a zebrafish platform, miR-145 knockdown resulted in underdeveloped gut and heart [60]. We conclude that miR-145 and, to a minor extent, miR-143 regulate the development and integrity of corneal epithelium and corneal homeostasis.

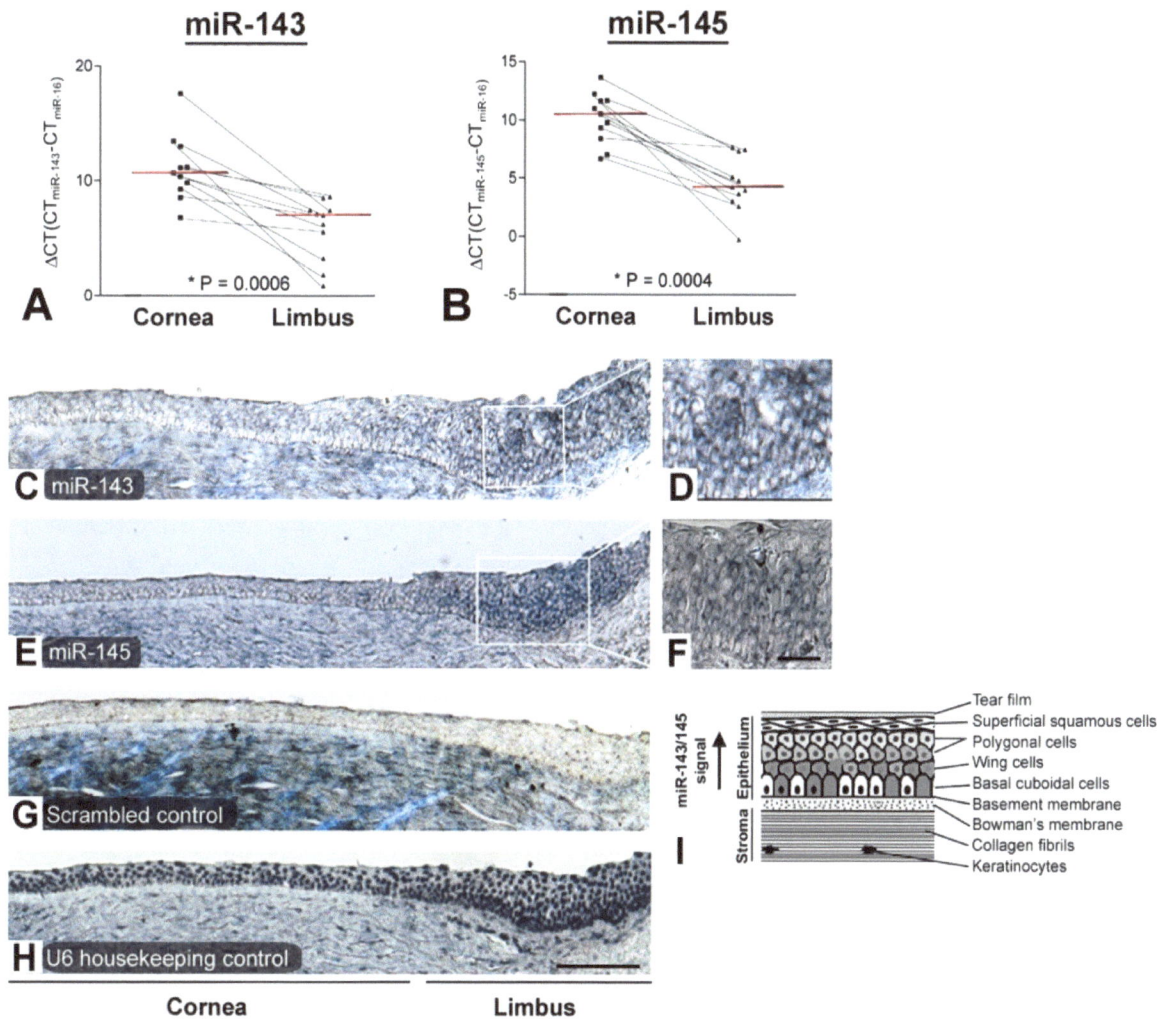

Figure 2: MicroRNA (miR-143 and -145) expression in the limbal epithelium. (A and B) Quantitative real-time PCR analysis of RNA samples from limbal and corneal epithelia showed significant up-regulation of (**A**) miR-143 and (**B**) miR-145 in the limbal epithelia when compared to the corneal epithelia (P<0.005, Mann Whitney U-test). The dots represented Δ values, which are the CT of tested microRNA subtracted by CT of housekeeping U6. The red horizontal lines indicated the mean CT values. (**C to F**) *In situ* hybridization analysis of microRNA localization in human corneal specimen. Cryosections were hybridized with digoxigenin (DIG)-labeled LNA-miRCURY oligo probe for (**C**) miR-143, (**E**) miR-145, (**G**) scrambled sequences and (**H**) housekeeping U6 and signals were detected by anti-DIG-alkaline phosphatase followed by substrate reaction. The expression of miR-143 and -145 were clearly observed in the limbal epithelium, but not corneal epithelium. Under higher magnifications (**D**, miR-143 and **F**, miR-145), both miRNAs were predominant in the parabasal layers, with signal decreasing towards the superficial squamous layers. (**I**) A schematic diagram to show the localization of miR-143 and -145 in limbal epithelial layers. Scale bars: 150 μm (**C, E, G and H**); 40 μm (**D and F**).

THERAPEUTIC POTENTIALS OF CEPC

Ocular Surface Pathology

CEPCs are imperative for corneal homeostasis. CEPC deficiency leads to corneal opacification, surface morbidity and vision loss. CEPC deficiency may be caused by primary etiologies, such as heritable genetic disorder aniridia, idiopathic conditions like Mooren's ulcer. There are also secondary or acquired causes, like chemical or thermal injury, Steven-Johnson syndrome, contact lens-induced keratopathy and limbitis. Clinical manifestations include epithelial erosion and ulcer, opacification, inflammation, corneal neovascularization, conjunctivalization, and unstable corneal surface. These conditions can cause pain, severe photophobia, reduced visual acuity and even blindness to the patients.

Surgical Approaches

1. Limbal Transplantation

Different approaches to reconstruct damaged cornea surfaces have been attempted for more than a century. Cornea transplantation, first conducted in 1905 by Dr Eduard Zirm, has been widely used to repair the failed cornea [61]. However, patients with CEPC deficiency have high risk of corneal graft failure since CEPCs are not included in the graft and only transient amplifying cells are transplanted. Hence, restoration of the CEPC population and a stable ocular surface is essential for successful transplantation. In 1989, transplantation of a limbal rim containing CEPCs was first introduced [9]. Since then, autologous and allogenic grafting of tissues composed of limbus with either cornea (keratolimbal graft) or conjunctiva (conjunctival limbal graft) have been performed to treat corneal surface wounds with success [62]. Usually the corneal surface is completely epithelialized within 2 weeks and there is a substantial improvement of visual acuity. However, there is no evidence of long-term donor cell survival. In autografting for unilateral CEPC deficiency, there is a risk of secondary CEPC deficiency in the healthy donor eye when large-sized graft or repeated surgery is required. For allografting to treat bilateral CEPC deficiency there are problems of donor tissue availability, graft rejection and long-term immuno-suppression. There are reports of limbal grafting failures, especially in the long-term, due to difficulty of prolonged maintenance of donor cells on the recipient corneal surface [63, 64]. The failed cases had persistent or recurrent epithelial defects, ocular complications and corneal vascularization. Among other factors, nuclear changes occur in defective donor limbal epithelial cells. The loss of most essential nuclear matrix proteins, including lamin A/C and proliferating cell nuclear antigen could affect the continuous growth and viability of limbal cells and the epithelial integrity after transplantation [65].

2. *Ex Vivo* Corneal Cell Therapy

Based on the pioneering work by Rheinwald on the cultivation of epidermal keratinocytes [66], *ex vivo* expansion of human CEPCs was developed [67], which was also the first report of cultured stem cell therapy for chemical burns of cornea surfaces. Autologous limbal cells were isolated from 1x2 cm^2 limbal biopsy and expanded in culture for transplantation. Two patients were treated and both improved visual acuity for more than 2 years. Since then, this technique has been widely adopted for the treatment of CEPC deficiency [68, 69]. However, there is so far no standard method for CEPC expansion. The culture techniques vary between explant or suspension cultures. Conditions differ in culture medium composition, growth factor supplementation, duration of culture period, use of feeder layers and air-lifting. The carriers can be fibrin gel or intact or denuded amniotic membrane. Cell sources vary from autologous or allogenic limbal cells.

In explant culture, limbal tissue is adhered to a carrier substrate prior to submerging in culture medium, which stimulates the proliferating limbal epithelial cells to migrate out of the biopsy. With rapid cell divisions, a confluent cell monolayer of 3x3 cm^2 in area can be achieved between 14 to 21 days [68]. An additional step of airlifting promotes stratification and differentiation of epithelium. This process requires the culture medium to be leveled to the lower surface of the epithelium, giving a polarized direction of nutrient supply from the basal epithelium [70]. In suspension culture, the basement membrane collagen is digested by dispase to loosen the epithelium from stroma tissue. Subsequently trypsin dissociates the epithelium into single cells [67, 71, 72], which are allowed to become confluence before air-lifting for stratification. Since dispase digestion takes 18 hours at 4°C, pH changes and free radicals in the tissue incubation would greatly affect the proliferative capacity of CEPCs. Supplementation of ascorbic acid as an anti-oxidative agent is thus required [73].

Ex vivo cultivated corneal cell therapy has advantages over the limbal graft treatment. Smaller sizes of healthy biopsy are required, the risk of causing CEPC deficiency in the healthy donor eye is thus minimized and repeated biopsy taking is possible. Also, risk of allograft rejection is reduced due to the absence of antigen-presenting Langerhan's cells in culture [37].

3. Alternative Cell Sources

Autologous oral or nasal mucosal epithelium can serve as effective substitutes for limbal allografts to reconstruct bilateral CEPC deficiency [74, 75]. There are potential advantages: (1) averting the risk of allogenic immuno-rejection and immuno-suppression; (2) less differentiated than epidermal keratinocytes and can be maintained and survive in culture for longer period of time without keratinization; (3) having similar keratin expression as corneal epithelial cells [76], and (4) quick healing of surgical wound of oral mucosa without scarring. Very recently, ex vivo culture of human immature dental pulp stem cells is used to treat CEPC deficiency caused by chemical burns in rabbits [77, 78]. When compared to the control corneas showing total conjunctivalization and opacification, the treated corneas regained the transparency and reduced neovascularization. The regenerated epithelium expressed CEPC markers including ABCG2, integrin β1, vimentin, connexin-43 and cytokeratin 3/12 [78]. Successful reconstruction of corneal surface had been reported by transplantation with cultured mesenchymal stem cells in a rat model [79].

Carrier Scaffold

1. Human Amniotic Membrane as a Scaffold and a Natural Substrate

Besides being a carrier to transfer the epithelial cell sheet to the damaged corneal surface, a surrogate niche is required also for the survival, expansion and post-transplantation functioning of donor corneal epithelial cells. Human amniotic membrane (HAM) has been used for this purpose. It is the innermost layer of the fetal membrane characterized by a thick distinct basement membrane overlaid by a monolayer epithelium with an underneath avascular stroma. HAM is devoid of blood vessels due to its close proximity to the highly vascularized chorionic membrane. It is widely used as a surgical material on its anti-angiogenic, anti-inflammatory, anti-scarring and anti-apoptotic properties [80]. The translucent HAM is a popular biological substrate for ocular reconstruction in ophthalmic surgeries to restore conjunctival defects without the risk of immunogenicity [81]. Protocols have been devised to explant limbal biopsy or even culture single cells in suspension directly on HAM for transfer to patients. Good clinical outcomes of corneal clarity and surface stability were often [68, 70-72, 82-85]. HAM basement membrane contains collagen IV and VII and laminin 1 and 5, which are important for basal epithelial cell adhesion, proliferation and migration. They also promote epithelial differentiation and prevent apoptosis [86, 87]. TGF-β associated scarring and myofibroblast differentiations are reduced. Growth factors, including EGF, TGF-α, KGF, HGF and bFGF are produced to stimulate epithelialization [88]. Our group had reported the increased expression of tissue inhibitor metalloproteinase 1 and reduced TGF-β1 and 2 to facilitate corneal epithelial cell proliferation on HAM [89].

2. Alternative Substrates

Despite the popular use of HAM in ocular reconstruction, serious issues remain: availability of good quality HAM, costly donor screening, risk of viral disease transmission and incomplete transparency of HAM. Various alternative substrates from natural biopolymers to artificial synthetic matrices have been tested as biodegradable template for cell attachment and growth. A high surface area is required for cell-polymer interactions, sufficient space for extracellular matrix regeneration and minimal diffusional constraints for nutrients. The substrates should attain sufficient tensile strength for cell/epithelium transfer and flexibility to match the contour of corneal surface. They should be resorbed once the epithelium is regenerated, and must not cause toxic effects or any immunologic or inflammatory reactions to the host tissue. Fibrin gel substrate produced from autologous blood can be used as a 3-dimensional scaffold with no toxic or inflammatory reactions [90]. Fibrin culture of limbal stem cells grafted to patients with chemically burned corneas had yielded successful re-epithelialization, regressed inflammation and vascularization, with clinically and cytologically stable corneal surfaces [91]. A new carrier-free cell sheet transfer technology using temperature-responsive culture surface has also generated corneal epithelial cell sheet grafts on damaged corneas [74, 92]. The temperature-sensitive biopolymer is deposited on culture surface and serves as the substrate for epithelial cell culture. The intact cell sheet is harvested by reducing the temperature, without the use of proteases and transferred without any carrier to the recipient cornea surface. The cell sheet is readily adhesive to the stromal tissue and no suturing is required. Another substrate source is acrylic acid plasma. It could maintain a serum free co-culture of corneal epithelial cells and growth-arrested fibroblasts [93]. This coating in the inner surface of a bandage contact lens could help cell delivery and immobilization on to patient's corneal surface. The use of autologous plasma substrate allows a serum-free culture condition, which could be a safer way of CEPC delivery when actually used clinically in future.

FUTURE PROSPECTS

Currently there is active research on the use of stem/progenitor cell-based replacement for ocular repair and regeneration. Cornea repair by limbal/CEPC transplantation has been applied to eye patients for over a decade. In patients when only the epithelium is damaged, donor CEPCs are responsible for repopulating the cornea. The tissue or cell grafts are mostly seeded on prepared HAM, fibrin substrates or synthetic, cross-linked human recombinant collagen substrate and are allowed to form fully stratified epithelia for transplantation. In cases where healthy CEPCs are inadequate, autologous epithelial precursors from oral or nasal mucosal epithelium or dental pulp stem cells can be a potential cell source for transdifferentiation. This should be safer for ocular resurfacing than with allogenic grafts. Similar stem cell-based therapy is being tested for corneal endothelial replacement, but is less reported than epithelial replacement. Corneal equivalent using immortalized primary cells (corneal epithelial, stromal keratocytes and corneal endothelial cells) seeded in a glutaraldehyde cross-linked collagen-chondroitin sulfate matrix scaffold to reconstruct all 3 corneal cell layers has proven potential for the development of implantable corneal tissues. The use of progenitor cells instead of immortalized primary cells towards a clinically applicable model is highly promising.

The biological mechanisms by which CEPCs regulate their pluripotency, undifferentiation as well as being stimulated to proliferation-competent cells in regenerating the corneal epithelium remain elusive. The search for specific markers of CEPCs would significantly aid the isolation and identification of these cells. A further understanding of the niche biochemistry would also contribute to control CEPC maintenance and differentiation. Moreover, identification of specific microRNAs involved in early differentiating CEPCs should aid the discovery of intrinsic regulation of these cells, in particular upon stimulation by injury, and devise new strategies to use them for therapeutic treatments.

REFERENCES

[1]   Dua HS, Shanmuganathan VA, Powell-Richards AO, *et al.* Limbal epithelial crypts: a novel anatomical structure and a putative limbal stem cell niche. Br J Ophthalmol 2005; 89(5):529-532.

[2]   Yeung AM, Schlotzer-Schrehardt U, Kulkarni B, *et al.* Limbal epithelial crypt: a model for corneal epithelial maintenance and novel limbal regional variations. Arch Ophthalmol 2008; 126(5):665-669.

[3]   Davanger M, Evensen A. Role of the pericorneal papillary structure in renewal of corneal epithelium. Nature 1971; 229(5286):560-561.

[4]   Dua HS, Kulkarni B, Singh R. Quest for limbal stem cells. Clin Exp Ophthalmol 2006; 34(1):1-2.

[5]   Cotsarelis G, Cheng SZ, Dong G, *et al.* Existence of slow-cycling limbal epithelial basal cells that can be preferentially stimulated to proliferate: implications on epithelial stem cells. Cell 1989; 57(2):201-209.

[6]   Umemoto T, Yamato M, Nishida K, *et al.* Limbal epithelial side-population cells have stem cell-like properties, including quiescent state. Stem Cells 2006; 24(1):86-94.

[7]   Lavker RM, Dong G, Cheng SZ, *et al.* Relative proliferative rates of limbal and corneal epithelia. Implications of corneal epithelial migration, circadian rhythm, and suprabasally located DNA-synthesizing keratinocytes. Invest Ophthalmol Vis Sci 1991; 32(6):1864-1875.

[8]   Park KS, Lim CH, Min BM, *et al.* The side population cells in the rabbit limbus sensitively increased in response to the central cornea wounding. Invest Ophthalmol Vis Sci 2006; 47(3):892-900.

[9]   Kenyon KR, Tseng SC. Limbal autograft transplantation for ocular surface disorders. Ophthalmology 1989; 96(5):709-722.

[10]   Reya T, Morrison SJ, Clarke MF, Weissman IL. Stem cells, cancer, and cancer stem cells. Nature 2001; 414(6859):105-111.

[11]   Romano AC, Espana EM, Yoo SH, *et al.* Different cell sizes in human limbal and central corneal basal epithelia measured by confocal microscopy and flow cytometry. Invest Ophthalmol Vis Sci 2003; 44(12):5125-5129.

[12]   Schlotzer-Schrehardt U, Kruse FE. Identification and characterization of limbal stem cells. Exp Eye Res 2005; 81(3):247-264.

[13]   Shortt AJ, Secker GA, Munro PM, *et al.* Characterization of the limbal epithelial stem cell niche: novel imaging techniques permit in vivo observation and targeted biopsy of limbal epithelial stem cells. Stem Cells 2007; 25(6):1402-1409.

[14] Pellegrini G, Golisano O, Paterna P, *et al.* Location and clonal analysis of stem cells and their differentiated progeny in the human ocular surface. J Cell Biol 1999; 145(4):769-782.

[15] Buck RC. Measurement of centripetal migration of normal corneal epithelial cells in the mouse. Invest Ophthalmol Vis Sci 1985; 26(9):1296-1299.

[16] Barrandon Y. Crossing boundaries: stem cells, holoclones, and the fundamentals of squamous epithelial renewal. Cornea 2007; 26(9 Suppl 1):S10-12.

[17] Zhou S, Schuetz JD, Bunting KD, *et al.* The ABC transporter Bcrp1/ABCG2 is expressed in a wide variety of stem cells and is a molecular determinant of the side-population phenotype. Nat Med 2001; 7(9):1028-1034.

[18] Budak MT, Alpdogan OS, Zhou M, *et al.* Ocular surface epithelia contain ABCG2-dependent side population cells exhibiting features associated with stem cells. J Cell Sci 2005; 118(8):1715-1724.

[19] Sarkadi B, Ozvegy-Laczka C, Nemet K, *et al.* ABCG2 - a transporter for all seasons. FEBS Lett 2004; 567(1):116-120.

[20] Brown CJ, Lain S, Verma CS, *et al.* Awakening guardian angels: drugging the p53 pathway. Nat Rev Cancer 2009; 9(12):862-873.

[21] Belyi VA, Levine AJ. One billion years of p53/p63/p73 evolution. Proc Natl Acad Sci USA 2009; 106(42):17609-17610.

[22] Mills AA, Zheng B, Wang XJ, *et al.* p63 is a p53 homologue required for limb and epidermal morphogenesis. Nature 1999; 398(6729):708-713.

[23] Beaudry VG, Attardi LD. SKP-ing TAp63: stem cell depletion, senescence, and premature aging. Cell Stem Cell 2009; 5(1):1-2.

[24] Di Iorio E, Barbaro V, Ferrari S, *et al.* Q-FIHC: Quantification of fluorescence immunohistochemistry to analyse p63 isoforms and cell cycle phases in human limbal stem cells. Microsc Res Tech 2006; 69(12):983-991.

[25] Barbaro V, Testa A, Di Iorio E, *et al.* C/EBPdelta regulates cell cycle and self-renewal of human limbal stem cells. J Cell Biol 2007; 177(6):1037-1049.

[26] Quelle DE, Zindy F, Ashmun RA, *et al.* Alternative reading frames of the INK4a tumor suppressor gene encode two unrelated proteins capable of inducing cell cycle arrest. Cell 1995; 83(6):993-1000.

[27] Leung C, Lingbeek M, Shakhova O, *et al.* Bmi1 is essential for cerebellar development and is overexpressed in human medulloblastomas. Nature 2004; 428(6980):337-341.

[28] Park IK, Morrison SJ, Clarke MF. Bmi1, stem cells, and senescence regulation. J Clin Invest 2004; 113(2):175-179.

[29] Thomas PB, Liu YH, Zhuang FF, *et al.* Identification of Notch-1 expression in the limbal basal epithelium. Mol Vis 2007; 13:337-344.

[30] Varnum-Finney B, Xu L, Brashem-Stein C, *et al.* Pluripotent, cytokine-dependent, hematopoietic stem cells are immortalized by constitutive Notch1 signaling. Nat Med 2000; 6(11):1278-1281.

[31] Wang XD, Leow CC, Zha J, *et al.* Notch signaling is required for normal prostatic epithelial cell proliferation and differentiation. Dev Biol 2006; 290(1):66-80.

[32] Lyngholm M, Hoyer PE, Vorum H, Nielsen K, Ehlers N, Mollgard K. Immunohistochemical markers for corneal stem cells in the early developing human eye. Exp Eye Res 2008; 87(2):115-121.

[33] Lyle S, Christofidou-Solomidou M, Liu Y, *et al.* The C8/144B monoclonal antibody recognizes cytokeratin 15 and defines the location of human hair follicle stem cells. J Cell Sci 1998; 111 (21):3179-3188.

[34] Figueira EC, Di Girolamo N, Coroneo MT, *et al.* The phenotype of limbal epithelial stem cells. Invest Ophthalmol Vis Sci 2007; 48(1):144-156.

[35] Harkin DG, Barnard Z, Gillies P, *et al.* Analysis of p63 and cytokeratin expression in a cultivated limbal autograft used in the treatment of limbal stem cell deficiency. Br J Ophthalmol 2004; 88(9):1154-1158.

[36] Chen Z, Evans WH, Pflugfelder SC, *et al.* Gap junction protein connexin 43 serves as a negative marker for a stem cell-containing population of human limbal epithelial cells. Stem Cells 2006; 24(5):1265-1273.

[37] Notara M, Daniels JT. Biological principals and clinical potentials of limbal epithelial stem cells. Cell Tissue Res 2008; 331(1):135-143.

[38] Schlotzer-Schrehardt U, Dietrich T, Saito K, *et al.* Characterization of extracellular matrix components in the limbal epithelial stem cell compartment. Exp Eye Res 2007; 85(6):845-860.

[39] Wilson SE, He YG, Lloyd SA. EGF, EGF receptor, basic FGF, TGF beta-1, and IL-1 alpha mRNA in human corneal epithelial cells and stromal fibroblasts. Invest Ophthalmol Vis Sci 1992; 33(5):1756-1765.

[40] Li DQ, Tseng SC. Three patterns of cytokine expression potentially involved in epithelial-fibroblast interactions of human ocular surface. J Cell Physiol 1995; 163(1):61-79.

[41] Sotozono C, Kinoshita S, Kita M, Imanishi J. Paracrine role of keratinocyte growth factor in rabbit corneal epithelial cell growth. Exp Eye Res 1994; 59(4):385-391.

[42] Wilson SE, He YG, Weng J, Zieske JD, Jester JV, Schultz GS. Effect of epidermal growth factor, hepatocyte growth factor, and keratinocyte growth factor, on proliferation, motility and differentiation of human corneal epithelial cells. Exp Eye Res 1994; 59(6):665-678.

[43] Finch PW, Rubin JS, Miki T, Ron D, Aaronson SA. Human KGF is FGF-related with properties of a paracrine effector of epithelial cell growth. Science 1989; 245(4919):752-755.

[44] Cheng CC, Wang DY, Kao MH, *et al.* The growth-promoting effect of KGF on limbal epithelial cells is mediated by upregulation of DeltaNp63alpha through the p38 pathway. J Cell Sci 2009; 122(24):4473-4480.

[45] Werner S, Smola H, Liao X, *et al.* The function of KGF in morphogenesis of epithelium and reepithelialization of wounds. Science 1994; 266(5186):819-822.

[46] Lambiase A, Rama P, Bonini S, *et al.* Topical treatment with nerve growth factor for corneal neurotrophic ulcers. N Engl J Med 1998; 338(17):1174-1180.

[47] You L, Kruse FE, Volcker HE. Neurotrophic factors in the human cornea. Invest Ophthalmol Vis Sci 2000; 41(3):692-702.

[48] Lambiase A, Bonini S, Micera A, *et al.* Expression of nerve growth factor receptors on the ocular surface in healthy subjects and during manifestation of inflammatory diseases. Invest Ophthalmol Vis Sci 1998; 39(7):1272-1275.

[49] Touhami A, Grueterich M, Tseng SC. The role of NGF signaling in human limbal epithelium expanded by amniotic membrane culture. Invest Ophthalmol Vis Sci 2002; 43(4):987-994.

[50] Brennecke J, Hipfner DR, Stark A, *et al.* Bantam encodes a developmentally regulated microRNA that controls cell proliferation and regulates the proapoptotic gene hid in Drosophila. Cell 2003; 113(1):25-36.

[51] Chen CZ, Li L, Lodish HF, *et al.* MicroRNAs modulate hematopoietic lineage differentiation. Science 2004; 303(5654):83-86.

[52] Reinhart BJ, Slack FJ, Basson M, *et al.* The 21-nucleotide let-7 RNA regulates developmental timing in Caenorhabditis elegans. Nature 2000; 403(6772):901-906.

[53] Huang KM, Dentchev T, Stambolian D. MiRNA expression in the eye. Mamm Genome 2008; 19(7-8):510-516.

[54] Yu J, Ryan DG, Getsios S, *et al.* MicroRNA-184 antagonizes microRNA-205 to maintain SHIP2 levels in epithelia. Proc Natl Acad Sci USA 2008; 105(49):19300-19305.

[55] Cordes KR, Sheehy NT, White MP, *et al.* miR-145 and miR-143 regulate smooth muscle cell fate and plasticity. Nature 2009; 460(7256):705-710.

[56] Xu N, Papagiannakopoulos T, Pan G, *et al.* MicroRNA-145 regulates OCT4, SOX2, and KLF4 and represses pluripotency in human embryonic stem cells. Cell 2009; 137(4):647-658.

[57] Boettger T, Beetz N, Kostin S, *et al.* Acquisition of the contractile phenotype by murine arterial smooth muscle cells depends on the Mir143/145 gene cluster. J Clin Invest 2009; 119(9):2634-2647.

[58] Cheng Y, Liu X, Yang J, *et al.* MicroRNA-145, a novel smooth muscle cell phenotypic marker and modulator, controls vascular neointimal lesion formation. Circ Res 2009; 105(2):158-166.

[59] Xin M, Small EM, Sutherland LB, *et al.* MicroRNAs miR-143 and miR-145 modulate cytoskeletal dynamics and responsiveness of smooth muscle cells to injury. Genes Dev 2009; 23(18):2166-2178.

[60] Zeng L, Carter AD, Childs SJ. miR-145 directs intestinal maturation in zebrafish. Proc Natl Acad Sci USA 2009; 106(42):17793-17798.

[61] Armitage WJ, Tullo AB, Larkin DF. The first successful full-thickness corneal transplant: a commentary on Eduard Zirm's landmark paper of 1906. Br J Ophthalmol 2006; 90(10):1222-1223.

[62] Dua HS, Azuara-Blanco A. Allo-limbal transplantation in patients with limbal stem cell deficiency. Br J Ophthalmol 1999; 83(4):414-419.

[63] Rao SK, Rajagopal R, Sitalakshmi G, *et al.* Limbal allografting from related live donors for corneal surface reconstruction. Ophthalmology 1999; 106(4):822-828.

[64] Basti S, Rao SK. Current status of limbal conjunctival autograft. Curr Opin Ophthalmol 2000; 11(4):224-232.

[65] Yam HF, Lam DS, Pang CP. Changes of nuclear matrix in long-term culture of limbal epithelial cells. Cornea 2002; 21(2):215-219.

[66] Rheinwald JG, Green H. Serial cultivation of strains of human epidermal keratinocytes: the formation of keratinizing colonies from single cells. Cell 1975; 6(3):331-343.

[67] Pellegrini G, Traverso CE, Franzi AT, *et al.* Long-term restoration of damaged corneal surfaces with autologous cultivated corneal epithelium. The Lancet 1997; 349:990-993.

[68] Tsai RJ, Li LM, Chen JK. Reconstruction of damaged corneas by transplantation of autologous limbal epithelial cells. N Engl J Med 2000; 343(2):86-93.

[69] Shortt AJ, Secker GA, Rajan MS, *et al.* Ex vivo expansion and transplantation of limbal epithelial stem cells. Ophthalmology 2008; 115(11):1989-1997.

[70] Nakamura T, Koizumi N, Tsuzuki M, *et al.* Successful regrafting of cultivated corneal epithelium using amniotic membrane as a carrier in severe ocular surface disease. Cornea 2003; 22(1):70-71.

[71] Koizumi N, Cooper LJ, Fullwood NJ, *et al.* An evaluation of cultivated corneal limbal epithelial cells, using cell-suspension culture. Invest Ophthalmol Vis Sci 2002; 43(7):2114-2121.

[72] Nakamura T, Inatomi T, Sotozono C, *et al.* Transplantation of autologous serum-derived cultivated corneal epithelial equivalents for the treatment of severe ocular surface disease. Ophthalmology 2006; 113(10):1765-1772.

[73] Espana EM, Romano AC, Kawakita T, *et al.* Novel enzymatic isolation of an entire viable human limbal epithelial sheet. Invest Ophthalmol Vis Sci 2003; 44(10):4275-4281.

[74] Nishida K, Yamato M, Hayashida Y, *et al.* Functional bioengineered corneal epithelial sheet grafts from corneal stem cells expanded ex vivo on a temperature-responsive cell culture surface. Transplantation 2004; 77(3):379-385.

[75] Ang LP, Nakamura T, Inatomi T, *et al.* Autologous serum-derived cultivated oral epithelial transplants for severe ocular surface disease. Arch Ophthalmol 2006; 124(11):1543-1551.

[76] Juhl M, Reibel J, Stoltze K. Immunohistochemical distribution of keratin proteins in clinically healthy human gingival epithelia. Scand J Dent Res 1989; 97(2):159-170.

[77] Gomes J, Monteiro BG, Melo GB, et al. Corneal Reconstruction With Tissue-Engineered Cell Sheets Composed Of Human Immature Dental Pulp Stem Cells. Invest Ophthalmol Vis Sci 2009; in press.

[78] Monteiro BG, Serafim RC, Melo GB, *et al.* Human immature dental pulp stem cells share key characteristic features with limbal stem cells. Cell Prolif 2009; 42(5):587-594.

[79] Ma Y, Xu Y, Xiao Z, *et al.* Reconstruction of chemically burned rat corneal surface by bone marrow-derived human mesenchymal stem cells. Stem Cells 2006; 24(2):315-321.

[80] Hao Y, Ma DH, Hwang DG, *et al.* Identification of antiangiogenic and antiinflammatory proteins in human amniotic membrane. Cornea 2000; 19(3):348-352.

[81] Gomes JA, Romano A, Santos MS, *et al.* Amniotic membrane use in ophthalmology. Curr Opin Ophthalmol 2005; 16(4):233-240.

[82] Grueterich M, Tseng SC. Human limbal progenitor cells expanded on intact amniotic membrane ex vivo. Arch Ophthalmol 2002; 120(6):783-790.

[83] Shimazaki J, Aiba M, Goto E, *et al.* Transplantation of human limbal epithelium cultivated on amniotic membrane for the treatment of severe ocular surface disorders. Ophthalmology 2002; 109(7):1285-1290.

[84] Koizumi N, Rigby H, Fullwood NJ, *et al.* Comparison of intact and denuded amniotic membrane as a substrate for cell-suspension culture of human limbal epithelial cells. Graefes Arch Clin Exp Ophthalmol 2007; 245(1):123-134.

[85] Shortt AJ, Secker GA, Notara MD, *et al.* Transplantation of ex vivo cultured limbal epithelial stem cells: a review of techniques and clinical results. Surv Ophthalmol 2007; 52(5):483-502.

[86] Dua HS, Gomes JA, King AJ, *et al.* The amniotic membrane in ophthalmology. Surv Ophthalmol 2004; 49(1):51-77.

[87] Cheng CY, Sun CC, Yu WH, *et al.* Novel laminin 5 gamma 2-chain fragments potentiating the limbal epithelial cell outgrowth on amniotic membrane. Invest Ophthalmol Vis Sci 2009; 50(10):4631-4639.

[88] Koizumi NJ, Inatomi TJ, Sotozono CJ, *et al.* Growth factor mRNA and protein in preserved human amniotic membrane. Curr Eye Res 2000; 20(3):173-177.

[89] Yam HF, Pang CP, Fan DS, *et al.* Growth factor changes in ex vivo expansion of human limbal epithelial cells on human amniotic membrane. Cornea 2002; 21(1):101-105.

[90] Lim JY, Min BH, Kim BG, *et al.* A fibrin gel carrier system for islet transplantation into kidney subcapsule. Acta Diabetol 2009; 46(3):243-248.

[91] Rama P, Bonini S, Lambiase A, *et al.* Autologous fibrin-cultured limbal stem cells permanently restore the corneal surface of patients with total limbal stem cell deficiency. Transplantation 2001; 72(9):1478-1485.

[92] Nishida K, Yamato M, Hayashida Y, *et al.* Corneal reconstruction with tissue-engineered cell sheets composed of autologous oral mucosal epithelium. N Engl J Med 2004, 351(12):1187-1196.

[93] Notara M, Bullett NA, Deshpande P, *et al.* Plasma polymer coated surfaces for serum-free culture of limbal epithelium for ocular surface disease. J Mater Sci Mater Med 2007; 18(2):329-338.

INDEX

A

Adult stem cells	9-12,17
Age	10-15, 36, 41, 45, 66, 112, 113
Angiogenesis	65-71
Articular cartilage	41-44

C

Cellular Therapy	24, 25, 108, 123
Cord Blood	9, 12, 26, 52, 101, 107, 123, 125
Corneal progenitor cells	149
Coronary artery disease	65-68
Cytokines	16-18, 23-25, 29-36, 52, 69, 71, 108, 149, 152
Compressive force	29-31

D

Dental stem cells	140-148
Diabetes	120-125
Diabetes Type 1	120-124
Differentiation	

E

Embryonic stem cells	9-13, 29, 30, 51- 54, 100-107, 114-116, 122-125, 140, 143
Epithelial Progenitor cells	15, 149
Ethics	1-3

F

Fibroblast Growth factor	16, 33, 66, 80, 152,
Functional tissue engineering	29, 36, 44, 50

G

Growth factors	65-71

H

Hematopoietic stem cells	11, 23-25, 103, 124
Hemodynamic force	34- 36

I

Immunity	120-125
Immunomodulation	16, 17
Insulin	120-125
Islet cells	25, 79, 125

J

Justice	1-7

L

Limbus	149-151, 154

M

Mechanical Forces	29-36
Microenvironments	23-27
MicroRNA	149-156
MSC	14, 16-19, 24-27, 31, 40, 47-53, 101, 105, 107, 123

N

Neural Stem Cells	9, 14, 15, 79, 82, 100-109, 114-116, 141
NSC Animal Model	100, 108

P

Pancreas	13, 14, 120-125
Pain	75-91
Pain Animal Models	77, 82
Paracrine effect	16, 17
Progenitor cells	75-91, 149, 156

R

Red blood cell	23

S

Strain	32-34
Stromal Cells	11, 23, 25

T

Tissue repair Therapy	9, 12, 15, 24, 27,

V

VEGF	16, 66-71, 107, 115,
Vulnerability	1, 3, 5